D·

[

ADVANCES IN VIRAL ONCOLOGY

Volume 1

Oncogene Studies

Advances in Viral Oncology
Volume 1

Oncogene Studies

Editor

George Klein, M.D., D.Sc.
Department of Tumor Biology
Karolinska Institutet
Stockholm, Sweden

Raven Press ■ New York

Raven Press, 1140 Avenue of the Americas, New York, New York 10036

Made in the United States of America

Library of Congress Cataloging in Publication Data
Main entry under title:

Advances in viral oncology.

Includes bibliographies and index.
Contents: v. 1. Oncogene studies.
1. Viral carcinogenesis.   2. Cell transformation.
3. Gene expression.   I. Klein, George, 1925-   .
[DNLM: 1. Oncogenic viruses—Periodical.   W1 AD888]
RC268.57.A3   1982   616.99'40194   82-10167
ISBN 0-89004-692-1

Preface

Viral oncology has always been a field of protean changes and surprises. At first, viral oncogenes were thought of as readily identifiable viral genes that would code for a single protein, responsible for transformation. With the discovery that all RNA tumor viruses had the previously unsuspected habit of reverse transcription to proviral DNA, the gap between the RNA and the DNA tumor viruses appeared to narrow, and unifying mechanisms—the ever-tempting mirage of the cancer field—appeared on the horizon once again. By now, the oncogenes of the RNA and DNA tumor viruses have again parted company. Or have they? New surprises may be in store.

For the DNA tumor viruses, the transforming information is an inalienable part of the viral genome. Not so for the directly transforming retroviruses: They pick up cellular sequences that bear the full responsibility for transformation. The cell-derived oncogenes replace large portions of the viral genome in most cases, making it defective and in need of a helper for replication. More than a dozen different cell-derived oncogenes have been identified so far. With a few exceptions, they are unrelated to each other. All correspond to unique and highly conserved cellular sequences. Their protein product was found to have an unusual kinase activity in several but not all cases, with preferential tyrosine phosphorylation as the distinctive feature. Their mechanism of action is not yet clear; several candidates for a natural substrate such as a 36K protein, vinculin, and other cytoskeleton components are currently in the forefront for consideration. This volume deals with the retrovirus-carried oncogenes, their products, and functional aspects.

If virally transduced cellular genes can transform normal into tumor cells, it ought to be possible to transform directly, with the corresponding cell derived DNA sequences, without any viral help. This was achieved by coupling one of the cell-derived sequences corresponding to a murine sarcoma virus-transmitted oncogene, with the appropriate parts of a nontransforming retroviral genome required for integration, activation, and transcription. The transforming activity of this artificially constructed virus provides the formal proof for the functional identity of the virus carried and the cell-derived oncogene.

This logic also requires that the DNA of nonvirally induced tumors should have transforming activity in direct transfection experiments. This was actually shown by Weinberg as summarized in this volume. So far, transformability is largely restricted to a long-established, aneuploid target cell. Despite the somewhat artificial nature of this test system, it was possible to identify oncogenes from chemically induced and spontaneous animal and human tumors. They appear to belong to distinct families, may be quite limited in number, have characteristic restriction enzyme sensitivities, and, perhaps most surprisingly, are not restricted in their transforming activity by either tissue or species barriers.

If oncogenes are originally normal cellular genes, it should be possible to transform them with normal cell-derived DNA. This has been achieved by Cooper et al., as summarized in this volume, but only after the DNA has been sheared to pieces 10 times smaller than the DNA of chemically-induced tumors in Weinberg's experiment. Also, transformation with normal cell-derived DNA occurred with a much lower efficiency. It is believed that the shearing of the normal DNA is needed to separate the cellular oncogene from linked regulation-sensitive controlling elements. The low efficiency of transformation would follow from the requirement to integrate the oncogene within the direct neighborhood of an active region of the cellular genome.

In contrast to the rapid and sometimes spectacular progress in the area of the directly transforming retroviruses there has been less progress in the understanding of the oncogenicity of the slow-acting, helper-independent leukemia viruses. Recently, an important new approach appears to have broken the ice, as summarized by Hayward. In ALV-induced chicken lymphomas, the long terminal repeat (LTR) at the 3' end of the viral genome, known to carry a viral promoter, was found to integrate in the neighborhood of a known oncogene *(myc)*, leading to a 50- to 100-fold increase in its transcription activity. This startling discovery reemphasizes the promiscuity of the oncogenes (because the *virally* carried *myc* gene induces a variety of nonlymphoid tumors), and the occurrence of multiple oncogenes in the same cell (since Cooper et al.'s transfection experiment identified an oncogene in the ALV-induced tumors that was not *myc*).

Intense efforts are now under way in many laboratories to test whether Hayward's model can explain the action of other slow acting retroviruses. The model may also throw new light on the long latency period that characterizes the action of these viruses. Retroviruses integrate indiscriminately at many different sites. The long latent period may be necessary for integration to occur in the proper location where it can activate the appropriate cellular oncogene. The need for a sufficiently large number of "hits" to achieve this may also explain why viremia is an important prerequisite for leukemia induction.

The chapters so far mentioned deal with the mechanisms of retroviral transformation and some of its consequences, as reflected by the DNA transfection studies. But what can we say about DNA virus-induced transformations? Is there any common denominator between the two "oncoviral kingdoms?"

We plan to return to this question in a later volume that will deal with DNA virus-reduced transformation. However, the temptation to suggest one of many possible bridges between the two fields could not be resisted entirely, as reflected by the second volume in this series which will discuss the p53 cellular protein emerging as a plural, if not general, transformation-related component.

The purpose of this volume is to summarize the recent information that has emerged on the nature and mode of action of the oncogenes (transforming genes, cancer genes), carried by the directly transforming RNA tumor viruses. Although amalgamated with the virus genome, these oncogenes have all turned out to be of cellular origin. This book is written for the specialist in cancer research and/or viral oncology who wishes to be informed about the recent developments in this area.

George Klein

Contents

Acknowledgment

I would like to express my gratitude to all authors for their painstaking work.

George Klein

Contributors

Susan M. Astrin
Institute for Cancer Research
Fox Chase Cancer Center
Philadelphia, Pennsylvania 19111

David Baltimore
Center for Cancer Research and
Department of Biology
Massachusetts Institute of Technology
Cambridge, Massachusetts 02139

Peter Bentvelzen
Radiobiological Institute TNO
Lange Kleiweg 151
2280 HV Rijswijk
The Netherlands

Klaus Bister
Department of Molecular Biology and
Virus Laboratory
University of California, Berkeley
Berkeley, California 94720

D. G. Blair
Laboratory of Molecular Oncology
National Cancer Institute
National Institutes of Health
Bethesda, Maryland 20205

C. Bruce Boschek
Institute of Virology
Justus-Liebig University
6300 Giessen
Federal Republic of Germany

Geoffrey M. Cooper
Sidney Farber Cancer Institute and
Department of Pathology
Harvard Medical School
Boston, Massachusetts 02115

Peter H. Duesberg
Department of Molecular Biology and
Virus Laboratory
University of California, Berkeley
Berkeley, California 94720

Ronald W. Ellis
Virus and Cell Biology Research
Merck Sharp & Dohme Research
Laboratories
West Point, Pennsylvania 19486

R. L. Erikson
Department of Pathology
University of Colorado Health Sciences
Center
Denver, Colorado 80262

Robert C. Gallo
Laboratory of Tumor Cell Biology
National Cancer Institute
National Institutes of Health
Bethesda, Maryland 20205

Louis Gazzolo
Virology Unit
INSERM-U.51
Groupe de Recherche CNRS 33
69371 Lyon Cedex 2, France

Stephen P. Goff
Center for Cancer Research and
Department of Biology
Massachusetts Institute of Technology
Cambridge, Massachusetts 02139

Gerard Goubin
Sidney Farber Cancer Institute and
Department of Pathology
Harvard Medical School
Boston, Massachusetts 02115

William S. Hayward
Sloan-Kettering Institute for Cancer
Research
New York, New York 10021

Theodore G. Krontiris
Sidney Farber Cancer Institute and
Department of Pathology
Harvard Medical School
Boston, Massachusetts 02115

Mary-Ann Lane
Sidney Farber Cancer Institute and
Department of Pathology
Harvard Medical School
Boston, Massachusetts 02115

Douglas R. Lowy
Dermatology Branch
National Cancer Institute
National Institutes of Health
Bethesda, Maryland 20205

Carlo Moscovici
Tumor Virology Laboratory
Veterans Administration Medical Center,
 and
Department of Pathology
College of Medicine
University of Florida
Gainesville, Florida 32602

Benjamin G. Neel
Rockefeller University
New York, New York 10021

A. F. Purchio
Department of Pathology
University of Colorado Health Sciences
 Center
Denver, Colorado 80262

Edward M. Scolnick
Virus and Cell Biology Research
Merck Sharp & Dohme Research
 Laboratories
West Point, Pennsylvania 19486

John R. Stephenson
Laboratory of Viral Carcinogenesis
National Cancer Institute
National Institutes of Health
Frederick, Maryland 21701

George J. Todaro
Laboratory of Viral Carcinogenesis
National Cancer Institute
National Institutes of Health
Frederick, Maryland 21701

G. F. Vande Woude
Laboratory of Molecular Oncology
National Cancer Institute
National Institutes of Health
Bethesda, Maryland 20205

Robert A. Weinberg
Center for Cancer Research and
Department of Biology
Massachusetts Institute of Technology
Cambridge, Massachusetts 02139

Flossie Wong-Staal
Laboratory of Tumor Cell Biology
National Cancer Institute
National Institutes of Health
Bethesda, Maryland 20205

Oncogene Studies

Advances in Viral Oncology, Volume 1,
edited by George Klein. Raven Press,
New York © 1982.

Genetic Structure and Transforming Genes of Avian Retroviruses

*Klaus Bister and Peter H. Duesberg

*Department of Molecular Biology and Virus Laboratory, University of California,
Berkeley, California 94720*

Recent biochemical and genetic analyses of acutely oncogenic retroviruses of different taxonomic groups have identified over a dozen different transforming *onc* genes and *onc* gene products (3,10,12,39,127–129,135,136,138,142). These *onc* genes are different from the essential virion genes *gag*, *pol*, and *env* (2) and are not essential for virus replication (39). Most retroviruses with *onc* genes lack part or all of the three essential virion genes and are, therefore, replication-defective. They can be considered as viral parasites of replication-competent helper viruses. Helper viruses carry complete complements of the three essential virion genes and are always found in infectious stocks of defective oncogenic viruses. Helper viruses typically do not contain *onc* genes. However, in some oncogenic viruses, notably in Rous sarcoma virus (RSV), *onc* genes are part of the genome of a replication-competent virus. Hence, RSV may be viewed as a retrovirus with a parasitic *onc* gene. It is not clear whether association with an *onc* gene confers any selective advantage to the virus. The only known function of retroviral *onc* genes is to transform host cells. To date, such *onc* genes have not been found in any other group of viruses but retroviruses (39).

The identification of *onc* genes, which began about 12 years ago with *src*, the *onc* gene of RSV has been a turning point in retrovirus research. It has divided retroviruses into those which are acutely and inevitably oncogenic and carry specific *onc* genes and those which lack *onc* genes and cause chronic viremia and occasionally leukemia and other tumors after long, latent periods. *Onc* gene analysis has also demonstrated that certain *onc* genes have very specific oncogenic spectra, like, for example, *src*, which almost exclusively causes sarcomas, or the *onc* gene of avian myeloblastosis virus (AMV), which almost exclusively causes acute leukemias. Others have broad oncogenic spectra, like the *onc* genes of fibroblast-transforming, acute leukemia viruses such as avian myelocytomatosis virus MC29 or avian erythroblastosis virus (AEV), which cause leukemia, carcinoma, and sarcoma (4,5,39,62,116). Further *onc* gene analysis has proven that structurally unrelated *onc* genes of viruses from the same taxonomic group may cause the same

---

Present address: Max-Planck-Institut für Molekulare Genetik, D-1000 Berlin 33, West Germany.

cancers. For example, RSV, Fujinami-, Y73-, and UR2-sarcoma viruses, as well as MC29 and AEV, all may cause sarcomas, or AEV, MC29, and E26 (an acute leukemia virus related to AMV) may all cause erythroblastosis (see below) (4,5, 39,82,116,137). That totally different *onc* genes nevertheless cause the same cancers suggests that different primary mechanisms may generate the same type of neoplasm.

However, the identification of retroviral *onc* genes has also raised a number of questions:

1. For example, in the absence of known epidemics or horizontal spread of retroviruses with *onc* genes, it remains unclear where these viruses come from and why viruses with related *onc* genes are sporadically and independently isolated from different animal tumors (see below) (4,5,39,62,69,82,87,109,116).

2. Another question is that of the role of lymphatic or chronic leukemia viruses in cancer. Owing to their almost ubiquitous distribution in many animal species (53, 58,64,83,95,124,147,160), these viruses appear as the most plausible causative agents of retroviral cancers. Yet, despite their names, these viruses are only rarely leukemogenic and lack known *onc* genes (29,39,40,53,58,64,83,95,147,160). This underscores the question of how such viruses cause cancer, and why they cause cancers inefficiently. Speculative models suggest that these viruses become oncogenic by transduction of cellular genes, related to viral *onc* genes, or indirectly by induction of certain cellular genes with transforming potential. The existence of cellular transforming genes, termed oncogenes, which may be joint with virion genes of retroviruses, has been postulated in 1969 by Huebner and Todaro (77). The identification of viral *onc* genes has since provided an experimental basis to test the hypothesis that viral *onc* genes are present in normal cells, and whether they can be transduced by retroviruses without *onc* genes (144,145). Indeed, structural homologs of most viral *onc* genes have been detected in DNA of normal cells (see below) (9,10,35,56,57,60,111,115,122,128,129,142,143,149). However, the products encoded by the cellular *onc*-related sequences and their functions remain to be determined, a task that has yet to be completed for most viral *onc* genes.

3. This leads us to the ultimate question, which is whether retroviral *onc* genes and/or their cellular homologs are relevant to natural cancers—excepting the few cases from which retroviruses with *onc* genes have been isolated.

To answer these questions, retroviral *onc* genes and their products must first be defined. Once the structure and function of viral *onc* genes are known, it will be possible to determine whether functional homologs of such genes are present in normal cells and play a role in natural cancers. Here we describe first the definition of *onc* genes and *onc* gene products of viruses from the avian tumor virus group. At this time, seven subgroups of oncogenic tumor viruses can be distinguished in this virus group based on different classes of *onc* genes and their protein products. Subsequently, we will review the relationship between viral *onc* genes and cellular DNA homologs including evidence from both the avian and mammalian systems.

DETECTION AND DEFINITION OF RETROVIRAL *ONC* GENES AND OF THEIR PROTEIN PRODUCTS

The chronicle of viral *onc* gene analysis starts with *src*, the *onc* gene of RSV. *Src* was genetically and physically identified in 1970 as a specific region of RSV RNA with a mass of 1.6 kb (46,98). Because of its unique linkage in RSV with a complete complement of essential virion genes, it became and has remained to date the only one that is defined by classic deletion (47,89,99,152,154) and recombinant analyses (7,49,152,155). The quest for the function of *src* could only start in 1977 when its product was first identified as a phosphoprotein of 60 kd that is serologically unrelated to essential virion proteins (21). A first result of this quest was that the protein has an intrinsic or associated phosphokinase function (52).

Until 1977, *onc* gene analysis of avian tumor viruses had been concerned exclusively with *src*, mainly because the availability of the focus assay developed by Temin and Rubin in 1958 (146) afforded a fast and quantitative measure of *src* gene function in cell culture. Later on it was realized that the oncogenic potential of MC29, a replication-defective acute leukemia virus, could also be measured by the focus assay (81,90). The discovery in 1977 that MC29, which belongs to the same taxonomic group of avian leukosis/sarcoma viruses as RSV (4,5), codes for a unique nonstructural protein and that the defectiveness of MC29 is apparently due to deletions in all three essential virion genes initiated the molecular analysis of the genetic structure of this virus (14,19,43). Identification and structural analysis of the MC29 RNA revealed that it contains specific sequences that proved to be unrelated to virion genes and, most significantly, unrelated to the *src* gene of RSV (43). This was the first evidence that the oncogenic potential of acute avian leukemia viruses was indeed encoded by unique genetic information of the viral RNA and that it was not due to the presence of a possibly modified *src* gene or even due to indirect mechanisms of oncogenicity without involvement of authentic viral *onc* genes. In the light of the genetic structure of the genome and its protein product (14), the *onc* gene of MC29 was defined as a hybrid of a *gag*-related and a specific RNA sequence that jointly encode the probable transforming protein (103). The detection of the MC29 *onc* gene product, a protein of 110 kd later shown to be a phosphoprotein (15), was aided by its serological relationship to the group-specific antigens (*gag* gene products) of the core proteins of retroviruses. The peculiar hybrid structure and mode of expression of the MC29 *onc* gene emerged to be the basic model for many other *onc* genes of acutely transforming retroviruses of avian and mammalian systems (see below).

The impact of the discoveries of a unique *onc* gene in MC29 and of additional unique *onc* genes in other sarcomagenic avian acute leukemia viruses, like AEV, was that the oncogenic spectra of different *onc* genes, even in viruses of the same taxonomic group, may strongly overlap (11). The findings of *onc* genes with hybrid structures like that of MC29 in many other viruses of different taxonomic groups, e.g., in murine Abelson leukemia virus (3) and in feline sarcoma viruses (135), lend credence to the functional significance of the hybrid *onc* gene structure diagnosed in MC29.

Sarcoma Viruses:

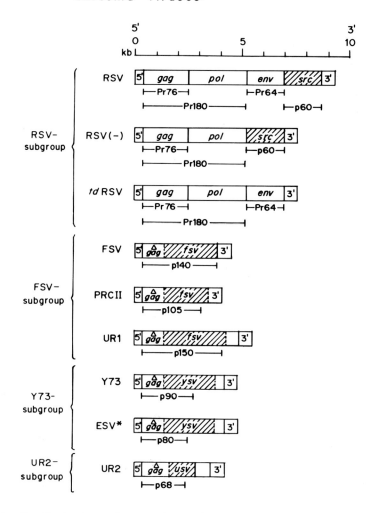

FIG. 1. Genetic structures of oncogenic retroviruses of the avian leukosis/sarcoma group. *Boxes* indicate the mass of viral RNAs in kilobases and *segments within boxes* indicate map locations in kilobases of complete or partial (Δ) complements of the three essential virion genes *gag, pol,* and *env,* of the *onc*-specific sequences, and of the noncoding regulatory sequences at the 5' and 3' end of viral RNAs. *Dotted lines* indicate that borders between genetic elements are uncertain. Based on *onc* gene-specific RNA sequences *(hatched boxes),* four subgroups of sarcoma viruses and three subgroups of acute leukemia viruses can be distinguished. The three-letter code for *onc*-specific RNA sequences extends the one used previously by the authors—*src* represents the *onc*-specific sequence of the RSV-subgroup of avian sarcoma viruses; *fsv* that of the Fujinami-subgroup, *ysv* that of the Y73-subgroup, and *usv* that of the UR2-subgroup of avian sarcoma viruses; *mcv* that of the MC29-subgroup and *aev* that of the AEV-subgroup of sarcomagenic, acute leukemia viruses; and *amv* that of the AMV-subgroup of acute leukemia viruses. Recently, a different nomenclature has been proposed by others, i.e., *myc* (= *mcv*), *erb* (= *aev*), *myb* (= *amv*), *fps* (= *fsv*), and *yes* (= *ysv*). *Lines and numbers* under the boxes symbolize the complexities in kilodaltons of the precursors *(Pr)* for viral structural proteins and of the transformation-specific polyproteins *(p).* For some viruses (*) complete genetic maps are not yet available, and some protein products (**) have only been identified in cell-free translation assays.

Acute Leukemia Viruses:

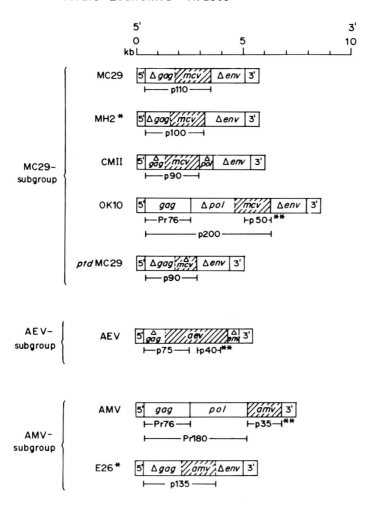

FIG. 1. (contd.) See legend on facing page.

Initiated by the unexpected discovery early in 1980 that Fujinami sarcoma virus (FSV) contained yet another unique sarcomagenic *onc* gene unrelated to *src* (16,93), three additional classes of unique *onc* genes have since been identified in avian sarcoma viruses (Fig.1). The discoveries of these unique *onc* genes extended the notion that there are totally different *onc* genes in the avian tumor virus group that may cause very similar or even identical cancers. The *onc* genes of all of these sarcoma viruses were shown to have a general genetic structure like the sarcomagenic acute leukemia viruses MC29 and AEV (68,76,93,156,157a,160a,162).

At about the same time another class of specific *onc* genes, those associated with acute leukemia viruses that do not cause sarcomas or transform fibroblasts in culture, like AMV, were first described (42,138,139). The relatively late entry of the *onc* genes of acute leukemia viruses that do not transform fibroblasts into the arena of *onc* gene analysis reflects once more the very difficulties of propagating and assaying these viruses in cell culture. The *onc* genes of these viruses can only be assayed in cultured hemopoietic cells or directly in the animal (105; C. Moscovici and L. Gazzolo, *this volume*).

The identification of *onc* genes has since provided a rational basis for the acute oncogenicity of viruses carrying such genes and for the lack of acute oncogenicity in leukosis or chronic leukemia viruses without *onc* genes. The multiplicity and structural diversity of presently known *onc* genes, however, dispels the prospect for one general mechanism of retroviral oncogenesis.

Src, the *onc* Gene of RSV

The only *onc* gene of retroviruses for which nearly complete genetic and biochemical definitions are available is the *src* gene of nondefective (nd) RSV. The genome of nd RSV contains, in addition to *src*, the three essential virion genes of retroviruses termed (2) *gag* (for internal core proteins with group-specific antigens), *pol* (for RNA-dependent DNA polymerase), and *env* (envelope glycoprotein), and terminal 5' and 3' regulatory RNA sequences in the following order: 5' *gag-pol-env-src* 3' (Fig. 1) (152–155). The *src* gene was functionally distinguished from the three essential virion genes of nd RSV by the isolation of a mutant that was temperature-sensitive in transformation but not in virus replication (98). At the same time, the *src* gene was also physically defined by the isolation of nonconditional *src* deletion mutants (46,89,99). These transformation-defective (td) *src* deletion mutants retain all virion genes and are physically and serologically like wild type RSV (Fig. 1) (46,49,89,153). However, the RNA of the wild type measures about 9.5 kb, whereas that of the td RSV measures only about 7.9 kb (Fig. 1) (47,49,99). On the basis of this difference, *src* gene-specific RNA sequences were first defined by subtracting from the 9.5 kb RNA of nd RSV the 7.9 kb RNA of the isogenic *src* deletion mutant (89). The genetic structure of td RSV has since been determined to be isogenic with that of nd RSV except for *src*, e.g., 5' *gag-pol-env* 3' (Fig. 1) (152,153). The 1.6 kb that set apart the RNAs of the wild type RSV from the *src* deletion mutant were shown to be a contiguous, *src*-specific sequence that mapped near but not at the 3' end of viral RNA (Fig. 1) (153,154).

The *src* gene was independently defined by recombination analysis in which a *src* deletion mutant with variant virion genes (5' *gag*-pol*-env** 3') was allowed to recombine with an nd RSV (5' *gag-pol-env-src* 3'). All sarcomagenic recombinants with variant virion genes had the genetic structure 5' *gag*-pol*-env*-src* 3' and, hence, had inherited the *src* gene from nd RSV (7,49,151,152,155) (Fig. 1). It followed that the 1.6 kb RNA sequence was *src*-specific and necessary for transformation.

Subsequently, a 60 kd protein product, termed p60, was identified in RSV-transformed cells that was serologically unrelated to the *gag*, *pol*, and *env* virion proteins (21). The p60 protein is phosphorylated and thought to be a phosphokinase (10,52) (see below). Since the genetic complexity of the 1.6 kb *src*-specific RNA sequence and that of p60 are about the same, the specific sequence of RSV must have encoded most or all of the protein (Fig. 1). This supposition and all of the above physical and chemical measurements of viral RNAs and *src*-specific RNA have recently been confirmed by direct analysis of the complete nucleotide sequences of the *src* genes of two RSV strains (34,126) and of the complete RNA genome of one RSV strain (126). These analyses have chemically defined that the coding sequence of *src* measures about 1,590 nucleotides. Hence, only 10 years after its detection, *src* had become the first retroviral *onc* gene and, in fact, the first retroviral gene altogether for which the complete coding sequence was known, and nd RSV had become one of the first retroviruses for which the complete nucleotide sequence is known.

With regard to the interrelationships of *src* genes from different RSV strains, it has recently been determined that the *src* genes of ten different RSV strains are 98% conserved with only scattered single nucleotide variations (94). This contrasts with the lower degrees of conservation associated with the *onc* genes of other oncogenic viruses of the avian tumor virus group (see below) and signals a close evolutionary and functional relationship among *src* genes. The same *src*-specific RNA sequence that has been identified in nd RSV is also present in an *env* deletion mutant of RSV, termed RSV($-$) (Fig. 1) (154) and in a *gag*-, *pol*-, and *env*-defective, sarcomagenic deletion mutant of RSV (100). Transformation by the *gag*-, *pol*-, and *env*-defective RSV is definitive proof that the *src* gene is not only necessary but is also sufficient for transformation (100). Expression of the *src* gene of RSV involves a mRNA that includes, besides *src*-specific RNA sequences, sequences derived from 5′ and 3′ ends of virion RNA (102). This implies that the *src* gene of RSV consists of a specific coding sequence unrelated to other virion genes and regulatory sequences shared with other retroviral genes. The particular combination and arrangement of the *src*-specific and the regulatory sequences in RSVs must be critical for transforming function, since the structural homologs of the *src*-specific sequence found in normal cells are not known to have transforming function (see below).

The *onc* Genes of Replication-Defective Acute Leukemia and Sarcoma Viruses

Defectiveness as an Obstacle for Genetic Analysis and Genome Identification

Since the genetic phenotype of most defective sarcoma and acute leukemia viruses is gag^-, pol^-, env^-, onc^+ (12,19,39,93), classic deletion and recombination analysis cannot be used to define their *onc* genes, as was the case with *src*. An *onc* deletion of such a virus (i.e., gag^-, pol^-, env^-, onc^-) would obviously be undetectable by classic techniques measuring viral gene expression. Likewise would the lack of secondary markers complicate or prevent recombination analysis of *onc* genes of defective viruses.

Defectiveness also complicates detection and identification of the viral RNA genomes. The genome of a nondefective retrovirus is essentially identified by extracting the RNA from purified virus. Since the defective virus is an obligatory parasite of a nondefective helper virus, typically a replication-competent lymphatic leukemia virus with a genetic design identical to that of td RSV (Fig. 1), it is only replicated as a virus complex. Although a defective/helper virus complex contains defective as well as helper viral RNAs, the ratio of the two RNAs in the virus complex released by a given infected cell is unpredictable, with the RNA of non-defective helper virus usually at an excess (39,41,48,93,96). The RNAs of such defective and helper virus complexes were first separated electrophoretically in the cases of defective murine sarcoma and leukemia viruses (96) and avian MC29 virus (43). Typically, the RNAs of such virus complexes yield one larger RNA species measuring 8 to 9 kb and a smaller one measuring 4 to 7 kb (43,96). The small RNA species were shown to be the genomes of defective transforming virus by their absence from pure preparations of nontransforming helper virus (43,96). Bio-chemical analysis directly identified the smaller RNA species, consistent with their low complexity, as the genome of the defective virus (39,96,103). The size of the helper virus RNA is invariably 8 to 9 kb as dictated by the requirement for complete *gag*, *pol*, and *env* genes in nondefective helper viruses (Fig. 1).

Given the RNA of a defective transforming virus, it can be determined whether a specific sequence, unrelated to essential virion genes, is present. In the avian system it has been asked whether such sequences were related to the genetically defined *src* gene standard. Experimentally, this is accomplished by comparing the RNAs or proviral DNAs of defective and helper virus by various nucleic acid techniques including hybridization of defective viral RNA with cDNA of helper viruses, comparative fingerprinting of RNase T_1-resistant oligonucleotides, com-parison of restriction enzyme sites of proviral DNAs, or RNA/DNA heteroduplex analyses. By these methods, two classes of sequences are distinguished in the RNAs of defective transforming viruses: helper virus-related or group-specific (103) se-quences and specific sequences (37,103). In all cases examined, the specific se-quences form contiguous internal map segments flanked by helper virus-related terminal segments (Fig. 1) (12,39,103). Although biochemical subtraction of helper virus-related sequences from the RNA of a defective, transforming virus is formally analogous to deletion analysis, the subtracted (shared) RNA is not the genome of a viable deletion mutant (Fig. 1). Therefore, it can only be inferred but cannot be rigorously deduced from this type of analysis that the resulting specific sequence of the defective oncogenic virus (hatched in Fig. 1) is sufficient or even necessary for transformation. Furthermore, it cannot be deduced whether such a specific sequence is identical with or only part of a transforming gene.

The genomic RNAs of all acutely transforming retroviruses investigated to date have since been shown to contain such specific sequences, also termed *onc*-specific, transformation-specific, or *x*-sequences, which are unrelated to essential virion genes (3,10,12,35,39,127,132,135,136,142). Such *onc*-specific RNA sequences appear to be the hallmark of highly oncogenic viruses and they represent most or at least part of their *onc* genes (see below). However, due to the defectiveness of all highly oncogenic viruses other than RSV, their *onc* genes are less completely defined than *src*.

onc Genes of Sarcomagenic Acute Leukemia Viruses of the MC29- and AEV-Subgroups

MC29 and AEV, the prototypes of sarcomagenic, acute leukemia viruses, have the broadest oncogenic potential among avian tumor viruses (see below) (4,5,12,39,62). Besides acute leukemias, these viruses cause carcinomas and sarcomas and transform fibroblasts in tissue culture. Their ability to transform fibroblasts makes it possible to assay their oncogenicity by the same focus assay technique that had been developed for RSV (4,11,14,62,81,90). It is probably for this reason that these viruses became, after RSV, the next targets of *onc* gene analysis among oncogenic avian retroviruses. Initial analyses of the *onc* genes of the sarcomagenic, acute leukemia viruses, modeled on the analysis of *src*, searched for a specific sequence, analogous or perhaps homologous to *src*. Indeed, specific sequences were found in such viruses. However, they turned out to differ from *src* both in their primary sequence and in their arrangement within the viral genetic structure.

The first steps in these analyses were the identification of viral genomes and the search for helper virus-unrelated, MC29- or AEV-specific RNA sequences. The most difficult variable to control in the quest for the physical and biochemical identification of the genome and gene products of a defective virus proved to be the availability of an infected culture that produces defective virus at a higher titer compared to its helper virus (11,41,48). An excess of helper virus components of defective oncogenic virus in mixed virus stocks often completely obscures the presence of defective oncogenic virus-specific components. Using virus stocks with high ratios of defective transforming to helper virus, a MC29-specific RNA with a mass of 5.7 kb and an AEV-specific RNA with a mass of 5.5 kb were identified (11,43). By way of comparison with helper viral RNAs, MC29 RNA was shown to contain an internal specific sequence of 1.6 kb (103) and AEV RNA, one of about 3 kb (11) (Fig. 1).

Once identified, it was necessary to collect genetic evidence that the specific sequences of these viruses were indeed necessary for transformation. Since, due to the absence of selective markers other than *onc*, suitable viral recombinants have not as yet been experimentally prepared, different isolates of closely and distantly related avian, acute leukemia viruses were used as substitutes of recombinants. The RNAs of these viral isolates were compared to each other by electrophoretic size analyses, by hybridization with cDNAs of various avian retroviruses, and by mapping RNase T_1-resistant oligonucleotides (12,17,18,48,103).

Such comparisons showed that four different isolates of the MC29-subgroup of avian acute leukemia viruses whose oncogenic spectra are closely related (4,5,62)— namely MC29 (103), MH2 (48), CMII (17), and OK10 (18)—also have closely related genetic structures (Fig. 1). The hallmark of each viral RNA is the internal, helper virus-unrelated sequence termed *mcv*, which measures about 1.6 kb in MC29 (103). Despite close sequence homology, the oligonucleotide composition of the *mcv* sequences of different members of the MC29-subgroup shows some variation in primary sequence (17,18,41,48). Unilateral, RNA-cDNA cross hybridization experiments between different virus strains of the MC29-subgroup signal differences, e.g., up to 30% between MC29 and MH2, in the complexities or primary structures of different *mcv* sequences (18,48,123,142). Reciprocal cross hybridizations between different strains need to be done to determine whether these differences reflect variations in the complexities of one set of specific sequences or strain-specific subsets or perhaps in both of these variables. In MC29, CMII, and MH2, the *mcv* sequence is flanked at the 5′ end by a partial (Δ) *gag* gene, termed Δ*gag*, and in OK10 by a complete *gag* followed by a Δ*pol* (Fig. 1). It is not clear as yet whether the Δ*gag* sequences of MC29, MH2, and CMII have the same complexities but they all share common 5′ *gag* oligonucleotides and their products share p19 and some p27 antigenic determinants (12). At the 3′ end, the *mcv* of MC29 and OK10 is flanked by a Δ*env* gene and that of CMII by a Δ*pol* followed by Δ*env* (Fig. 1). MH2 RNA also contains *env* sequences, but the RNA has not been analyzed sufficiently to determine whether its *mcv* sequence borders at *env* (Fig. 1) (48). In summary, comparative analyses of the four MC29-subgroup viral RNAs show: (a) that the 5′ terminal Δ*gag* sequences and most of the internal *mcv* sequences are highly conserved; (b) that their specific sequences vary in complexity and/or primary structure; (c) that the *env*-related sequences are related by hybridization but are variable in terms of complexity and at the level of shared and specific T_1-oligonucleotides; and (d) that the RNAs may have optional sequence elements such as the 3′ half of *gag* and the Δ*pol* at the 5′ end of *mcv* in OK10, or the Δ*pol* at the 3′ end of *mcv* in CMII (Fig. 1).

The notion of optional parts of the *mcv* sequence itself has recently been directly demonstrated with partially transformation-defective (ptd) *mcv* deletion mutants of MC29 isolated by focus cloning of virus released by a transformed quail cell line (120). These *mcv* deletion mutants lack an internal region of the *mcv* sequence of up to 0.6 kb (17b). Although these mutants have lost most of their ability to transform haematopoietic cells *in vitro* or to cause tumors *in vivo* (120; G. M. Ramsay and L. N. Payne, *personal communication*), they still transform cultured fibroblasts with an efficiency equal to that of wild type MC29.

As described above, the genetic structure of AEV was found to be very similar to that of MC29 (11). However, AEV RNA carries an internal specific sequence, termed *aev*, of about 3 kb that is about twice as large as *mcv* and, more importantly, is not sequence-related to *mcv* (11). The *aev* sequence is flanked by 5′ terminal Δ*gag* and 3′ terminal Δ*env*-related sequences (Fig. 1). Since AEV is the only known member of its subgroup, comparative genetic analyses analogous to those of the MC29-subgroup viruses are not available. Nevertheless, based on very similar general genetic structures (Fig. 1) and similar oncogenic properties, AEV- and MC29-subgroup viruses appear to form an analogous series of acute leukemia viruses. This suggests that homologous group-specific and analogous specific elements of the two subgroups of acute leukemia viruses have similar functions (Fig. 1).

A survey of the genetic structures of the sarcomagenic acute leukemia viruses of the MC29- and AEV-subgroups allows then the following deductions. Since in all viruses studied 5' Δ*gag* and internal specific sequences are present, both of these sequences may be necessary for oncogenicity. However, since not all viruses of the MC29-subgroup contain and express the same complement of their specific sequence, not all of *mcv* appears necessary for oncogenicity. Hence, the *mcv* sequence includes optional and essential elements. Future genetic analyses would have to distinguish between essential and strain-specific elements of *mcv* and would have to determine whether the optional *mcv* elements affect the oncogenic spectrum of the virus. This is suggested because the ptd MC29 strains were observed to lack leukemogenicity in animals (G. M. Ramsay and L. N. Payne, *personal communication*) and because different members of the MC29-subgroup vary in oncogenicity (4,5,62). Since congruent (but not identical) 5' Δ*gag* elements are conserved in all MC29-related viruses and in AEV, it would appear that the respective specific sequence alone may not be sufficient for oncogenicity. However, since all of these viruses are selected, in addition to transforming function, for the ability to replicate with helper viruses, we cannot on the basis of RNA analyses alone distinguish between either essential replicative or oncogenic or both functions of Δ*gag* in these viruses (see below). By contrast, the variability of the 3' terminal sequences in primary structure, complexity, and relationship to either *pol* or *env* suggests that these sequences may not be essential for oncogenicity.

A direct involvement of the 5' Δ*gag* sequences in the expression of specific sequences is demonstrated by the analysis of *onc* gene protein products. In MC29-transformed cells, a phosphoprotein of 110 kd (p110) was found, which by serological analysis was shown to contain the 5' part of *gag* gene-coded protein sequences and additional sequences unrelated to known virion proteins (14,15). Similar *gag* gene-related, nonstructural proteins, ranging in size from 75 kd in AEV to 200 kd in OK10, have been found in cells transformed by all viruses of the MC29- (12,17,70,71,76,121) and AEV- (70,72) subgroups of acute leukemia viruses (Fig. 1). That these proteins are coded for by the specific as well as the *gag*-related RNA sequences of these oncogenic viruses was deduced from *in vitro* translation of viral RNAs of known genetic structure (103,113) and from peptide analysis of these proteins (70,88). This directly demonstrates that the specific sequences of these viruses are not independently expressed, but function together with at least the 5' part of *gag* (or all of *gag* and part of Δ*pol* in OK10) as one genetic unit that may be the *onc* gene of these viruses (Fig. 1) (11,12,17,18,41,103). Like the *src* gene product p60 (10,52), all of these *gag*-related proteins were shown to be phosphorylated in the cell (15,18).

In vitro translation experiments using purified AEV RNA suggest that, in addition to a *gag*-related 75 kd protein, the specific AEV sequence may encode a second protein that is not *gag*-related (113) (Fig. 1). However, assessment of the possible biological relevance of this observation must wait until it is known whether the virus encodes a similar or identical counterpart in infected cells. Possibly consistent with a coding capacity of two proteins, AEV was found to express a subgenomic mRNA of 3.5 to 4.3 kb (134).

Given the similar oncogenic spectra of the viruses of the MC29-subgroup and assuming transforming function for the *gag*-related proteins, we deduce that the size differences among the 90, 100, 110, and 200 kd *gag*-related proteins of CMII, MH2, MC29, and OK10 directly confirm the point made above, on the basis of RNA analysis, that the Δ*gag*/*gag*-Δ*pol*-*mcv* units include optional elements (see Fig. 1).

The optional nature, at least for fibroblast transformation, of an internal region of the *mcv* sequence has been most directly illustrated by the MC29-deletion mutants described above, which code for smaller *gag*-related proteins (120) and have lost *mcv*-specific RNA- and peptide-sequences (17b,121a). Similarly, genetic analyses involving Δ*gag* deletion mutants would be necessary to define the role of Δ*gag* in the oncogenicity of these hybrid genes. Because the genetic units of the MC29-subgroup viruses that consist of Δ*gag*-*mcv* or *gag*-Δ*pol*-*mcv* share conserved 5' Δ*gag*-elements and most of *mcv* but differ in optional, internal sequences, it has been proposed that these genes and their protein products have two essential domains, one consisting of the conserved *gag*-related, the other of the conserved *mcv*-related sequences (18).

Since the known proteins coded for by the acute leukemia viruses described above do not account for *env*- and *pol*-related genetic information of the 3' half of the viral RNAs, it cannot be excluded that 3' terminal sequences are also necessary for transformation. Nevertheless, the variability of the 3' terminal sequences, both in terms of oligonucleotide composition and in relationship to *env* and *pol* genes (Fig. 1) as well as the lack of detectable protein products, argue that these sequences may not be essential for oncogenicity (12,39,41).

We conclude that the *onc* genes of the sarcomagenic, acute leukemia viruses are transforming genes that differ from *src* not only in their primary structure, but also in their basic genetic structure. The hallmarks of the *onc* genes of sarcomagenic, acute leukemia viruses are that they are hybrids of specific sequences and sequences related to the structural virion gene, *gag*, and that (in the MC29-subgroup) they are variable in primary sequence and/or complexity.

onc *Genes of Sarcoma Viruses of the FSV-, Y73-, and UR2-Subgroups*

The basic genetic structure of the sarcomagenic acute leukemia viruses and the basic difficulties in resolving it were encountered again in three different subgroups of sarcoma viruses: the FSV-subgroup, which includes FSV (16,68,93), PRCII (108,160b), and UR1 (156); the Y73-subgroup, which includes Y73 (86,161,162) and Esh virus (59); and the UR2-subgroup (1a,157a). The sizes and known or estimated genetic structures of the RNAs of FSV-, Y73-, and UR2-subgroup viruses are depicted in Fig. 1. The RNA of each subgroup is characterized by a distinct, internal specific sequence that is flanked by 5' terminal Δ*gag* (Fig. 1). As shown in Fig. 1, the specific sequence of FSV, termed *fsv*, the best studied example of these sarcoma viruses, maps close to the 3′ terminal regulatory *c*-region present in all avian retroviruses (93). However, recently a molecular clone of FSV has been found to contain a small *env*-related segment between *fsv* and the 3′ terminal *c*-region (Fig. 1,93a). This element represents the 3′ half of gp85, a glycoprotein which maps in the 5′ region of *env* (126). Likewise, UR2 has been shown to contain oligonucleotides of gp37 (157a), a glycoprotein which maps at the 3′ end of *env* (126). This underscores the similarity among the genetic structures of these sarcoma viruses and sarcomagenic acute leukemia viruses (Fig. 1).

Comparative analyses among different viruses of the FSV-subgroup indicate that the complexity and/or the primary structure of the specific sequence in different viruses of the subgroup varies. Specifically, it was found by hybridization that PRCII RNA lacks about half of the specific 3 kb sequence of FSV (135a). The 1.5 kb of the *fsv* sequence that is shared by FSV and PRCII maps at the 5′ end of the sequence in FSV (W-H. Lee and P. H. Duesberg, *unpublished data*). Likewise does PRC II lack about 1 to 1.5 kb of the specific sequence of a variant termed PRCIV (160a,160b).

Each of the sarcoma viruses of the FSV-, Y73-, and UR2-subgroups encodes a nonstructural, *gag*-related phosphoprotein (15,16,59,92,93,108). The sizes of the respective proteins encoded by a given virus are diagrammed in Fig. 1. Assuming that a protein is required for transformation and that the viral RNA is translated in only one reading frame, it has been argued that in the case of FSV the 140 kd Δ*gag-fsv* protein is not only necessary but also sufficient for transformation, since the genetic complexities of the 4.5 kb FSV RNA and of the 140 kd protein are about the same (Fig. 1) (93). As with the MC29-subgroup viruses, there is considerable variation among the sizes of nonstructural proteins encoded by FSV- and Y73-subgroup viruses (Fig. 1). Thus, the protein of FSV measures 140 kd and that of PRCII of the same subgroup measures only 105 kd (108). After subtracting about 50 kd for *gag*-related sequences (corresponding to about 1 kb of *gag*-related coding RNA sequences), the masses of the specific protein sequences of the two viral proteins differ by about 40%. This is in good agreement with differences estimated to exist between the masses of their specific RNA sequences based on hybridization. Hence, the Δ*gag-fsv* genes of different virus strains of the FSV-subgroup, like the Δ*gag-mcv* genes of different virus strains of the MC29-subgroup, must include optional strain-specific and conserved, essential elements. The same appears to be true for *gag*-related proteins of the Y73-subgroup, since Y73 and Esh sarcoma viruses also encode proteins of different sizes, namely proteins of 90 and 80 kd, respectively (Fig. 1) (59,86,161,162). There is as yet no information whether the size differences of the specific RNA sequences and proteins of any of these sarcoma viruses correlate with differences in their oncogenic spectra.

We conclude that the *onc* genes of the FSV-, Y73-, and URII-subgroups of sarcoma viruses are structurally and possibly also functionally analogous to those of sarcomagenic, acute leukemia viruses and include optional and conserved elements.

onc *Genes of the AMV-Subgroup of Acute Leukemia Viruses*

AMV and E26 are replication-defective acute leukemia viruses that generally fail to transform fibroblasts and cause essentially only leukemias in fowl signaling a unique class of *onc* genes (4,5,62,82,105,106,116). Until recently, biochemical analysis of AMV-related viruses has been slow because AMV stocks typically contained very little defective transforming virus and a large excess of helper virus and thus made the biochemical detection of AMV-specific components present as a minority very difficult and indirect. The discoveries of defective AMV particles released by AMV-transformed, nonproducer myeloblasts free of helper virus (42) and molecular cloning of proviral AMV DNA (138,139) have since allowed the first direct analyses of the viral genome. Defective AMV particles contain a 7.5 kb viral RNA (Fig.1) (42) which agrees with size estimates of molecularly cloned AMV proviral DNA (138,139). In addition, an AMV-specific RNA component of about 7.5 kb was found in infectious AMV stocks (24,25).

The RNA of defective AMV particles was found to contain a complete *gag* and also a *pol* gene, and AMV-transformed nonproducer myeloblasts express the corresponding primary gene products, namely the 76 kd *gag* (Pr76) and 180 kd *gag-pol* (Pr180) precursor proteins (42) (Fig. 1). This is consistent with the ability of AMV to produce defective virus particles for the following reasons. Based on genetic and biochemical analysis of defective virus particles released by cell cultures transformed by defective viruses in the absence of helper viruses, such as RSV(–) (154), AMV (42), and OK10 (18,121), it has been concluded that a functional *gag* gene is sufficient for virus particle formation. However, there is no evidence for *gag-* or *gag-* and *pol*-related nonstructural, possible transforming proteins in AMV-transformed cells (42). Between *pol* and a unique 3' terminal *c*-region, which is unrelated to the *c*-region of most other viruses of the avian tumor virus group (42), AMV RNA contains a specific sequence, of about 1.0 to 1.5 kb (42,115,139), termed *amv*. The *amv* sequence is unrelated to those of any other acutely transforming avian tumor virus except E26 (Fig. 1) (42,123). It appears then that the genetic structure of AMV resembles closely that of RSV(–) (Fig. 1). From this genetic structure it may be expected that the *amv* sequence codes possibly for a specific protein unrelated to *gag* and *pol* genes, by a spliced mRNA generated similarly to that coding for the *src* protein of RSV (102). Indeed, such a mRNA species has been found in AMV-transformed myeloblasts (24,61). Preliminary evidence indicates that a 35 kd protein is translated *in vitro* from AMV RNA (Fig. 1) (W-H. Lee, P. Duesberg, and M. Baluda, *unpublished data*).

Although the specific sequence of E26 is closely related to that of AMV (42,123,142), its genetic structure is similar to that of MC29 virus (17a). This would appear then to be the first example of a specific sequence that can be part of two different types of transforming genes (see below), e.g., as a Δ*gag-amv* hybrid gene in E26 and as a coding sequence by itself in AMV (Fig. 1). The differences in the genetic structures and products of these two acute leukemia viruses may explain their different oncogenic spectra; AMV causing predominately myeloid and E26 predominately erythroid leukemia (see below and 17a,106,137).

Seven Different Subgroups of Oncogenic Retroviruses in the Avian Tumor Virus Group Defined by onc-*Specific RNA Sequences*

At this time, seven different species of specific RNA sequences have been identified in oncogenic viruses of the avian tumor virus group. These *onc*-specific sequences are unique and unrelated to each other. Since most of the oncogenic viruses carrying these sequences lack functional complements of all essential virion genes, their specific sequences are the only structural markers for their classification into subgroups (39,40). On this basis, the following seven subgroups of oncogenic viruses can be distinguished (Fig. 1): (a) the RSV-subgroup of sarcoma viruses, including nd RSVs and RSV(–) (39,94); (b) the FSV-subgroup of sarcoma viruses, including FSV (16,68,93), PRCII and PRCIV (108,135a,160b), and UR1 (156); (c) the Yamaguchi 73 (Y73)-subgroup of sarcoma viruses including Y73 (86,161,162) and Esh sarcoma virus (59); (d) the UR2-subgroup of sarcoma viruses with UR2 sarcoma virus as its only presently known member (1a,157a); (e) the MC29-subgroup of acute leukemia viruses, including MC29, CMII, MH2, and OK10 (12,17, 18,43,48,123,132,142); (f) the AEV-subgroup of acute leukemia viruses (11,12, 123,142); and (g) the AMV-subgroup of acute leukemia viruses, including AMV and E26 (17a,42,123,139).

The *onc* gene of the RSV-subgroup has been termed *src* to signal that the oncogenic specificity, i.e., sarcoma induction, is encoded by this sequence (154). The same term *src* is commonly used in the literature to denote either the transforming gene or the specific sequence of RSV. Nevertheless, there is a difference between the functional and specific sequences of *src* since *src* expression involves spliced 5' and adjacent 3' regulatory elements (34,102,126). To avoid prejudging the oncogenic specificities of other *onc* genes and *onc* gene-specific RNA sequences, we have since adopted a trivial three letter code for the specific sequence, but not for the *onc* genes, of the other oncogenic viruses (18,40,42). This code is derived from the name of that virus of a given subgroup in which it was first identified and hence is easy to recognize and to remember, e.g., *fsv* for the FSV-subgroup, *ysv* for the Y73-subgroup, *usv* for the UR2-subgroup, *mcv* for the MC29-subgroup, *aev* for the AEV-subgroup, and *amv* for the AMV-subgroup (Fig. 1).

We have described above that the specific sequences do not represent complete genetic units of *onc* genes. Instead, they represent in type I *onc* genes (see below) all coding sequences minus regulatory sequences *(src, amv)* and in type II or hybrid *onc* genes (see below) only a part of the coding sequences of the respective *onc* genes. Moreover, it is emphasized that the coding sequences of *onc* genes of some subgroups are highly conserved in their complexity, e.g., 98% in different RSV strains (see above) (94), whereas those of the MC29-subgroup and of the FSV-subgroup vary over 30% in complexities and/or primary sequence as estimated from the mass of their protein products and of their specific and group-specific RNA sequences (Fig. 1). Hence, in order to define absolute, subgroup-specific sequences, as a basis of subclassification, essential *onc* gene sequences need to be distinguished from optional and strain-specific sequences by genetic analyses. Until absolute, subgroup-specific *onc* sequences are known, not all of the specific sequence of one given virus can be considered as representative of a subgroup.

Alternative codes have been chosen for both the specific sequences as well as for the *onc* genes of acute leukemia viruses. One of these mainly reflects oncogenic specificity (63). Because the *onc* genes of acute leukemia viruses, in particular, have been shown to have multiple specificities, and because different sarcoma viruses with completely different *onc* genes but very similar or identical specificities have since been identified, the use of oncogenic specificity as a basis to name specific sequences or *onc* genes, and hence to classify viruses, has outlived its usefulness. Another comprehensive code, deriving from trivial virus nomenclature as well as oncogenic specificity, has recently been proposed (30), and appropriate translation of symbols are shown in the legend of Fig. 1.

Although some of the subgroups now distinguished on the basis of specific sequences had been defined and characterized previously solely on the basis of the oncogenic properties encoded by these RNA sequences, several can only be distinguished by biochemical techniques (see below) (4,5,62,116). For example, based on histological and biological analyses, the sarcoma viruses of the RSV- and FSV-subgroups have been virtually indistinguishable. Although isolated independently, these two avian sarcoma viruses have long been considered as variants of the same strain, supported by reports that certain stocks of Fujinami virus contained *src*-related RNA sequences (141,158). The unique identity of FSV was only recognized recently by biochemical analyses of the viral genome and its specific p140 protein product (16,93). The case of FSV for the first time clearly demonstrated that biochemical resolution of *onc* genes is the only unambiguous basis for classification of sarcomagenic retroviruses. Biological resolution based on available pathological markers is ambiguous. Reliance on biochemical markers will also be essential in order to distinguish between sarcomagenic, fibroblast-transforming acute leukemia viruses of the MC29- and AEV-subgroups on the one hand and the sarcoma viruses on the other, and among sarcomagenic and nonsarcomagenic acute leukemia viruses.

Two Distinct Types of *onc* Gene-Design

Among the *onc* genes described here, two different types can be distinguished: those with a coding sequence that is specific and unrelated to essential virion genes (type I) and those with a coding sequence that is a hybrid of genetic elements derived from essential virion genes, typically including a partial (Δ) *gag* gene, and a specific or *x*-sequence (type II) (13,18,40). Examples for type I are the *src* gene of RSV and possibly the *onc* gene of AMV (125a). Examples for type II are the Δ*gag-x onc* genes of MC29, AEV, FSV, Y73, and UR2. The specific sequences of the type II hybrid *onc* genes are all linked at their 5' ends to partially deleted *gag* or *pol* genes (Fig. 1). By contrast, the specific sequences of type I *onc* genes, whose coding sequences lack genetic elements of essential virion genes, either replace *env* genes [RSV($-$), AMV] or are inserted between *env* and the 3' terminus of viral RNA as in nd RSV (Fig. 1).

Based on available analyses of type I *src* genes and type II *onc* genes of the MC29 and FSV-subgroups, the two types of *onc* genes appear to differ also in conservation of primary sequence and sequence-complexity. The *src* genes of different RSV strains are 98% conserved in terms of primary sequence and complexity (94) whereas the complexities of the type II *onc* genes of the MC29- and FSV-subgroup may vary over 30% (see above). In the case of the MC29-subgroup viruses there is tenuous evidence that optional elements of *mcv* influence the oncogenic spectrum of the virus, e.g., compare known differences among the oncogenic spectra of the four members of the MC29-subgroup (4,5,62,116) and in particular the difference between the wild type and ptd strains, which lack leukemogenic potential (17b,120,121a). It is not known as yet whether the complexity differences among the sarcoma viruses of the FSV-subgroup also influence the oncogenic spectra of the respective viruses.

The two types of *onc* genes also differ in their mechanism of gene expression: the hybrid *onc* genes, whose specific sequences replace *gag*- or *pol*-genetic elements, are translated from genome-size viral RNA into *gag*- or *gag*- and *pol*-related proteins like the Pr76 *gag* or Pr180 *gag-pol* proteins of nontransforming viruses that they replace (Fig. 1). However, there is no evidence that the hybrid gene products are subsequently processed (12,14,70). By contrast, the *src* gene of RSV and possibly the *onc* gene of AMV (125a) are translated from spliced subgenomic mRNAs (Fig. 1) (24,61,73,102). Their expression follows the pattern established for the *env* genes of nondefective retroviruses (73,102). Hence, the mechanism of gene expression of the two different types of *onc* genes closely follows that of the 5' most virion gene that is partially or completely replaced by the specific sequences (Fig. 1).

The role of Δ*gag* in the type II *onc* genes may be to provide a functional domain to these *onc* genes or to provide signals for the expression of the adjacent specific sequences, which appear to lack splice acceptor sites, or perhaps to perform both of these functions. Since RNA splicing is a common mechanism in retroviral gene expression (73,102) yet is apparently not used to express specific sequences of type II *onc* genes, it may be argued that the protein translated from the 5' Δ*gag*-related sequences of about 1 kb in type II *onc* genes serves a direct function rather than to compensate for a missing splice acceptor site in the adjacent specific sequences. The conservation of the Δ*gag-x* hybrid *onc* gene design in mammalian retroviruses, totally unrelated to the avian tumor viruses, namely in Abelson murine leukemia virus (3) and in the feline sarcoma viruses (53,135), supports this notion. Also consistent with this view are the different oncogenic spectra of AMV and E26 (see below), in which a closely related specific RNA sequence is expressed as type I *onc* gene in AMV and probably as type II *onc* gene in E26 (17a). If expression of the *gag*-related coding sequences were not essential for type II *onc* function, it appears plausible that splice acceptor sites would have evolved which allow expression without Δ*gag*. A decision about the role of Δ*gag* in type II *onc* genes may be reached if Δ*gag* deletion mutants become available.

Conversely, it would be interesting to know whether *src* would have transforming function as type II *onc* gene, that is, as a genetic unit that includes *gag*- and/or *pol*-related elements. There is indirect evidence that one given virus may employ both types of *onc* gene expression. In AEV- and OK10-transformed cells, subgenomic mRNA species containing specific sequences have been described (26,134) and the synthesis by cell-free translation of AEV or OK10 RNA of 40 and 50 kd proteins, respectively, unrelated to virion genes, has been reported (113; G. H. Ramsay and M. J. Hayman, *personal communication*).

In summary, known type I *onc* genes encode virion gene-unrelated proteins, highly conserved in terms of complexity. Type II *onc* genes encode virion gene-related proteins with conserved and variable, specific and group-specific elements, and thus may include several functional domains. Plasticity in terms of sequence complexity is a hallmark of type II *onc* genes.

Possible Functions of *onc* Gene Protein Products

Very little is known about the function of the *onc* gene products, i.e., the transforming proteins of retroviruses, and the molecular mechanisms leading to transformation of the host cell. Most studies have examined the function of the *src* gene product p60. It has been proposed that it functions catalytically as a phosphokinase, a property discovered by the *in vitro* phosphorylation of the heavy chain of IgG in immunoprecipitates of p60 incubated with γ-[^{32}P] labeled ATP (10,52). *In vivo*, the kinase activity associated with p60 is thought to phosphorylate certain cellular proteins, in particular a 36 kd protein (52,119) preferentially at tyrosine residues (32,33,80). There is still some uncertainty as to whether the kinase activity of p60 is intrinsic or an associated cellular enzyme. Expression of tyrosine specific kinase activity by *src* molecularly cloned in bacterial plasmids is considered as evidence in favor of intrinsic kinase activity (59a,100a). However, the specific activity of the cloned *src* protein was reported to be between 10- (59a) and over 100-fold (A. P. Levinson and J. M. Bishop, *personal communication*) lower than the authentic viral protein.

The search for possible functions of the *gag*-related phosphoproteins encoded by type II *onc* genes of the MC29-, AEV-, FSV-, and Y73-subgroups has been modeled on the work with the *src* protein. Results obtained to date again suggest association with a phosphokinase activity in some cases (6,15,55,59,86,92,108,112). The kinase activity associated with these proteins in immunoprecipitates is directed primarily to the phosphorylation of the viral proteins themselves. However, it does not appear to be an intrinsic activity of these proteins but may instead be due to associated cellular enzymes (15,92). The observation that phosphorylation of the *gag*-related nonstructural p140 of FSV is temperature-sensitive in cells infected by virus, that is temperature-sensitive for cell transformation, may be interpreted as direct support for the view that this protein is a temperature-sensitive kinase (112). However, additional evidence that p140 of temperature-sensitive FSV is a substrate of fast, reversible phosphorylation, which rapidly loses, but fails to accept phosphate at the nonpermissive temperature, offers as an alternative explanation the view that the protein may be a temperature-sensitive substrate of phosphorylation (92). A direct demonstration of *in vivo* enzymatic activities of the viral proteins has not been provided. Nevertheless, increased levels of phosphorylation of cellular proteins at tyrosine residues in cells transformed by the sarcoma viruses of the FSV- and Y73-subgroups have been taken as evidence that the transforming proteins of these viruses may function in a manner similar to p60 of RSV (33,80).

It is possible that products of type II *onc* genes have, in addition to a possible catalytic function, a physical function involving their *gag*-related elements. Analogous to the function of virion *gag* proteins, the *gag* portions of the nonstructural proteins of these viruses may function by binding to specific cellular and also to intracellular viral nucleic acid sequences (37a) or by directing the transforming proteins to specific subcellular compartments, like cellular membranes. This specific binding may represent a regulatory function for a cellular catalytic activity or perhaps of a yet-to-be-discovered catalytic activity of the *gag*-related proteins themselves. This function would then correspond to one of the two domains proposed for the proteins of the MC29-subgroup viruses (18), described above.

The structural plasticity of type II *onc* genes of the MC29- and FSV-subgroups may in fact signal multiple functional domains: one associated with conserved *gag*-related elements, one associated with conserved elements of the respective, specific sequence, and others associated with variable elements. The variable elements of these *onc* genes might represent physical domains, which assist enzymatic or structural functions associated with the conserved elements of these genes.

RETROVIRUSES AS VECTORS FOR *ONC* GENES OR *ONC* GENES AS PARASITES OF RETROVIRUSES

Retroviruses with *onc* genes are selected for two functions: a transitive function, which is to transform cells, and an intransitive or vector function, which is to replicate or to be replicated. A survey of the genetic structures of oncogenic retroviruses (Fig. 1) indicates that most oncogenic viruses lack most or all of the essential virion genes and hence have only minimal replicative functions. The residual essential viral sequences of oncogenic retroviruses may be viewed as vectors of *onc* genes that can only replicate as parasites of helper viruses. The survey in Fig. 1 suggests that after subtracting variable transformation-specific sequences, the minimal vector for a viral transforming gene consists of 5' terminal sequences of 1.5 kb, which include the noncoding (34,126) 5' terminus of about 0.5 kb and about 1 kb of the coding sequence of *gag*, and the noncoding (34,126) 3' terminal sequences of about 0.7 kb including the heteropolymeric *c*-region of 0.5 kb and 0.2 kb of poly (A) (42,148,153). The noncoding terminal sequences are essential for replication of viral RNA via proviral DNA. The coding sequences of the 5' half of the *gag* gene may then serve two additional RNA vector functions: one is to be packaged by viral coat proteins, the other to form 60 to 70S dimer complexes typical of all infectious retroviruses (38,97). The location of these vector functions in the 5' half of *gag* and possibly part of the noncoding 5' sequence is based on two considerations. Subgenomic viral mRNAs share with virion RNAs noncoding 5' and 3' terminal sequences (102), yet mRNAs are not regularly packaged by viral coat proteins, neither do they appear to form RNA dimer structures. This leaves these 5' sequences as site for these vector functions, since all other coding virion sequences including *onc*-specific sequences may vary without affecting these two vector functions (Fig. 1). This is also supported by the finding that a self-complementary RNA sequence, the possible RNA dimer linkage site, is indeed found in the 5' coding region of the *gag* gene (126), and by the observation that packaging of defective viral RNAs by helper viral coat proteins must involve specific protein-RNA interactions. In the avian retrovirus group, packaging of defective viral genomes by helper virus proteins is exclusively group-specific (19), the group being defined by shared *gag*-related sequences (39,151). This does not exclude that the noncoding terminal sequences are also necessary vector elements, since all viruses defective or nondefective also share these sequences (see note page 42).

There is no clear evidence that *onc* genes confer any selective advantage to retroviruses (39). Indeed, this is not to be expected since, with the exception of nd RSV, the *onc* genes of all avian and mammalian oncogenic retroviruses are not united with replication-competent viruses. Instead they are replication-defective, nonessential viral satellites of nondefective viruses without *onc* genes (Fig. 1). The rule (with the one exception of nd RSV) that retroviruses with *onc* genes are defective appears to vindicate the proposal that defectiveness is fundamentally linked with the ability of retroviruses to cause direct transformation (125). In the following, we suggest reasons why retroviruses with *onc* genes are defective.

The *onc* genes or, more precisely, the specific sequences of retroviruses may be viewed as selfish parasites of retroviruses. They use elements of retroviruses as replication vectors and, in the case of type II hybrid *onc* genes, even as part of their coding sequence since Δ*gag* functions as part of the type II *onc* genes (see above). Such parasitic sequences may be replicated in two ways, either as part of a nondefective or partially defective retrovirus, which retains three, two, or one intact virion gene as in the cases of nd RSV, AMV, and OK10, respectively or, more typically, as genetic hybrid structures, which lack expression of all virion genes (Fig. 1). If *onc* genes are parasites of nondefective retroviruses, like *src* in nd RSV, they are assured replication with the rest of the viral genome; however, they are then subject to restrictive host responses directed against all virion genes. By contrast, if *onc* genes only use the minimal vector elements from retroviruses, they may persist and function in cells independent of helper viruses, i.e., non-producer cells, and may switch helper viruses in the case that a given helper virus becomes subject to host restriction. The price for this degree of freedom for the defective oncogenic viruses is to depend on the helper virus for replication. As a consequence, the defective virus in the coat of helper viruses is subject to viral interference and must compete with the helper virus for replication. The preponderance of defective oncogenic retroviruses suggests that for *onc* genes the existence as part of a defective virus must be an advantage over an existence as part of a nondefective virus.

DIFFERENT *ONC* GENES WITH OVERLAPPING SPECIFICITIES SIGNAL DIFFERENT MECHANISMS OF TRANSFORMATION

Despite insufficiencies in the definition of *onc* genes, it is clear that at least seven different classes of specific sequences (*src, mcv, aev, fsv, ysv, usv,* and *amv*) and hence probably seven different *onc* genes exist in the avian tumor virus group alone. This number is likely to increase as more oncogenic viruses are analyzed. Some of these distinct *onc* genes cause specific cancers like those of the sarcoma viruses and that of AMV; others have broad oncogenic spectra like those of the sarcomagenic, acute leukemia viruses. However, there is considerable overlap among the oncogenic spectra of unrelated *onc* genes.

For example, four subgroups of sarcoma viruses cause essentially only sarcomas in the animal, although they have completely (or partially, excepting shared *gag* elements) unrelated *onc* genes. Nevertheless, there are relative histological differences between sarcomas caused by RSV and FSV. The RSV sarcomas tend to be frequently fibrosarcomas and rarely myxosarcomas, whereas the FSV sarcomas tend to be myxosarcomas (64,93). However, the structural differences among the type II *onc* genes of the defective sarcoma viruses of the FSV-, Y73-, and UR2-subgroups are not known to correlate with any differences in their oncogenic spectra.

By contrast, the structural differences between the *onc* genes of the MC29- and AEV-subgroups of sarcomagenic, acute leukemia viruses do correlate with differences in oncogenicity. Multiple leukemias, including myelocytomatosis and erythroblastosis, are caused by MC29-subgroup viruses but predominantly erythroblastosis by AEV (4,5; C. Moscovici, *personal communication*). AEV rarely causes carcinomas and frequently sarcomas; by contrast, MC29 viruses frequently cause carcinomas and less frequently sarcomas (4,5,39,62,116). Clearly, the *onc* genes of the sarcomagenic acute leukemia viruses have the broadest spectra among known avian *onc* genes, and consequently also overlap with those of most other more specific *onc* genes, such as the *onc* genes of the sarcoma viruses and of the acute leukemia viruses of the AMV-subgroup (39,40). In addition, avian sarcoma and acute leukemia viruses overlap with mammalian sarcoma viruses in their ability to transform mammalian cells in the animal and in culture (39,64,117).

Despite some overlaps, the structural differences between the *onc* genes of the acute leukemia viruses of the AMV-subgroup and those of the sarcomagenic, acute leukemia viruses correspond to unambiguous differences in their oncogenic spectra. The most notable difference is the failure of the AMV-subgroup viruses to transform fibroblasts in cell culture and to cause sarcomas in the animal (4,5,62,82,105,106,116). The overlap includes erythroleukemias, which are caused readily by E26 of the AMV-subgroup and sometimes by AMV (4,5,82,105,137) and also by AEV and MC29 (4,5,62,116).

Since at least six different *onc* genes (*src, fsv, ysv, usv, mcv,* and *aev*) can cause sarcomas, at least three *(aev, mcv, amv)* erythroleukemias, and two *(mcv, aev)* carcinomas, we conclude that probably different mechanisms, and presumably different cellular targets, exist for a given form of oncogenic transformation. The overlap among the oncogenic spectra of different *onc* genes suggests that different *onc* genes either interact with different specific cellular targets or that *onc* genes interact with nonspecific targets. A unique and specific target for a given form of cancer would fail to explain why different *onc* genes may cause the same disease and why in some cases one *onc* gene may cause different cancers. Hence, different *onc* genes of viruses belonging to the same taxonomic group appear to transform the same target cells by different mechanisms.

It may be argued that *onc* genes with unrelated primary structures nevertheless encode functionally very similar or identical proteins as, for example, a kinase. Although this may be possible for structurally unrelated transforming proteins of viruses with very similar and very specific oncogenic spectra, like the sarcoma viruses of the four different subgroups, it fails to explain the multiple specificities of *onc* genes from viruses with broader oncogenic spectra, like those of the sarcomagenic, acute leukemia viruses. It would appear then that there is no substantial evidence for one common molecular mechanism by which retroviral *onc* genes and their products transform the host cell.

The findings that unrelated *onc* genes cause the same cancers argue against the hypothesis that the transforming proteins of these viruses closely resemble specific cellular differentiation proteins and that transformation is a consequence of a competition between a specific viral transforming protein and a specific, related cellular counterpart (63). The observations that AMV and MC29, two viruses with totally unrelated *onc* genes, both transform mature macrophages cultured *in vitro* (50,51) or that in the animal the unrelated *onc* genes of AEV and E26 both transform predominantly cells of the erythroid lineage (82,106,137) also contrast with the proposal that *onc* gene products of these acute leukemia viruses can only interact with targets in one specific type of differentiated cell (8,63). It has also recently been reported that feline sarcoma virus, a retrovirus with a type II *onc* gene as in MC29, can induce the malignant phenotype in cells from two different (i.e., mesodermal and neuroectodermal) germ layers (22).

The nature of viral *onc* gene products and of cellular targets that govern oncogenic specificity remain to be elucidated. These are believed to include factors determining susceptibility to virus infection and replication and unknown factors that control the number and location of proviruses in an infected cell as well as the ratio of defective-transforming to helper-virus RNAs produced by a given cell. In addition, intracellular substances that interact directly with viral transforming proteins, as for example the kinases that associate with some viral transforming proteins (see above) or the cellular proteins that become phosphorylated by the kinases associated with some viral transforming proteins, are considered to influence oncogenic specificity.

Although neoplastic transformation by *onc* genes apparently proceeds by direct and inevitable yet unknown mechanisms, retroviruses without *onc* genes also may cause cancers. However, these viruses transform inefficiently and only after considerable latent periods by presumably distinct mechanisms (see below). Some of the cancers caused by viruses without *onc* genes, like the lymphatic leukemia or leukosis viruses, are phenotypically very similar to those caused by viruses with *onc* genes. For example, besides lymphatic leukemias and osteopetrosis, leukemia viruses have been observed to cause kidney and liver carcinomas and even sarcomas (4,5,64,105,116). Hence, there may be mechanisms of carcinoma and sarcoma formation by retroviruses that do not use known viral *onc* genes (see below).

However, analysis of the apparently indirect mechanism of oncogenesis by these viruses is even more difficult than that by viruses with *onc* genes because tumor formation is a rare consequence of infection and only occurs after long latent periods in the animal and not simultaneous with virus replication (27,29,64,116,124,147,160). The nature of the 3′ terminal *c*-region has been implicated as at least one indirect cause of leukemogenesis by avian leukosis viruses (148). However, recent experiments with recombinants differing in *c*-regions have suggested that other unknown variables affecting other viral genetic elements might be critical determinants of leukemogenicity (29). (A relevant mechanism involving induction of cellular oncogenes is discussed below.) Most typical infections by lymphatic leukemia viruses fail to cause cancers altogether. Such infections may be latent, involving in particular endogenous avian or murine xenotropic viruses with little virus expression (29,95,147) or take the form of viremias without apparent leukemias or other forms of cancer (27,29,53,58,64,83,124,160).

RELATIONSHIP BETWEEN VIRAL *ONC* GENES AND CELLULAR PROTOTYPES

Retroviruses with *onc* genes are acutely and inevitably oncogenic in susceptible animals. However, such viruses are rarely found in natural cancers, indicating that they do not play a significant role in natural carcinogenesis. Several retroviruses with *onc* genes, like Harvey (69), Kirsten (87), and Moloney (104) murine sarcoma viruses (MSV) and the avian OK10 (109) and the murine Abelson acute leukemia virus (1), have been isolated from animals that developed tumors after inoculation with lymphatic leukemia viruses without *onc* genes (39,127). The rare, spontaneous or lymphatic leukemia virus-induced appearance of retroviruses with *onc* genes and the complete lack of evidence for an epidemic, horizontal spread of retroviruses with *onc* genes have raised several critical questions about the origin and cancer-relevance of these viruses. Are viral oncogenes stored in covert form in normal cells? How do viruses with related *onc* genes like the four members of the MC29-subgroup or Kirsten and Harvey MSV appear in seemingly independent spontaneous cancers? Are lymphatic leukemia viruses involved in the emergence of viral oncogenes? Since lymphatic leukemia viruses are almost ubiquitous in many animal species (see above) (64,147), in particular in chicken (124,160), mice (27,58,95), or cats (53,83), they could have been instrumental in the generation of viruses with *onc* genes, even in isolates from animals not inoculated with lymphatic leukemia viruses.

These questions were first addressed by the oncogene hypothesis of Huebner and Todaro (77). The oncogene hypothesis postulates that viral *onc* genes are present in normal cells and may cause cancer if induced by carcinogens or other oncogenic agents, including retroviruses without *onc* genes. Subsequently, it was proposed by Temin's protovirus hypothesis that cellular genetic elements with a potential of becoming viral genes including viral *onc* genes, termed proto-viruses, can evolve into authentic viral genes and can be transduced by existing or evolving retroviruses to generate oncogenic viruses (144,145).

Quantitative or Qualitative Model?

An experimental test of the oncogene hypothesis became possible with the identification of *onc* gene-specific sequences initially in RSV (46,89), then in murine Kirsten and Harvey sarcoma viruses (96,128,129) and later in many other avian and mammalian retroviruses (see above). The first direct evidence of sequence homology between cellular DNA and *onc*-specific sequences of viral *onc* genes was obtained by hybridization of *onc*-specific cDNA with cellular DNA or RNA in the cases of Kirsten and Harvey sarcoma viruses (128,129,149) and later also with those of Moloney MSV (57), RSV (143), MC29 (123,131,133,142), AMV (139), and other viruses. These results lend indirect support to the oncogene and transduction hypotheses. However, these hybridization experiments did not determine whether viral *onc* genes (referred to as the quantitative model) or structural relatives of viral *onc* genes with possibly different functions (referred to as the qualitative model) were detected in normal cells.

According to the quantitative model, cellular transformation by viruses with *onc* genes is thought to be due to enhanced dosage of *onc* gene products shared by viruses and cells (9,10). If correct, this hypothesis argues that normal cells must contain and express at a low level a number of transforming genes, all of which must be controlled to prevent spontaneous expression above a nonmalignant level (10). The number of *onc* genes in normal cells of a given species would be at least the same as the number of different *onc* genes found in the corresponding taxonomic groups of viruses, e.g., in chicken at least seven corresponding to those of the avian tumor virus group and at least one more corresponding to reticuloendotheliosis virus (23,75), a member of a distinct taxonomic group of avian retroviruses (151). By contrast, the qualitative model holds that viral *onc* genes and cellular homologs are qualitatively different and does not make any predictions on the function of the cellular *onc*-related DNAs.

Structural Homology Between Viral *onc* Genes and Cellular Prototypes

The first direct structural and functional comparisons between viral *onc* genes and cellular prototypes were carried out when cellular *onc*-related DNA sequences or proto-*onc* genes (9,10) became available as molecular clones in phage or plasmid vectors. These comparative analyses included heteroduplexes formed between viral RNA or proviral DNA and cloned cellular DNA, mapping restriction endonuclease-sensitive sites of cellular and proviral DNAs and fingerprinting viral RNA-cellular DNA hybrids. In addition, functional assays have been conducted to test whether, on transfection with cellular *onc*-related DNA, normal cells become transformed cells. In the following, we summarize briefly studies carried out to define the relation between the *onc* genes of three viral prototypes and their cellular homologs.

Cellular Prototypes of the onc *Genes of Moloney and Harvey Sarcoma Viruses*

The first such comparisons were conducted by Vande Woude and his collaborators with the cloned cellular homolog of the *onc*-specific 1.5 kb sequence of Moloney MSV (20,111). Using heteroduplex analyses and restriction endonuclease mapping, it was found that the 1.5 kb Moloney MSV-specific RNA sequence has a near identical, colinear counterpart in normal mouse cell DNA that is not linked to helper Moloney leukemia virus-related sequences. Transfection assays failed to show direct transforming potential of the cloned, cellular proto-MSV DNA but after ligation with terminal sequences of proviral Moloney MSV DNA, the proto-MSV DNA transformed mouse 3T3 fibroblasts (20). The terminal sequences of all proviral DNAs contain redundant elements transcribed from the 3' and 5' ends of viral RNA, which are termed long terminal repeats (LTR). These LTRs include promotors for transcription of viral RNA, which are thought to render the proto-MSV DNA biologically active in the 3T3 fibroblast transformation assay. Similar results have been reported with the cellular DNA of Harvey MSV (36).

It is consistent with the quantitative model that proto-MSV expression is not observed in normal cells (57). However, with regard to the relevance of these experiments for the quantitative model, one would have to know whether viral and related cellular sequences encode indeed the same transforming proteins. In addition, it would be critical to know whether only terminal sequences of MSV or also terminal sequences of Moloney leukemia virus could induce proto-MSV DNA sequences to transform cells, in order to exclude the possibility that besides promoter functions other functions are encoded in the terminal sequences of MSV. Structural analyses of Moloney leukemia and sarcoma virus RNAs have indeed detected sarcoma and leukemia virus-specific terminal markers, which may signal functional differences (54). Obviously, answers to these questions will depend on a more complete genetic definition of the *onc* genes and *onc* gene products of Moloney and Harvey MSVs than is available at this time (see Ellis et al., and Blair and Vande Woude, *this volume*). Finally, it would also be of interest to know whether cellular promotors could substitute for viral promotors in inducing transforming function of proto-MSVs.

The Cellular Prototype of the src *Gene of RSV, a Type I* onc *Gene*

The cellular *src*-related locus of chickens has recently been cloned and compared to molecularly cloned RSV DNA by heteroduplex analyses (130). As with Moloney MSV, most *src*-specific sequences appear to be present in the cloned cellular proto-*src* locus. Fingerprint analysis of viral RNA hybridized to proto-*src* DNA showed directly that all *src*-specific oligonucleotide sequences of RSV RNA have related counterparts in proto-*src* (44,94). However, the same analysis also showed that the cellular locus is not linked to other non-*src* virion oligonucleotides, even from noncoding sequences mapping directly adjacent to *src* in RSV and in particular not to those noncoding sequences of RSV that are part of viral *src* mRNA (102). In contrast to proto-MSV DNA, the proto-*src* DNA is interrupted by six sequences of nonhomology relative to viral *src* (130). There is no evidence to date for any biological activity of proto-*src* DNA, although the level of proto-*src* mRNA expression in normal cells is very similar to that of viral *src* expressed in some RSV-transformed rat cells but about 10- to 20-fold lower than in RSV-transformed chicken cells (10).

The Cellular Prototype of the Type II onc Gene of MC29

In addition to sequences related to *src*, normal cellular chicken DNA also contains sequences related to other type I and II *onc* genes of the avian tumor virus group including MC29 (123,131,133,142). A lambda phage carrying the cellular locus related to the specific *mcv* sequence of MC29, termed cellular *mcv* locus or proto-*mcv*, has been selected from a chicken DNA library in our laboratory (44,122). Based on fingerprinting RNA-DNA hybrids, the proto-*mcv* was found to contain a complete structural homolog of the viral *mcv* sequence. However, the locus was not linked to Δ*gag* or to any other virion sequences. Since Δ*gag* is not present in the *mcv* locus, the Δ*gag-mcv* hybrid of MC29 does not have a complete structural homolog in the cell. Moreover, the proto-*mcv* locus of the chicken was found to be interrupted by a 1 kb DNA sequence unrelated to viral *mcv*. As with the *src*-related locus, there is no evidence on the biological activity of proto-*mcv* DNA, although again proto-*mcv* RNA is expressed in normal chicken cells (123,131). The level of proto-*mcv* RNA expression in normal cells is only about 2- to 5-fold lower than that of MC29 virus RNA in transformed rat cells (118) and about 30- to 100-fold lower than in MC29-transformed quail cells (74,118).

Conclusions

It would appear that the *onc*-specific sequences of oncogenic retroviruses have complete or almost complete cellular homologs. Thus, the coding sequences of type I *onc* genes have complete structural counterparts in normal cells but not those of type II hybrid *onc* genes. Biological activity in assays measuring transformation of 3T3 fibroblasts has been observed with cellular DNA related to Moloney and Harvey MSV on ligation to terminal sequences of proviral MSV DNA, but not as yet with the cellular DNA related to *src* or *mcv* despite similar efforts (*personal communications and unpublished observations*).

In conclusion, available evidence supports the qualitative model in the case of type II *onc* genes, like that of MC29, since only a part of the hybrid *onc* gene is found in uninfected cells, but does not at this time distinguish between the two models in the case of type I *onc* genes, like *src* or the specific sequences of MSVs. To distinguish further between the two models, it would be necessary to determine: (a) whether the gene products of cellular, structural homologs of viral *onc* sequences are also functional homologs of viral *onc* gene products—in particular in cells where viral *onc* expression and cellular proto-*onc* expression are at similar levels, as in the cases of some RSV- and MC29-transformed rat cells and normal chicken cells; (b) whether the intervening sequences that set apart most cellular *onc*-related sequences (23,35,36,56,60,115,122,149a) from their viral counterparts are noncoding introns or perhaps coding sequences of the cell; in the second case cellular proto-*onc* sequences would encode products that are structurally and possibly functionally different from viral transforming proteins; and (c) whether experimental transduction of cellular *onc*-related sequences by molecularly cloned retroviruses without functional *onc* genes generates oncogenic viruses (see below).

If the cellular *onc*-related sequences do represent functional homologs of viral *onc* genes and are cellular transforming genes as postulated by the quantitative model, it follows that all normal chicken cells must regularly prevent expression of potential cancer genes over a critical level. These potential cancer genes would correspond to at least 0.01% of the genome of the chicken. This is estimated as follows. Chicken cellular DNA sequences related to eight known viral *onc* genes, e.g., the seven of the avian tumor virus group (Fig. 1) and one of reticuloendotheliosis virus group (23,75) together represent at least 15 kb. In the cases where the respective cellular loci have been analyzed—e.g., *src* (130), *mcv* (44,122), *aev* (149a), *amv* (115), *rel* (reticuloendotheliosis-specific sequence) (23)—the *onc*-related cellular DNA sequences are separated by one *(mcv, amv)* or more *(src, aev, rel)* intervening sequences unrelated to viral counterparts representing up to 10 times as much DNA as that related to viral *onc* genes (130,149a). Hence, the total contiguous, chicken cellular DNA regions flanked by and including *onc*-related DNA represent at least about 100 kb. This represents about 0.01% of the haploid chicken genome of 1×10^6 kb. This number would go up if more *onc* genes were discovered and if chicken DNA would contain sequences related to *onc* genes of mammalian retrovirus, as has been suggested in one case (60). It appears then that a prediction of the quantitative model would be that a substantial number of normal cellular genes are potential transforming genes.

Induction and Transduction of Cellular Sequences Related to Viral Oncogenes—Evidence for the Quantitative Model?

In accord with the quantitative model, it was proposed that viruses without viral *onc* genes, like the lymphatic leukemia viruses, cause cancer by inducing the expression of cellular genes related to viral *onc* genes (74,107,114,148). This is thought to work as follows. During reverse transcription, identical LTRs are generated at both ends of proviral DNA. These LTR sequences contain viral promotor signals, which initiate RNA synthesis from the 5' LTR (148). Since the promotor of the 3' terminal LTR does not promote viral transcription, it may instead promote transcription of adjacent cellular sequences. Specifically, it was concluded that "downstream promotion", resulting in an increased transcription of cellular *mcv*-related sequences from a background of 2 to 10 copies of RNA per normal cell

(74,123,131) to about 100 to 200 copies of hybrid mRNA that includes viral LTR elements and cellular *mcv*-related sequences, is the cause for viral lymphomas in chicken (74). Thus, the level of cellular proto-*mcv* RNA in lymphoma cells is similar to that of viral MC29 RNA in nonproducer quail fibroblasts transformed by MC29, e.g., 100 to 200 copies (74,118).

Although these experiments are compatible with the quantitative model they raise a number of critical questions. It remains to be explained why expression of 10 to 20 copies of MC29 virus RNA per cell appears to be sufficient to transform rat fibroblasts (118) when 2 to 10 copies of presumably functionally identical proto-*mcv* do not transform chicken fibroblasts or lymphoid cells. A corollary is that *src* expression in some RSV-transformed mammalian cells is also not higher than the level of cellular proto-*src* expression in normal chicken cells (10). Further, downstream promotion fails to explain the long, latent periods of tumor formation by viruses without *onc* genes in view of the following. Retroviruses have no apparent specificity in the nucleotide sequence of the cellular DNA integration site (145), yet the downstream promotion model postulates site-specific or at least region-specific integration as a cause of cancer (74). Tumor formation is thought to reflect clonal selection from cells with randomly integrated proviruses. This selection has been suggested to explain the long, latent periods associated with leukemogenesis by lymphatic leukemia viruses (74). Yet in view of the large number of susceptible cells and viruses in viremic animals and the relatively large regions surrounding proto-*mcv* that are targets for downstream promotion (74,113a), short, latent periods could be expected in some cases. In addition, it remains to be explained why other investigators have isolated from such lymphomas DNA with transforming potential for 3T3 mouse fibroblasts (that is thought to represent a causative cellular transforming gene), which is not linked to proviral DNA of lymphatic leukemia viruses (31,74). The data available to date also do not explain why induction of the cellular *mcv* locus is not observed in 15% of the lymphomas analyzed and why the cancer presumably induced by the endogenous *mcv* locus seems limited to B-cell lymphomas (74). Induction of the *mcv* locus would be expected to cause sarcomas and carcinomas and acute leukemias, in particular, since MC29 virus causes these diseases rather than lymphomas (4,5,62,116). It has also not been excluded that induction of cellular *mcv*-related sequences in lymphomas may be a consequence rather than the cause of cell transformation, and that induction of other cellular genes might be detectable with suitable DNA probes. This would be compatible with the observation that transformation by RSV induces expression of numerous cellular genes in transformed fibroblasts (65). A recent analysis of bursal lymphomas in chicken has suggested that lymphatic leukemia viruses may activate proto-*mcv* by mechanisms other than downstream promotion (113a). Viral promotors integrated downstream of proto-*mcv* and in the opposite polarity were found to enhance expression of proto-*mcv* involving proto-*mcv* mRNAs not linked to viral RNA. A similar analysis of leukemogenesis by bovine leukemia virus designed to test downstream promotion failed to support this model. Proviral integration was found not to be adjacent to a unique cellular locus and viral-cellular hybrid mRNAs were not detected (86a). Finally, a recent investigation of different human tumor cells as well as of normal human cells for the expression of proto-*mcv* and other viral *onc*-related sequences has failed to detect a consistent correlation between the expression of proto-*onc* genes and neoplastic transformation (53a). In view of these uncertainties, induction of cellular proto-*onc* sequences by viruses without *onc* genes or other substances is not as yet regarded as proof for the quantitative model.

Different models have been proposed to explain induction of lymphomas in mice by murine leukemia viruses withoug *onc* genes. These models postulate that chronic mitotic stimulation of responsive T-cell populations by virus infection or virus-induced proteins is the cause of the viral lymphomas (91,101). The relevance of these models to chicken lymphoma has not yet been tested.

Clearly, transduction of cellular *onc*-related sequences by viruses without *onc* genes would be direct support for the quantitative model. Recently, experimental transduction of *src* has been claimed to occur at a frequency of over 50% within two months after inoculation of chicken with *src* deletion mutants lacking over 75% of the *src* gene (66,67,150,157). Deletions lacking one *src* terminus were reported to transduce *src* at the same, rather high, frequencies as deletions which retained both termini (66,67,157). In view of evidence that cellular proto *src* appears not linked to other virus-related sequences (78,79,94,130), this is surprising since transduction by deletions lacking one *src* terminus would require rare, illegitimate recombination and should, therefore, be much less frequent than transduction by deletions retaining both residual *src* termini requiring asymmetric, homologous recombination, which is known to occur in retroviruses (94,100). Proof for the transductional origin of the *src* genes of the resulting RSVs has been based on presumably host-derived *src*-oligonucleotide and peptide markers (84,85,150,157,158). However, subsequent analyses have not confirmed the existence of unambiguous host-markers in recovered *src* genes because these markers were indistinguishable from point mutations of parental counterparts (94). Since the *src* deletions used in these transduction experiments were not molecularly cloned, it cannot be excluded that the complete *src* genes of recovered RSVs originated by cross reactivation of nonoverlapping *src* deletions, possibly present in the *src* deletion stocks used to generate recovered RSVs. The point mutations could have been consequences of the reactivation process or could have been spontaneous, as retroviral genes undergo mutation at frequencies of about 10^{-3} to 10^{-4} on clonal selection (28,94,110). Further, the number of different *src* oligonucleotide or peptide markers reportedly recovered from the cell (66,67,150,157) is too large to be derived from the single *src*-related locus of the cell (78,79,130), unless one assumes that cellular *src*-related loci are as variable as recovered *src* genes (94). In this case, however, the variable *src* oligonucleotides and peptides could not be used to prove a cellular origin. Finally, the largest and most distinctive *src* oligonucleotide of recovered RSVs considered to be a marker of transduction by two different laboratories (150,157) was not detected in molecularly cloned proto-*src* of chicken (94). Therefore, available evidence for experimental transduction of cellular *onc*-related sequences is not sufficient to support the quantitative model.

Origin of Retroviral *onc* Genes

The close relationship between viral and cellular *onc*-related sequences suggests that transduction of cellular DNA by retorviruses has occurred at some time during the evolution of oncogenic viruses, since the oncogenic viruses described above appear to be recombinants between retroviruses and cellular, *onc*-related sequences.

However, transduction of *onc*-related sequences by retroviruses without *onc* genes must be a complex process for the following three reasons. First, because the analysis of the genetic structures of acutely oncogenic retroviruses shows that *onc*-specific sequences are located within viral RNA genomes at very specific sites (see above and Fig. 1), and because the cellular proto-*onc* genes lack any detectable linkage to non-*onc* virion sequences, transduction must involve double illegitimate recombination. Second, the internal sequences of nonhomology observed in most proto-*onc* genes would have to be deleted in order to make these sequences colinear with known viral *onc* genes. It is conceivable that this is accomplished by a splicing mechanism during or after transcription. However, since, for example, the *src*-related mRNA of normal cells measures about 3.9 kb (10,140,159) but viral *src* mRNA only about 2 kb (73,102) and since the MC29-related mRNA of normal cells measures about 2.8 kb (10,133,134) but the *mcv*-sequence of MC29 only about 1.6 kb, it remains unclear whether cellular splicing removes all intervening sequences of nonhomology on transcription. Although it has been reported that normal cells contain a protein that is antigenically and structurally related to the viral *src* gene product and to have a kinase function (10,52), there is no evidence that the cellular protein has transforming function, and it has recently been shown that the viral p60 *src* protein and its presumed cellular counterpart differ in their phosphorylation patterns (136a). Third, in the case of type II *onc* genes, such as the Δ*gag-mcv* gene of MC29, specific deletions of the transducing retrovirus would have to occur to form the Δ*gag-x* hybrid *onc* genes (Fig. 1). All of these events must occur during the course of an infection of a single animal by a retrovirus in order for a transmissible recombinant virus to emerge.

Alternatively, the formation of an oncogenic virus could proceed via vertically transmissible, recombinant prototypes of oncogenic viruses such as the 30S defective retrovirus-like RNAs found in certain normal cells (39,45). These are transmitted like known replication-competent, endogenous retroviruses without *onc* genes, but have genetic structures similar to those of defective oncogenic viruses (39,45,127,136). If these defective viral genomes were immediate precursors of oncogenic viruses, only relatively minor genetic changes might be necessary to form an oncogenic virus by recombination with a helper virus or the cell. A case in point is the 30S defective retrovirus-like RNA closely related to Harvey and Kirsten sarcoma viruses that has been detected in untransformed rat cells (96,127,136). Hence, the evolutionary origin of defective retroviruses might have been a multiphase process starting from cellular sequences related to viral *onc* genes, or proto-*onc* genes and retroviruses without *onc* genes, which led to the generation of endogenous prototypes of oncogenic viruses like the 30S defective retrovirus-like RNAs. The formation of such proto-oncogenic viruses would involve rare, illegitimate recombinations and specific deletions. But their potential to be transmitted as endogenous viruses would provide ample time and opportunities for the evolution of their viral and oncogenic properties. The final step would be the conversion of these precursors into highly oncogenic viruses, involving mutation or further recombinations with retroviruses and, possibly, the cell. In this case, not all of the above events would have to occur during the infection of a single animal. Instead, an oncogenic virus could be generated by a relatively minor genetic change from a preexisting, transmissible precursor.

SUMMARY

In this chapter, we have reviewed the present knowledge about the structures, possible functions, and origins of mainly avian retroviral *onc* genes. We point out that the beginning of the last decade has brought to light the first *onc* gene, namely the *src* gene of RSV. The number of *onc* genes identified since then in other avian and mammalian retroviruses has by now exceeded a dozen. In the avian tumor virus group alone, seven different classes of *onc* genes have been defined based on different *onc* gene-specific RNA sequences of viral genomes. In addition, the transforming proteins encoded by many *onc* genes have been discovered and the genetic structures of many retroviruses with *onc* genes have been defined during this time. On this basis, *onc* gene-related cellular DNA sequences, predicted by the oncogene and protovirus hypotheses, and termed proto-*onc* genes, have then been detected in the DNA of normal cells.

The strategy of *onc* gene expression follows two basic designs: *onc* genes of type I, whose coding sequence is unrelated to essential virion genes like in RSV and AMV, utilize subgenomic mRNAs coding for transforming proteins unrelated to virion proteins; and hybrid *onc* genes of type II, consisting of specific and virion gene-related, in particular *gag* gene-related, sequences like in myelocytomatosis virus MC29, AEV, and Fujinami-, Y73-, and UR2-sarcoma viruses are expressed via genome-size mRNAs coding for *gag* gene-related transforming proteins. Type I *onc* genes appear to be highly conserved in primary structure and sequence complexity, but type II *onc* genes of different viruses of the same subgroup may vary over 30% in sequence complexity and/or in primary structure.

Despite extensive research, little is as yet known about the function of viral *onc* gene products. The quest for *onc* gene function is probably most advanced in the case of p60, the phosphoprotein coded for by the *src* gene of RSV. The *src* protein p60 has been shown to be closely associated with a tyrosine-specific kinase activity and cellular proteins phosphorylated by this enzyme have been found. Similar activities have been proposed for the transforming proteins of other sarcoma viruses, but it remains to be proven that these activities are intrinsic enzymatic activities of viral proteins. Nothing is known about any activities of the transforming proteins encoded by the acute leukemia viruses.

With the exception of RSV, all acutely oncogenic retroviruses are defective to various degrees. In the extreme cases, the viral genome contains only an *onc*-specific RNA sequence flanked by noncoding 5' and 3' terminal sequence elements and a coding 5' terminal Δ*gag*-element, which together appear to represent the minimal vector elements for *onc* genes to be replicated and packaged like retroviral RNAs by helper virus proteins. In the case of RSV, the *onc* gene has become an integral part of the genome of a replication-competent virus. Hence, *onc* genes can be viewed as integrated or separate parasites of replication-competent retroviruses.

Since several totally different *onc* genes of either type I or type II may cause the same cancers, e.g., sarcomas, or erythroblastoses, different mechanisms appear to be used by different viruses to transform a given target cell into a tumor cell. The absence of *onc* genes from leukosis and lymphatic leukemia viruses is consistent with the low oncogenic potential of these viruses. Infection by lymphatic leukemia viruses causes cancers only rarely and, in particular, not simultaneously with virus replication, implying an indirect mechanism of transformation.

The finding of *onc* gene-related sequences in the DNA of normal chicken cells, but also in other vertebrate species including humans, suggests that acutely oncogenic retroviruses have evolved by recombinational events between nontransforming retroviruses and cellular genetic information. However, since all known cellular DNAs related to *onc* genes of avian tumor viruses are not flanked by other virion sequences and are interrupted by intervening sequences unrelated to viral counterparts, illegitimate recombinations and specific deletions of intervening sequences must have occurred to generate known oncogenic viruses from cellular DNA and retroviruses without *onc* genes. In addition, it is pointed out that type II, hybrid *onc* genes do not have complete sequence counterparts in normal cells, since cellular *onc*-related sequences are not linked to sequences related to essential virion genes like *gag*. The function of the *onc*-related sequences in normal cells is unknown and experimentation on their possible involvement in natural cancers or their potential to function as transforming genes after transduction or induction by lymphatic leukemia viruses without *onc* genes has only just begun.

ACKNOWLEDGMENTS

Supported by a grant from the National Cancer Institute, CA11426.

REFERENCES

1. Abelson, H. T., and Rabstein, L. S. (1970): Lymphosarcoma: Virus-induced thymine-independent disease in mice. *Cancer Res.*, 30:2213–2222.
1a. Balduzzi, P. C., Notter, M. F. D., Morgan, H. R., and Shibuya, M. (1981): Some biological properties of two new avian sarcoma viruses. *J. Virol.*, 40:268–275.
2. Baltimore, D. (1975): Tumor viruses: 1974. *Cold Spring Harbor Symp. Quant. Biol.*, 39:1187–1200.
3. Baltimore, D., Shields, A., Otto, G., Goff, S., Besmer, P., Witte, O., and Rosenberg, N. (1980): Structure and expression of the Abelson murine leukemia virus genome and its relationship to a normal cell gene. *Cold Spring Harbor Symp. Quant. Biol.*, 44:849–854.

4. Beard, J. W. (1980): Avian oncorna viruses: Biology. In: *Viral Oncology*, edited by George Klein, pp. 55–87. Raven Press, New York.
5. Beard, J. W., Langlois, A. J., and Beard, D. (1973): Etiological stain specificities of the avian tumor virus. In: *Unifying Concepts of Leukemia, Biblioteca Haematologica 39*, edited by R. M. Dutcher and L. Chieco-Bianchi, pp. 31–44. Karger, Basel, Switzerland.
6. Beemon, K. (1981): Transforming proteins of some feline and avian sarcoma viruses are related structurally and functionally. *Cell*, 24:145–154.
7. Beemon, K., Duesberg, P. H., and Vogt, P. K. (1974): Evidence for crossing over between avian tumor viruses based on analysis of viral RNAs. *Proc. Natl. Acad. Sci. USA*, 71:4254–4258.
8. Beug, H., von Kirchbach, A., Döderlein, G., Conscience, J.-F., and Graf, T. (1979): Chicken hematopoietic cells transformed by seven strains of defective avian leukemia viruses display three distinct phenotypes of differentiation. *Cell*, 18:375–390.
9. Bishop, J. M. (1981): Enemies within: The genesis of retrovirus oncogenes. *Cell*, 23:5–6.
10. Bishop, J. M., Courtneidge, S. A., Levinson, A. D., Oppermann, H., Quintrell, N., Sheiness, D. K., Weiss, S. R., and Varmus, H. E. (1980): The origin and function of avian retrovirus transforming genes. *Cold Spring Harbor Symp. Quant. Biol.*, 44:919–930.
11. Bister, K., and Duesberg, P. H. (1979): Structure and specific sequences of avian erythroblastosis virus RNA: Evidence for multiple classes of transforming genes among avian tumor viruses. *Proc. Natl. Acad. Sci. USA*, 76:5023–5027.
12. Bister, K., and Duesberg, P. H. (1980): Genetic structure of avian acute leukemia viruses. *Cold Spring Harbor Symp. Quant. Biol.*, 44:801–822.
13. Bister, K., and Duesberg, P. H. (1981): Two different designs of transforming genes in retroviruses. In: *Antiviral Chemotherapy: Design of Inhibitors of Viral Function*, edited by K. K. Gauri, pp. 1–10. Academic Press, New York.
14. Bister, K., Hayman, M. J., and Vogt, P. K. (1977): Defectiveness of avian myelocytomatosis virus MC29: Isolation of long-term nonproducer cultures and analysis of virus-specific polypeptide synthesis. *Virology*, 82:431–448.
15. Bister, K., Lee, W-H., and Duesberg, P. H. (1980): Phosphorylation of the nonstructural proteins encoded by three avian acute leukemia viruses and by avian Fujinami sarcoma virus. *J. Virol.*, 36:617–621.
16. Bister, K., Lee, W-H., Robins, T., and Duesberg, P. H., (1980): Fujinami sarcoma virus and sarcomagenic avian acute leukemia viruses have similar genetic structures. In: *Animal Virus Genetics*, edited by B. Fields, R. Jaenisch, and C. F. Fox, pp. 527–539. Academic Press, New York.
17. Bister, K., Löliger, H-C., and Duesberg, P. H. (1979): Oligoribonucleotide map and protein of CMII: Detection of conserved and nonconserved genetic elements in avian acute leukemia viruses CMII, MC29, and MH2. *J. Virol.*, 32:208–219.
17a. Bister, K., Nunn, M., Moscovici, C., Perbal, B., Baluda, M. A., and Duesberg, P. H. (1982): E26 and AMV: Two acute leukemia viruses with related transformation-specific RNA sequences, but different genetic structures, gene products and oncogenic properties. *Proc. Natl. Acad. Sci. USA*, 79:3677–3681.
17b. Bister, K., Ramsay, G., and Hayman, M. J. (1982): Deletions within the transformation-specific RNA sequences of acute leukemia virus MC29 give rise to partially transformation-defective mutants. *J. Virol.*, 41:754–766.
18. Bister, K., Ramsay, G., Hayman, M. J., and Duesberg, P. H. (1980): OK10, an avian acute leukemia virus of the MC29 subgroup with a unique genetic structure. *Proc. Natl. Acad. Sci. USA*, 77:7142–7146.
19. Bister, K., and Vogt, P. K. (1978): Genetic analysis of the defectiveness in strain MC29 avian leukosis virus. *Virology*, 88:213–221.
20. Blair, D. G., Oskarsson, M., Wood, T. G., McClements, W. C., Fischinger, P. J., and Vande Woude, G. F. (1981): Activation of the transforming potential of a normal cell sequence: A molecular model for oncogenesis. *Science*, 212:941–943.
21. Brugge, J. S., and Erikson, R. L. (1977): Identification of a transformation-specific antigen induced by an avian sarcoma virus. *Nature*, 269:346–348.
22. Chen, A. P., Essex, M., Shadduck, J. A., Niederkorn, J. Y., and Albert, D. (1981): Retrovirus encoded transformation-specific polyproteins: Expression coordinated with malignant phenotype in cells from different germ layers. *Proc. Natl. Acad. Sci. USA*, 78:3915–3919.
23. Chen, I. S. Y., Mak, T. W., O'Rear, J. J., and Temin, H. M. (1981): Characterization of reticulonedotheliosis virus strain T DNA and isolation of a novel variant of reticuloendotheliosis virus strain T by molecular cloning. *J. Virol.*, 40:800–811.

24. Chen, J. H., Hayward, W. S., and Moscovici, C. (1981): Size and genetic content of virus-specific RNA in myeloblasts transformed by avian myeloblastosis virus (AMV). *Virology*, 110:128–136.
25. Chen, J. H., Moscovici, M. G., and Moscovici, C. (1980): Isolation of complementary DNA unique to the genome of avian myeloblastosis virus (AMV). *Virology*, 103:112–122.
26. Chiswell, D. J., Ramsay, G., and Hayman, M. J. (1981): Two virus specific RNA species are present in cells transformed by defective leukemia virus OK10. *J. Virol.*, 40:301–304.
27. Cloyd, M. W., Hartley, J. U., and Rowe, W. P. (1980): Lymphomagenicity of recombinant mink cell focus-inducing murine leukemia viruses. *J. Exp. Med.*, 151:542–552.
28. Coffin, J. M., Tsichlis, P. N., Barker, C. S., Voynow, S., and Robinson, H. L. (1980): Variation in avian retrovirus genomes. *Ann. N.Y. Acad. Sci.*, 54:410–425.
29. Coffin, J. M., Tsichlis, P. N., and Robinson, H. L. (1981): Genetics of leukemogenesis by avian leukosis viruses. In: *Haematology and Blood Transfusion, Vol. 26. Modern Trends in Human Leukemia IV*, edited by R. Neth, R. C. Gallo, T. Graf, K. Mannweiler, and K. Winkler, pp. 432–438. Springer, Berlin, Heidelberg.
30. Coffin, J. M., Varmus, H. E., Bishop, J. M., Essex, M., Hardy, W. D., Martin, G. S., Rosenberg, N. E., Scolnick, E. M., Weinberg, R. A., and Vogt, P. K. (1981): A proposal for naming host cell derived inserts in retrovirus genomes. *J. Virol.*, 40:953–957.
31. Cooper, G. A., and Neiman, P. E. (1981): Two distinct candidate transforming genes of lymphoid leukosis virus-induced neoplasms. *Nature*, 292:857–858.
32. Cooper, J. A., and Hunter, T. (1981): Changes in protein phosphorylation in Rous sarcoma virus-transformed chicken embryo cells. *Mol. Cell. Biol.*, 1:165–178.
33. Cooper, J. A., and Hunter, T. (1981): Four different classes of retroviruses induce phosphorylation of tyrosines present in similar cellular proteins. *Mol. Cell. Biol.*, 1:394–407.
34. Czernilofsky, A. P., Levinson, A. D., Varmus, H. E., and Bishop, J. M. (1980): Nucleotide sequences of an avian sarcoma virus oncogene *(src)* and proposed amino acid sequence for gene product. *Nature*, 287:198–203.
35. Dalla Favera, R., Gelmann, E. P., Gallo, R. C., and Wong-Staal, F. (1981): A human *onc* gene homologous to the transforming gene (v-sis) of simian sarcoma virus. *Nature*, 292:31–35.
36. DeFeo, D., Gonda, M. A., Young, H. A., Chang, E. H., Lowy, D. R., Scolnick, E. M., and Ellis, R. W. (1981): Analysis of two divergent rat genomic clones homologous to the transforming gene of Harvey murine sarcoma virus. *Proc. Natl. Acad. Sci. USA*, 78:3328–3332.
37. Dina, D., Beemon, K., and Duesberg, P. H. (1976): The 30S Moloney sarcoma virus RNA contains leukemia virus nucleotide sequences. *Cell*, 9:299–309.
37a. Donner, P., Greiser-Wilke, I., and Moelling, K. (1982): Nuclear localization and DNA binding of the transforming gene product of avian myelocytomatosis virus. *Nature*, 296:262–266.
38. Duesberg, P. H. (1968): Physical properties of Rous sarcoma virus RNA. *Proc. Natl. Acad. Sci. USA*, 60:1511–1518.
39. Duesberg, P. H. (1980): Transforming genes of retroviruses. *Cold Spring Harbor Symp. Quant. Biol.*, 44:13–29.
40. Duesberg, P. H., and Bister, K. (1981): Transforming genes of retroviruses: Definition, specificity and relation to cellular DNA. In: *Cancer: Achievements, Challenges and Prospects for the 1980s*, edited by J. H. Burchenal and H. F. Oettgen, pp. 111–136. Grune & Stratton, New York.
41. Duesberg, P. H., Bister, K., and Moscovici, C. (1979): Avian acute leukemia virus MC29: Conserved and variable RNA sequences and recombination with helper virus. *Virology*, 99:121–134.
42. Duesberg, P. H., Bister, K., and Moscovici, C. (1980): Genetic structure of avian myeloblastosis virus released from transformed myeloblasts as a defective virus particle. *Proc. Natl. Acad. Sci. USA*, 77:5120–5124.
43. Duesberg, P. H., Bister, K., and Vogt, P. K. (1977): The RNA of avian acute leukemia virus MC29. *Proc. Natl. Acad. Sci. USA*, 74:4320–4324.
44. Duesberg, P. H., Robins, T., Lee, W-H., Papas, T., Garon, C., and Bister, K. (1982): On the relationship between the transforming *onc* genes of avian Rous sarcoma and MC29 viruses and homologous loci of the chicken cell. In: *Expression of Differentiated Functions in Cancer Cells*, edited by R. Revoltella et al. pp. 471–484. Raven Press, New York.
45. Duesberg, P. H., and Scolnick, E. M. (1977): Murine leukemia viruses containing a 30S RNA subunit of unknown biological activity, in addition to the 38S subunit of the viral genome. *Virology*, 83:211–216.
46. Duesberg, P. H., and Vogt, P. K. (1970): Differences between the ribonucleic acids of transforming and nontransforming avian tumor viruses. *Proc. Natl. Acad. Sci. USA*, 67:1673–1680.

47. Duesberg, P. H., and Vogt, P. K. (1973): RNA species obtained from clonal lines of avian sarcoma and from avian leukosis virus. *Virology*, 54:207–219.

48. Duesberg, P. H., and Vogt, P. K. (1979): Avian acute leukemia viruses MC29 and MH2 share specific RNA sequences: Evidence for a second class of transforming genes. *Proc. Natl. Acad. Sci. USA*, 76:1633–1637.

49. Duesberg, P. H., Vogt, P. K., Beemon, K., and Lai, M. M-C. (1975): Avian RNA tumor viruses: Mechanism of recombination and complexity of the genome. *Cold Spring Harbor Symp. Quant. Biol.*, 39:847–857.

50. Durban, E. M., and Boettiger, D. (1981): Replicating, differentiated macrophages can serve as *in vitro* targets for transformation by avian myeloblastosis virus. *J. Virol.*, 37:488–492.

51. Durban, E. M., and Boettiger, D. (1981): Differential effects of transforming avian RNA tumor viruses on avian macrophages. *Proc. Natl. Acad. Sci. USA*, 78:3600–3604.

52. Erikson, R. L., Collet, M. S., Erikson, E., Purchio, A. F., and Brugge, J. S. (1980): Protein phosphorylation mediated by partially purified avian sarcoma virus transforming gene product. *Cold Spring Harbor Symp. Quant. Biol.*, 44:907–917.

53. Essex, M. (1980): Etiology and epidemiology of leukemia and lymphoma in outbred animal species. In: *Advances in Comparative Leukemia Research*, edited by D. A. Yohn, B. A. Lapin, and J. R. Blakeslee, pp. 423–430. Elsevier/North Holland, New York.

53a.Eva, A., Robbins, K. C., Andersen, P. R., Srinivasan, A., Tronick, S. R., Reddy, E. P., Ellmore, N. W., Galen, A. T., Lautenberger, J. A., Papas, T. S., Westin, E. H., Wong-Staal, F., Gallo, R. C., and Aaronson, S. A. (1982): Cellular genes analogous to retroviral *onc* genes are transcribed in human tumour cells. *Nature*, 295:116–119.

54. Evans, L. H., and Duesberg, P. H. (1982): Isolation of a transformation-defective *onc* gene deletion mutant of Moloney murine sarcoma virus. *J. Virol.*, 41:735–743.

55. Feldman, R. A., Hanafusa, T., and Hanafusa, H. (1980): Characterization of protein kinase activity associated with the transforming gene product of Fujinami sarcoma virus. *Cell*, 22:757–765.

56. Franchini, G., Even, J., Sherr, C. J., and Wong-Staal, F. (1981): *Onc* sequences (v-*fes*) of Snyder-Theilen feline sarcoma virus are derived from noncontiguous regions of a cat cellular gene (c-*fes*). *Nature*, 290:154–157.

57. Frankel, A. E., and Fischinger, P. J., (1976): Nucleotide sequences in mouse DNA and RNA specific for Moloney sarcoma virus. *Proc. Natl. Acad. Sci. USA*, 73:3705–3709.

58. Gardner, M. B., Henderson, B. E., Estes, J. D., Rongey, P. W., Casagrande, J., Pike, M., and Huebner, R. J. (1976): The epidemiology and virology of C-type virus-associated hematological cancers and related diseases in wild mice. *Cancer Res.*, 36:574–581.

59. Ghysdael, J., Neil, J. C., and Vogt, P. K. (1981): A third class of avian sarcoma viruses, defined by related transformation-specific proteins of Yamaguchi 73 and Esh sarcoma viruses. *Proc. Natl. Acad. Sci.*, 78:2611–2615.

59a.Gilmer, T. M., and Erikson, R. L. (1981): Rous sarcoma virus transforming protein, p60^{src}, expressed in *E. coli*, functions as a protein kinase. *Nature*, 294:771–773.

60. Goff, S. P., Gilboa, E., Witte, O. N., and Baltimore, D. (1980): Structure of the Abelson murine leukemia virus genome and the homologous cellular gene: Studies with cloned viral DNA. *Cell*, 22:777–785.

61. Gonda, T. D., Sheiness, D. K., Fanshier, L., Bishop, J. M., Moscovici, C., and Moscovici, M. G. (1981): The genome and the intracellular RNAs of avian myeloblastosis virus. *Cell*, 23:279–290.

62. Graf, T., and Beug, H. (1978): Avian leukemia viruses: Interaction with their target cells *in vivo* and *in vitro*. *Biochem. Biophys. Acta*, 516:269–299.

63. Graf, T., Beug, H., and Hayman, M. J. (1980): Target cell specificity of defective avian leukemia viruses: Haematopoietic target cells for a given virus type can be infected but not transformed by strains of a different type. *Proc. Natl. Acad. Sci. USA*, 77:389–393.

64. Gross, L. (1970): *Oncogenic Viruses*. Pergamon Press, New York.

65. Groudine, M., and Weintraub, H. (1980): Activation of cellular genes by avian RNA tumor viruses. *Proc. Natl. Acad. Sci. USA*, 77:5351–5354.

66. Hanafusa, H., Halpern, C. C., Buchhagen, D. C., and Kawai, S. (1977): Recovery of avian sarcoma virus from tumors induced by transformation-defective mutants. *J. Exp. Med.*, 145:1735–1737.

67. Hanafusa, H., Wang, L-H., Hanafusa, T., Anderson, S. M., Karess, R. E., and Hayward, W. S. (1980): The nature and origins of the transforming gene of avian sarcoma viruses. In: *Animal*

Virus Genetics, edited by B. Fields, R. Jaenisch, and C. F. Fox, pp. 483–497. Academic Press, New York.

68. Hanafusa, T., Wang, L-H., Anderson, S. M., Karess, R. E., Hayward, W. S., and Hanafusa, H. (1980): Characterization of the transforming gene of Fujinami sarcoma virus. *Proc. Natl. Acad. Sci. USA*, 77:3009–3013.

69. Harvey, J. J. (1964): An unidentified virus which causes the rapid production of tumors in mice. *Nature*, 204:1104–1105.

70. Hayman, M. J. (1981): Transforming proteins of avian retroviruses. *J. Gen. Virol.*, 52:1–14.

71. Hayman, M. J., Kitchener, G., and Graf, T. (1979): Cells transformed by avian myelocytomatosis virus strain CMII contain a 90K *gag*-related protein. *Virology*, 92:191–199.

72. Hayman, M. J., Royer-Pokora, B., and Graf, T. (1979): Defectiveness of avian erythroblastosis virus: Synthesis of a 75K *gag*-related protein. *Virology*, 92:31–45.

73. Hayward, W. S., (1977): The size and genetic content of viral RNAs in avian oncovirus-infected cells. *J. Virol.*, 24:47–64.

74. Hayward, W. S., Neel, B. G., and Astrin, S. M. (1981): Activation of a cellular *onc* gene by promoter insertion in ALV-induced lymphoid leukosis. *Nature*, 290:475–480.

75. Hu, S. S. F., Lai, M. M. C., Wong, T. C., Cohen, R. S., and Sevoian, M. (1981): Avian reticuloendotheliosis virus: Characterization of the genome structure by heteroduplex mapping. *J. Virol.*, 37:899–907.

76. Hu, S. S. F., Moscovici, C., and Vogt, P. K. (1978): The defectiveness of Mill Hill 2, a carcinoma-inducing avian oncovirus. *Virology*, 89:162–178.

77. Huebner, R. J., and Todaro, G. J. (1969): Oncogenes of RNA tumor viruses as determinants of cancer. *Proc. Natl. Acad. Sci. USA*, 64:1087–1094.

78. Hughes, S. H., Payvar, F., Spector, D., Schimke, R. T., Robinson, H., Payne, G. S., Bishop, J. M., and Varmus, H. E. (1979): Heterogeneity of genetic loci in chickens: Analysis of endogenous viral and nonviral genes by cleavage of DNA with restriction endonuclease. *Cell*, 18:347–359.

79. Hughes, S. H., Stubblefield, F., Payvar, F., Engel, J. D., Dodgson, J. B., Spector, D., Cordell, B., Schimke, R. T., and Varmus, H. E. (1979): Gene localization by chromosome fractionation: Globin genes are on at least two chromosomes and three estrogen-inducible genes are on three chromosomes. *Proc. Natl. Acad. Sci. USA*, 76:1348–1352.

80. Hunter, T., Sefton, B. M., and Beemon, K. (1980): Phosphorylation of tyrosine: A mechanism of transformation shared by a number of otherwise unrelated RNA tumor viruses. In: *Animal Virus Genetics*, edited by B. Fields, R. Jaenisch, and C. F. Fox, pp. 499–514. Academic Press, New York.

81. Ishizaki, R., Langlois, A. J., Chabot, J., and Beard, J. W. (1971): Component of strain MC29 avian leukosis virus with the property of defectiveness. *J. Virol.*, 8:821–827.

82. Ivanov, X., Mladenov, Z., Nedyalkov, S., and Todorov, T. G. (1962): Experimental investigation into avian leukosis. I. Transmission experiments of certain diseases of the avian leukosis complex in Bulgaria. *Bull. Inst. Pathol. Comp. Animaux*, 9:5–36.

83. Jarrett, O. (1978): Infectious leukemias in domestic animals. In: *Modern Trends in Human Leukemia III*, edited by R. Neth, R. C. Gallo, P. H. Hofschneider, and K. Mannweiler, pp. 439–444. Springer, Berlin, Heidelberg..

84. Karess, R. E., and Hanafusa, H. (1981): Viral and cellular *src* genes contribute to the structure of recovered avian sarcoma virus transforming protein. *Cell*, 24:155–164.

85. Karess, R. E., Hayward, W. S., and Hanafusa, H. (1980): Transforming proteins encoded by the cellular information of recovered avian sarcoma virus. *Cold Spring Harbor Symp. Quant. Biol.*, 44:765–771.

86. Kawai, S., Yoshida, M., Segawa, K., Sugiyama, H., Ishizaki, R., and Toyoshima, K. (1980): Characterization of Y73, an avian sarcoma virus: A unique transforming gene and its product, a phosphopolypeptide with protein kinase activity. *Proc. Natl. Acad. Sci. USA*, 77:6199–6203.

86a. Kettmann, R., Deschamps, J., Cleuter, Y., Couez, D., Burny, A., and Marbaix, G. (1982): Leukemogenesis by bovine leukemia virus: Proviral DNA integration and lack of RNA expression of viral long terminal repeat and 3' proximate cellular sequences. *Proc. Natl. Acad. Sci. USA*, 79:2465–2469.

87. Kirsten, W. H., and Mayer, L. A. (1967): Morphologic responses to a murine erythroblastosis virus. *J. Natl. Cancer Inst.*, 39:311–335.

88. Kitchener, G., and Hayman, M. J. (1980): Comparative tryptic peptide mapping studies suggest a role in cell transformation for *gag*-related proteins of avian erythroblastosis virus and avian myelocytomatosis virus strains CMII and MC29. *Proc. Natl. Acad. Sci. USA*, 77:1637–1641.

89. Lai, M. M. C., Duesberg, P. H., Horst, J., and Vogt, P. K. (1973): Avian tumor virus RNA: A comparison of three sarcoma viruses and their transformation-defective derivatives by oligonucleotide fingerprinting and DNA-RNA hybridization. *Proc. Natl. Acad. Sci. USA*, 70:2266–2270.

90. Langlois, A. J., and Beard, J. W. (1967): Converted-cell focus formation in culture by strain MC29 avian leukosis virus. *Proc. Soc. Exp. Biol. Med.*, 126:718–722.

91. Lee, J. C., and Ihle, J. N. (1981): Chronic immune stimulation is required for Moloney leukemia virus-induced lymphomas. *Nature*, 289:407–409.

92. Lee, W-H., Bister, K., Moscovici, C., and Duesberg, P. H. (1981): Temperature-sensitive mutants of Fujinami sarcoma virus: Tumorigenicity and reversible phosphorylation of the transforming p140 protein. *J. Virol.*, 38:1064–1076.

93. Lee, W-H., Bister, K., Pawson, A., Robins, T., Moscovici, C., and Duesberg, P. H. (1980): Fujinami sarcoma virus: An avian RNA tumor virus with a unique transforming gene. *Proc. Natl. Acad. Sci. USA*, 77:2018–2022.

93a.Lee, W-H, Liu, C-P., and Duesberg, P. (1982): A DNA clone of avian Fujinami sarcoma virus with temperature-sensitive transforming function in mammalian cells. *J. Virol. (in press)*.

94. Lee, W-H., Nunn, M., and Duesberg, P. H. (1981): *Src* genes of ten Rous sarcoma virus strains, including two reportedly transduced from the cell, are completely allelic; Putative markers of transduction are not detected. *J. Virol.*, 39:758–776.

95. Levy, J. A. (1978): Xenotropic type-C virus. *Curr. Top. Microbiol. Immunol.*, 79:111–213.

96. Maisel, J., Klement, V., Lai, M. M. C., Ostertag, W., and Duesberg, P. H. (1973): Ribonucleic acid components of murine sarcoma and leukemia viruses. *Proc. Natl. Acad. Sci. USA*, 70:3536–3540.

97. Mangel, W. F., Delius, H., and Duesberg, P. H. (1974): Structure and molecular weight of the 60-70S RNA and the 30-40S RNA of the Rous sarcoma virus. *Proc. Natl. Acad. Sci. USA*, 71:4541–4545.

98. Martin, G. S. (1970): Rous sarcoma virus: A function required for the maintenance of the transformed state. *Nature*, 227:1021–1023.

99. Martin, G. S., and Duesberg, P. H. (1972): The *a* subunit in the RNA of transforming avian tumor viruses: I. Occurrence in different virus strains. II. Spontaneous loss resulting in non-transforming variants. *Virology*, 47:494–497.

100. Martin, G. S., Lee, W-H., and Duesberg, P. H. (1980): Generation of nondefective Rous sarcoma virus by asymmetric recombination between deletion mutants. *J. Virol.*, 36:591–594.

100a.McGrath, J. P., and Levinson, A. D. (1982): Bacterial expression of an enzymatically active protein encoded by RVS *src* gene. *Nature*, 295:423–425.

101. McGrath, M. S., Pillemer, E., Kooistra, D. A., Jacobs, S., Jerabek, L., and Weissman, I. L. (1980): T-lymphoma retroviral receptors and control of T-lymphoma cell proliferation. *Cold Spring Harbor Symp. Quant. Biol.*, 44:1297–1304.

102. Mellon, P., and Duesberg, P. H. (1977): Subgenomic, cellular Rous sarcoma virus RNAs contain oligonucleotides from the 3' half and the 5' terminus of virion RNA. *Nature*, 270:631–634.

103. Mellon, P., Pawson, A., Bister, K., Martin, G. S., and Duesberg, P. H. (1978): Specific RNA sequences and gene products of MC29 avian acute leukemia virus. *Proc. Natl. Acad. Sci. USA*, 75:5874–5878.

104. Moloney, J. B. (1966): A virus-induced rhabdomyosarcoma of mice. In: *Conference on Murine Leukemia*, National Cancer Institute Monograph No. 22, pp. 139–142. U.S. Public Health Service, Bethesda, Maryland.

105. Moscovici, C. (1975): Leukemic transformation with avian myeloblastosis virus: Present status. *Curr. Top. Microbiol. Immunol.*, 71:79–101.

106. Moscovici, C., Samarut, J., Gazzolo, L., and Moscovici, M. G. (1981): Myeloid and erythroid neoplastic responses to avian defective leukemia viruses in chickens and in quail. *Virology*, 113:765–768.

107. Neel, B. G., Hayward, W. S., Robinson, H. L., Fang, J., and Astrin, S. M. (1981): Avian leukosis virus-induced tumors have common proviral integration sites and synthesize discrete new RNAs: Oncogenesis by promoter insertion. *Cell*, 23:323–334.

108. Neil, J. C., Delamarter, J. F., and Vogt, P. K. (1981): Evidence of three classes of avian sarcoma viruses: Comparison of the transformation-specific proteins of PRCII, Y73 and Fujinami viruses. *Proc. Natl. Acad. Sci. USA*, 78:1906–1910.

109. Oker-Blom, N., Hortling, L., Kallio, A., Nurmiaho, E. L., and Westermarck, H. (1978): OK10 virus, an avian retrovirus resembling the acute leukemia viruses. *J. Gen. Virol.*, 40:623–633.

110. O'Rear, J. J., and Temin, H. M. (1981): Mapping of alterations in noninfectious proviruses of spleen necrosis virus. *J. Virol.*, 39:138–149.

111. Oskarsson, M. K., McClements, W. L., Blair, D. S., Maizel, J. V., and Vande Woude, G. F. (1980): Properties of a normal mouse cell DNA sequence (sarc) homologous to the *src* sequence of Moloney sarcoma virus. *Science*, 207:1222–1224.

112. Pawson, T., Guyden, J., Kung, T-H., Radke, K., Gilmore, T., and Martin, G. S. (1980): A strain of Fujimami sarcoma virus which is temperature-sensitive in protein phosphorylation and cellular transformation. *Cell*, 22:767–776.

113. Pawson, T., and Martin, G. S. (1980): Cell-free translation of avian erythroblastosis virus RNA. *J. Virol.*, 34:280–284.

113a. Payne, G. S., Bishop, J. M., and Varmus, H. E. (1982): Multiple arrangements of viral DNA and an activated host oncogene in bursal lymphomas. *Nature*, 295:209–214.

114. Payne, G. S., Courtneidge, S. A., Crittenden, C. B., Faldy, A. M., Bishop, J. M., and Varmus, H. E. (1981): Analysis of avian leukosis virus DNA and RNA in bursal tumors: Viral gene expression is not required for maintenance of the tumor state. *Cell*, 23:311–322.

115. Perbal, B., and Baluda, M. (1982): The avian myeloblastosis virus transforming gene is related to unique chicken DNA regions separated by at least one intervening sequence. *J. Virol.*, 41:250–257.

116. Purchase, G. H., and Burmester, B. R. (1977): Leukosis sarcoma group. In: *Diseases of the Poultry*, edited by M. S. Hofstad, B. W. Calnek, C. F. Helmbold, W. M., Reid, and H. W. Yoder, Jr., pp. 502–568. Iowa State University Press, Ames, Iowa.

117. Quade, K. (1979): Transformation of mammalian cells by avian myelocytomatosis virus and avian erythroblastosis virus. *Virology*, 98:461–465.

118. Quade, K., Saule, S., Stehelin, D., Kitchener, G., and Hayman, M. J. (1982): Virus gene expression in rat cells transformed by avian myelocytomatosis virus strain MC29 and avian erythroblastosis virus. *J. Gen. Virol. (in press)*.

119. Radke, K., and Martin, G. S. (1979): Transformation by Rous sarcoma virus: Effect of *arc*-gene expression on the synthesis and phosphorylation of cellular polypeptides. *Proc. Natl. Acad. Sci. USA*, 76:5212–5216.

120. Ramsay, G., Graf, T., and Hayman, M. J., (1980): Mutants of avian myelocytomatosis virus with smaller *gag* gene-related proteins have an altered transforming ability. *Nature*, 288:170–172.

121. Ramsay, G., and Hayman, M. J. (1980): Analysis of cells transformed by defective leukemia virus OK10: Production of non-infectious particles and synthesis of Pr76 *gag* and an additional 200,000 dalton protein. *Virology*, 106:71–81.

121a. Ramsay, G. M., and Hayman, M. J. (1982): Isolation and biochemical characterization of partially transformation-defective mutants of avian myelocytomatosis virus strain MC29: Localization of the mutation to the *myc* domain of the 11OK *gag-myc* polyprotein. *J. Virol.*, 41:745–753.

122. Robins, T., Bister, K., Garon, C., Papas, T., and Duesberg, P. (1982): Structural relationship between a normal chicken DNA locus and the transforming gene of the avian acute leukemia virus MC29. *J. Virol.*, 41:635–642.

123. Roussel, M., Saule, S., Lagrou, C., Rommens, C., Beug, H., Graf, T., and Stehelin, D. (1979): Three new types of viral oncogenes of cellular origin specific for haematopoietic cell transformation. *Nature*, 281:452–455.

124. Rubin, H., Fanshier, C., Cornelius, A., and Hughes, W. F. (1962): Tolerance and immunity in chicken after congenital and contact infection with avian leukosis virus. *Virology*, 17:143–156.

125. Rubin, H., and Hanafusa, H. (1963): Significance of the absence of infectious virus in virus-induced tumors. In: *Viruses, Nucleic Acids and Cancer*, pp. 508–525. Williams and Williams, Baltimore.

125a. Rushlow, K. E., Lautenberger, J. A., Papas, T. S., Baluda, M. A., Perbal, B., Chirikjian, J. G., and Reddy, P. (1982): Nucleotide sequence of the transforming gene of avian myeloblastosis virus. *Science (in press)*.

126. Schwartz, D., Tizard, R., and Gilbert, W. (1982): The nucleotide sequence of Prague Rous sarcoma virus. *Cell (in press)*.

127. Scolnick, E. M. (1981): Transformation by rat-derived oncogenic retroviruses. *Microbiol. Rev.*, 45:1–8.

128. Scolnick, E. M., and Parks, W. P. (1974): Harvey sarcoma virus: A second murine type C sarcoma virus with rat genetic information. *J. Virol.*, 13:1211–1219.

129. Scolnick, E. M., Rands, E., Williams, D., and Parks, W. P. (1973): Studies on the nucleic acid sequences of Kirsten sarcoma virus: A model for the formation of a mammalian RNA-containing sarcoma virus. *J. Virol.*, 12:456–463.

130. Shalloway, D., Zelenetz, A. D., and Cooper, G. M. (1981): Molecular cloning and characterization of the chicken gene homologous to the transforming gene of Rous sarcoma virus. *Cell*, 24:531–542.

131. Sheiness, D. K., and Bishop, J. M. (1979): DNA and RNA from uninfected vertebrate cells contain nucleotide sequences related to the putative transforming gene of avian myelocytomatosis virus. *J. Virol.*, 31:514–521.

132. Sheiness, D. K., Bister, K., Mosocvici, C., Fanshier, L., Gonda, T., and Bishop, J. M. (1980): Avian retroviruses that cause carcinoma and leukemia: Identification of nucleotide sequences associated with pathogenicity. *J. Virol.*, 33:962–968.

133. Sheiness, D. K., Hughes, S. H., Varmus, H. E., Stubblefield, E., and Bishop, J. M. (1980): The vertebrate homolog of the putative transforming gene of avian myelocytomatosis virus: Characteristics of the DNA locus and its RNA transcript. *Virology*, 105:415–424.

134. Sheiness, D. K., Vennstrom, B., and Bishop, J. M. (1981): Virus specific RNAs in cells infected by avian myelocytomatosis virus and avian erythroblastosis virus: Modes of oncogene expression. *Cell*, 23:291–300.

135. Sherr, C. J., Fedele, L. A., Oskarsson, M., Maizel, J., and Vande Woude, G. (1980): Molecular cloning of Snyder-Theilen feline leukemia and sarcoma virus: Comparative studies of feline sarcoma virus with its natural helper virus and with Moloney murine sarcoma virus. *J. Virol.*, 34:200–212.

135a.Shibuya, M., Hanafusa, T., Hanafusa, H., and Stephenson, J. R. (1980): Homology exists among the transforming sequences of avian and feline sarcoma viruses. *Proc. Natl. Acad. Sci. USA*, 77:6536–6540.

136. Shih, T. Y., and Scolnick, E. M. (1980): Molecular biology of mammalian sarcoma viruses. In: *Viral Oncology*, edited by George Klein, pp. 135–160. Raven Press, New York.

136a.Smart, J. E., Oppermann, H., Czernilofsky, A. P., Purchio, A. F., Erikson, R. L., and Bishop, J. M. (1981): Characterization of sites for tyrosine phosphorylation in the transforming protein of Rous sarcoma virus (pp60^{v-src}) and its normal cellular homologue (pp60^{c-src}). *Proc. Natl. Acad. Sci. USA*, 78:6013–6017.

137. Sotirov, N. (1981): Histone H5 in the immature blood cells of chickens with leukosis induced by avian leukosis virus strain E26. *J. Natl. Cancer Inst.*, 66:1143–1147.

138. Souza, L. M., Komaromy, M. C., and Baluda, M. A. (1980): Identification of a proviral genome associated with avian myeloblastic leukemia. *Proc. Natl. Acad. Sci. USA*, 77:3004–3008.

139. Souza, L. M., Strommer, J. N., Hillyard, R. L., Komaromy, M. C., and Baluda, M. A. (1980): Cellular sequences are present in the presumptive avian myeloblastosis virus genome. *Proc. Natl. Acad. Sci. USA*, 77:5177–5181.

140. Spector, D. H., Smith, K., Padgett, T., McCombe, P., Roulland-Dussoix, D., Moscovici, C., Varmus, H. E., and Bishop, J. M. (1978): Uninfected avian cells contain RNA related to the transforming gene of avian sarcoma viruses. *Cell*, 13:371–379.

141. Stehelin, D., Guntaka, R., Varmus, H. E., and Bishop, J. M. (1976): Purification of DNA complementary to nucleotide sequences required for neoplastic transformation of fibroblasts by avian sarcoma viruses. *J. Mol. Biol.*, 101:349–365.

142. Stehelin, D., Saule, S., Roussel, M., Sergeant, A., Lagrou, C., Rommens, C., and Raes, M. B. (1980): Three new types of viral oncogenes in defective avian leukemia viruses: I. Specific nucleotide sequences of cellular origin correlate with specific transformation. *Cold Spring Harbor Symp. Quant. Biol.*, 44:1215–1223.

143. Stehelin, D., Varmus, H. E., Bishop, J. M., and Vogt, P. K. (1976): DNA related to the transforming gene(s) of avian sarcoma viruses is present in normal avian DNA. *Nature*, 260:170–173.

144. Temin, H. M. (1971): The protovirus hypothesis: Speculations on the significance of RNA directed DNA synthesis for normal development and for carcinogenesis. *J. Natl. Cancer Inst.*, 46:3–7.

145. Temin, H. M. (1980): Origin of retroviruses from cellular movable genetic elements. *Cell*, 21:599–600.

146. Temin, H. M., and Rubin, H. (1958): Characteristics of an assay for Rous sarcoma virus and Rous sarcoma cells in tissue culture. *Virology*, 6:669–688.

147. Tooze, J. (1973): *The Molecular Biology of Tumour Viruses.* Cold Spring Harbor Laboratory, Cold Spring Harbor, New York.

148. Tsichlis, P. N., and Coffin, J. M. (1980): Role of the c-region in relative growth rates of endogenous and exogenous avian oncoviruses. *Cold Spring Harbor Symp. Quant. Biol.*, 44:1123–1132.

149. Tsuchida, N., Gilden, R. V., and Hatanaka, M. (1974): Sarcoma virus-related RNA sequences in normal rat cells. *Proc. Natl. Acad. Sci. USA*, 71:4503–4507.

149a. Vennström, B., and Bishop, J. M. (1982): Isolation and characterization of chicken DNA homologous to the two putative oncogenes of avian erythroblastosis virus. *Cell*, 28:135–143.

150. Vigne, R., Neil, J. C., Breitman, M. L., and Vogt, P. K. (1980): Recovered *src* genes are polymorphic and contain host markers. *Virology*, 105:71–85.

151. Vogt, P. K. (1977): Genetics of RNA tumor viruses. In: *Comprehensive Virology*, edited by H. Fraenkel-Conrat and R. R. Wagner, pp. 341–455. Plenum, New York.

152. Wang, L-H. (1978): The gene order of avian RNA tumor viruses derived from biochemical analyses of deletion mutants and viral recombinants. *Annu. Rev. Microbiol.*, 32:561–593.

153. Wang, L-H., Duesberg, P. H., Beemon, K., and Vogt, P. K. (1975): Mapping RNase T_1-resistant oligonucleotides of avian tumor virus RNAs: Sarcoma specific oligonucleotides are near the poly(A) end and oligonucleotides common to sarcoma and transformation-defective viruses are at the poly(A) end. *J. Virol.*, 16:1051–1070.

154. Wang, L-H., Duesberg, P. H., Kawai, S., and Hanafusa, H. (1976): Location of envelope-specific and sarcoma-specific oligonucleotides in RNA of Schmidt-Ruppin Rous sarcoma virus. *Proc. Natl. Acad. Sci. USA*, 73:447–451.

155. Wang, L-H., Duesberg, P. H., Mellon, P., and Vogt, P. K. (1976): Distribution of envelope-specific and sarcoma-specific nucleotide sequences from different parents in the RNAs of avian tumor virus recombinants. *Proc. Natl. Acad. Sci. USA*, 73:1073–1077.

156. Wang, L-H., Feldman, R., Shibuya, M., Hanafusa, H., Notter, M. F. D., and Balduzzi, P. E. (1981): Genetic structure, transforming sequence and gene product of avian sarcoma virus, UR1. *J. Virol.*, 40:258–267.

157. Wang, L-H., Halpern, C. C., Nadel, M., and Hanafusa, H. (1978): Recombination between viral and cellular sequences generates transforming sarcoma virus. *Proc. Natl. Acad. Sci. USA*, 75:5812–5816.

157a. Wang, L-H., Hanafusa, H., Notter, M. F. J., and Balduzzi, P. C. (1982): Genetic structure and transforming sequence of avian sarcoma virus UR2. *J. Virol.*, 41:833–841.

158. Wang, L-H., Snyder, P., Hanafusa, T., Moscovici, C., and Hanafusa, H. (1980): Comparative analysis of cellular and viral sequences related to sarcomagenic cell transformation. *Cold Spring Harbor Symp. Quant. Biol.*, 44:755–764.

159. Wang, S. Y., Hayward, W. S., and Hanafusa, H. (1977): Genetic variation in the RNA transcripts of endogenous virus genes in uninfected chicken cells. *J. Virol.*, 24:64–73.

160. Weyl, K. S., Dougherty, R. M. (1977): Contact transmission of avian leukosis virus. *J. Natl. Cancer Inst.*, 58:1019–1025.

160a. Wong, T-C., Hirano, A., Lai, M. M. C., and Vogt, P. K. (1982): Genome structure of the defective avian sarcoma virus PRCIV. *Virology*, 117:156–164.

160b. Wong, T-C., Lai, M. M. C., Hu, S. S. F., Hirano, A., and Vogt, P. K. (1982): Class II defective avian sarcoma viruses: Comparative analysis of genome structure. *Virology (in press)*.

161. Yoshida, M., Kawai, S., and Toyoshima, K. (1980): Uninfected avian cells contain structurally unrelated progenitors of avian sarcoma genes. *Nature*, 287:633–654.

162. Yoshida, M., Kawai, S., and Toyoshima, K. (1981): Genome structure of avian sarcoma virus Y73 and unique sequence coding for polyprotein p90. *J. Virol.*, 38:430–437.

Note added in proof

Recently H. M. Temin et al. have found that reticuloendotheliosis virus RNA, from which all *gag* sequences were deleted, is still packaged by helper virus (H. M. Temin, *personal communication*).

Advances in Viral Oncology, Volume 1,
edited by George Klein. Raven Press,
New York © 1982.

Avian Sarcoma Viruses, Protein Kinases, and Cell Transformation

R. L. Erikson and A. F. Purchio

*Department of Pathology, University of Colorado Health Sciences Center,
Denver, Colorado 80262*

ROUS SARCOMA VIRUS

The Transforming Gene, *src*, and Its Origin

Because it is such an efficient transforming virus, Rous sarcoma virus (RSV), among all the RNA tumor viruses available for study, has received a great deal of attention and has been the subject of numerous investigations (5,27,69). The attention directed toward this virus appears justified because it has proven to be a useful and interesting agent for the study of biochemical aspects of malignant transformation. The molecular description of cell transformation by RSV has developed rapidly over the past several years. More recently, however, studies on other avian sarcoma viruses (ASVs) have yielded equally interesting information.

Beginning in 1970, mutants of RSV that had an altered capacity to transform cells in culture and to produce fibrosarcomas in infected animals were isolated (34,41,68). These viral mutants were either temperature sensitive (ts), being unable to transform chicken cells at 41° C but able to transform cells at 35° C, or transformation-defective (td) deletion mutants unable to transform cells under any conditions tested. Gel electrophoresis and oligonucleotide mapping showed that in the td mutants the deletions were about 2,000 nucleotides in length and occurred very near the 3′ end of the RNA genome of the virus (69). Moreover, the ts mutations were found to occur in the region of the RSV genome that is missing in the deletion mutants. Studies such as these, which are described in more detail elsewhere, (*this volume*), led to the genetic definition of the RSV transforming gene, which was denoted *src* for sarcoma. Because viruses with either type of mutation replicate normally, the product of the *src* gene appears to play no role in the life cycle of the virus.

Studies with ts mutant-infected cells indicate that the product of the RSV *src* gene affects cytoskeletal structure, growth in soft agar, and rate of hexose uptake, characteristics that are phenotypic markers of transformation in culture. Avian or mammalian cells infected with a ts mutant can be reversibly switched to either the transformed or normal state within a few hours after the appropriate temperature shift. Inhibitors of protein synthesis do not affect the conversion from the transformed to normal state upon shift to the nonpermissive temperature (2), suggesting that all the components necessary for normal cellular function are present, but are perhaps modified in a readily reversible manner, in cells in which the *src* gene product is active.

Molecular hybridization analyses with radioactive DNA specific for the RSV *src* gene revealed that normal uninfected vertebrate cells contain DNA and RNA sequences closely related to *src* (65,66). These normal cellular sequences are denoted c-*src* (cell-*src*). Moreover, the fact that these *src*-like sequences were also present in poly A-containing, polyribosome-associated RNA indicated that the c-*src* DNA sequences are likely to be expressed in the form of a normal cellular protein (64,72).

The cellular DNA homologous to v-*src* (viral-*src*) has been obtained in the form of a molecular clone from a lambda library of chicken DNA (61,67). The library yielded four clones containing *src*-related DNA sequences from approximately 400,000 plaques. Analyses showed that the four independently isolated clones were generated from a single locus, and thus, if the chicken genome is uniformly represented in the library, it is unlikely that more than one c-*src* gene is present in uninfected chicken cells. Electron microscopic analyses of heteroduplexes formed between the DNA from these clones and from molecular clones of v-*src* DNA showed that 1.6 to 1.9 kb of the cellular *src*-containing DNA is homologous to v-*src* with seven nonhomologous regions that may represent intervening sequences in the c-*src* gene, which has a total length of 7 to 8 kb. The homologous sequences appear to represent the coding sequences for the c-*src* gene because, as described below, the v-*src* gene protein product and its putative cellular homologue are nearly identical in size (60,000 daltons) and in peptide composition, and a product of this size could be encoded by the approximately 1.8 kb of homologous sequences.

As described below, subgenomic viral RNA encompassing the *src* gene can be translated in cell-free extracts to yield a polypeptide indistinguishable from that produced in infected cells. Consequently, the v-*src* gene does not contain major intervening sequences requiring a splicing event to produce a functional mRNA. In contrast, c-*src* mRNA is about 4.4 kb in length and thus must have been spliced prior to expression in the cytoplasm. However, since its size is considerably greater than that required to produce the 60,000-dalton putative product of the gene, it may contain several nontranslated regions.

It is likely that RSV arose by recombination between a nontransforming avian retrovirus and the c-*src* gene and, indeed, this process has been duplicated, in part, under laboratory conditions. It has been shown that newly arising sarcoma viruses can be isolated from tumors of chickens and quails that were apparently induced by td RSV containing partial deletions of the *src* gene (28,33,71). During replication in the chicken, each of the newly recovered sarcoma viruses has reacquired an intact and functional *src* gene, at least 75% of which was obtained from cellular sequences. Transformation and tumors result when *src* mRNA is generated, under control of the integrated viral DNA, at levels at least 100-fold greater than the level of c-*src* mRNA (5) in uninfected cells. Takeya et al. (67) have suggested two possible mechanisms for the generation of transforming RSV. One is homologous recombination at the DNA level where normal c-*src* might be inserted at and replace the residual v-*src* sequences, producing a large recombinant. During transcription, the intervening sequences in c-*src* would be spliced to produce the RSV genome. A second possibility is recombination at the RNA level if c-*src* mRNA were incorporated into virions. Recombination may occur during reverse transcription or between proviral DNA intermediates. These investigators also point out that substantial evidence has accumulated that the transforming genes of several other RNA tumor viruses have been derived from normal cellular sequences and that the RSV system is potentially very useful for the elucidation of the events that give rise to transforming viruses.

The Transforming Gene Product, pp60$^{v\text{-}src}$, and Its Normal Cell Homologue pp60$^{c\text{-}src}$

As described above, by the mid-1970s it was clear from genetic and biochemical studies of the RSV genome that the product of the *src* gene was unlikely to be related to any polypeptides necessary for viral replication and, thus, any protein product of the gene was unlikely to be present in significant quantities in purified virions or to be an essential component of the infectious virus. The RSV transforming-gene product was originally identified by the use of serum from rabbits bearing RSV-induced tumors (TBR serum) to immunoprecipitate radiolabeled proteins from RSV-transformed cells of both avian and mammalian origin. This approach led to the identification of a transformation-specific antigen of 60,000 daltons (8). Furthermore, cell-free translation of the subgenomic 3′-third of the RSV genome, the region containing the *src* gene, also yielded a 60,000-dalton product (51). Not only did the transformation-specific antigen and the *src*-specific cell-free translation product have the same molecular weight, they proved to have similar methionine-containing tryptic peptides, thus showing with near certainty that this polypeptide was indeed the product of the RSV *src* gene (49). Tumor-bearing rabbits therefore recognized the *src* gene product and responded by producing antibody. The polypeptide immunoprecipitated from transformed cells proved to be a phosphoprotein and was by convention denoted pp60^{src} (9,39). More recently, the sequence of the *src* gene has been determined and an amino acid sequence of its product predicted (D. Schwartz, *personal communication*) (15). The results show a single open reading frame of substantial length and indicate that only a single product consisting of 526 amino acids could be produced.

When pp60^{src} was characterized as a phosphoprotein, it was observed that partial digestion of the molecule with the proteolytic enzyme V8 from *Staphylococcus aureus* generated two large fragments, both of which contained phosphorous radiolabel. Experiments showed that these two fragments corresponded to the amino and carboxy terminal portions of the molecule, and it was reported that pp60^{src} had two major sites of phosphorylation (11). Phosphoamino acid analysis revealed that the amino-terminal fragment contains a phosphoserine residue(s), whereas the carboxy-terminal fragment contains a phosphotyrosine residue (14,31).

The initial studies also demonstrated that the serine residue is phosphorylated by a cyclic AMP (cAMP)-stimulated protein kinase activity in cell-free extracts (11). This is of considerable importance because precedent established with other substrates of the cAMP-dependent protein kinase indicates that their function is influenced by their phosphorylation state (36), and the same may prove true for $pp60^{src}$. Thus, the cAMP-dependent protein kinase, an enzyme that is potentially able to regulate the activity of the transforming gene product of RSV, is present in both normal and transformed cells.

In contrast to the serine residue, cell-free phosphorylation studies showed that the tyrosine residue is phosphorylated by a cAMP-independent protein kinase activity. Furthermore, this same series of experiments revealed that the phosphotyrosine residue on the carboxy-terminal V8 fragment is not significantly phosphorylated in $pp60^{src}$ encoded by ts transformation mutants of RSV when ts mutant-transformed cells are grown at the nonpermissive temperature (normal morphology), whereas phosphorylation is similar to that of $pp60^{src}$ encoded by wild-type virus when ts mutant-transformed cells are grown and radiolabeled at the permissive temperature (transformed morphology) (11).

At relatively low levels, $pp60^{v-src}$ proved to be located in the cytoplasm of transformed cells (54), apparently associated with the plasma membrane (37,73), in contrast to the DNA tumor virus-encoded proteins implicated in transformation, which are largely confined to the nucleus. In addition, $pp60^{v-src}$ seems to be associated with the cellular adhesion plaques (56). Although it is closely associated with the plasma membrane after synthesis, the protein is synthesized on membrane-free polyribosomes and thus does not appear to be translated with the conventional leader sequence found for many membrane proteins (52).

Studies with ts mutants showed that on temperature shifts of transformed cells the morphological and some of the biochemical changes mentioned above occurred rapidly whether moving from normal to transformed or transformed to normal conditions. The appearance of surface ruffles is detectable as early as 30 min after a shift to the permissive temperature (1). It might be inferred from such behavior that the single *src* gene product biochemically modifies several cellular substrates in a readily reversible manner. Many unrelated studies on the role of protein phosphorylation in the regulation of diverse cellular functions (for review, see ref. 26) suggested a possible function for $pp60^{src}$ that could help explain the transformed cell phenotype. Initial studies directed at detecting a protein kinase activity associated with $pp60^{src}$ produced an unexpected result. When specific immunoprecipitates containing $pp60^{src}$ were tested for protein kinase activity, they were found to catalyze the transfer of radiolabel from $[\gamma-^{32}P]ATP$ to the heavy chain of IgG but not to any exogenously added common substrates of protein kinases (13,39,57). In addition, similar activity was found to be associated with $pp60^{src}$ generated by cell-free translation of that region of subgenomic viral RNA that contained the *src* gene

(17). A number of experiments showed that the presence of pp60[src] was an obligatory requirement for the IgG kinase activity. Hunter and Sefton (31) have identified the amino acid phosphorylated in IgG as tyrosine (as was the case for the carboxy terminus of pp60[src]), a previously undetected and relatively rare (as compared to serine and threonine) phosphoamino acid. Subsequently, during conventional phosphotransferase reactions, partially purified preparations of pp60[src] were shown to phosphorylate tyrosine residues in a variety of protein substrates such as tubulin and casein (14).

Until recently, the best evidence that the protein kinase activity is encoded by *src* comes from studies that show that the enzymatic activity purified from cells infected with a mutant ts for transformation is more thermolabile than a comparable preparation from cells infected with wild-type virus (19,20,40). Although the increased thermolability of the protein kinase activity *in vitro* is in accord with the expression of the transforming function in the infected cell, such a result does not eliminate the possibility of a second function associated with pp60[src].

Because the eukaryotic host cells transformed by RSV express a variety of protein kinases, it was of interest to obtain expression of pp60[src] in an environment devoid of these enzymatic activities, and the availability of molecular clones of the *src* gene carried in prokaryotes suggested a potentially useful source of the enzyme. Earlier studies failed to detect covalent protein phosphorylation in bacteria, but, more recently, distinct protein kinases and phosphoprotein phosphatases have been detected in *Salmonella typhimurium* (70). Despite this observation, because of evolutionary distance, the reactions are likely to be carried out by enzymes unrelated to those expressed in eukaryotic cells, and characterization of p60[src] expressed in *Escherichia coli* would be of value.

To obtain expression, the *lac* UV5 promoter-operator DNA fragment that had been used previously as a "portable promoter" (3) was ligated to the 5′ end of the RSV *src* gene by the use of *Eco* RI linkers (25). *E. coli*, containing plasmids with *src* under the control of the *lac* promoter, were screened for the expression of a 60,000-dalton protein by immunoprecipitation of ^{35}S-labeled extracts with antibody directed against pp60[src]. Clones expressing a protein immunologically and structurally related to the pp60[src] were detected, whereas bacteria carrying identical plasmids lacking the *src* gene yielded no detectable protein of this sort.

The p60[v-src] produced in *E. coli* was partially purified by immunoaffinity chromatography and characterized with regard to protein kinase functions (24). The results show that the protein from bacteria possesses a phosphotransferase activity that is *src*-specific based on the following criteria: (a) anti-*src* IgG is phosphorylated, (b) protein substrates such as tubulin and casein are phosphorylated at tyrosine residues, and (c) anti-*src* IgG inhibits the phosphorylation of exogenous substrates. No protein kinase activity is detectable in immunoaffinity-purified preparations from an identical amount of bacteria that lack the *src* gene. These data strongly support the previous conclusions that the enzymatic activity observed in preparations of pp60[src] from eukaryotic cells is actually encoded by the *src* gene and is not the result of the co-purification of one of the cell-encoded protein kinases expressed in eukaryotic cells.

The availability of a prokaryotic source of p60[v-src] that is qualitatively a protein kinase may serve to resolve a currently unsettled issue. Others (40) have purified pp60[v-src] to near homogeneity, and although these preparations retain their capacity to phosphorylate exogenous proteins, pp60[v-src] does not become phosphorylated during the reaction, whereas pp60[v-src] partially purified in this laboratory becomes phosphorylated under similar conditions (19,20). We have shown that the apparent autophosphorylation occurs on the same tyrosine residue as is phosphorylated in virus-infected cells (20). Moreover, as mentioned above, this tyrosine site is not phosphorylated when ts mutants of RSV are grown at the nonpermissive temperature, whereas it is phosphorylated at the permissive temperature (11). To gain additional insight concerning the phosphorylation of this tyrosine residue, pp60[src] was purified from cells infected with a mutant ts for transformation as described in the legend to Fig. 1. The thermolability of the capacity of this enzyme preparation to carry out self-phosphorylation was measured and compared to a similar preparation from wild-type virus-infected cells. As can be seen, the "autophosphorylation" *in vitro* of pp60[v-src] prepared from ts mutant-infected cells showed increased thermolability as compared to wild-type enzyme. Thus, the *in vivo* and *in vitro* results are consistent with an autophosphorylation function for pp60[v-src]. However, these data do not establish the case conclusively because phosphorylation of the ts mutant protein may not occur because, when pp60[v-src] is denatured, configurational changes render it a poor substrate for the putative pp60[src] kinase. Careful examination of p60[v-src] produced in *E. coli*, presumably in the absence of such a kinase activity, may resolve this puzzle.

As described above, the RSV *src* gene is derived from normal avian cells, and the normal cellular gene (c-*src*) is expressed as poly A-containing polyribosome-associated RNA. When a protein product of the c-*src* gene was sought, it was found that a 60,000-dalton phosphoprotein could be immunoprecipitated from normal avian and mammalian cells with certain cross-reactive sera derived from RSV tumor-bearing mammals (10,47,56,59). This protein has been designated pp60[c-src], although its genetic origin has not been proven by appropriate translation experiments. In addition to being antigenically related, viral, avian cell, and mammalian cell p60s are structurally very similar. Comparative studies on the sites of phosphorylation have shown that the normal cell *src*-related proteins contain both phosphoserine and phosphotyrosine with the former located in the protease V8 amino-terminal peptide and the latter in the protease V8 carboxy-terminal fragment. Furthermore, the phosphoserine residue(s) is located in tryptic peptide(s) similar or identical to that from viral pp60[src] (13), suggesting that pp60[c-src] may also be a substrate for cAMP-dependent protein kinase in normal cells.

The close structural relationship of viral and cellular p60s initially raised the possibility of a functional relationship and studies soon showed that the presence of pp60[c-src] correlated with the presence of a protein kinase activity specific for tyrosine residues in the immune complex assay (14). The results from the laboratory

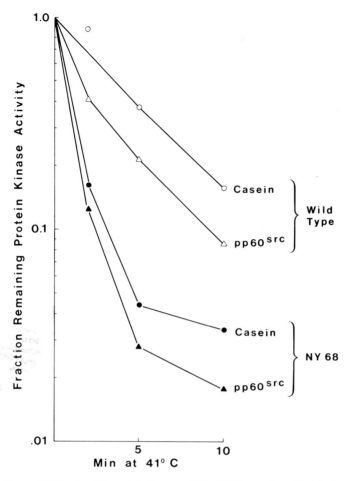

FIG. 1. Thermolability of pp60^{src} protein kinase activity. Chicken embryo fibroblasts were transformed with either wild-type Schmidt-Ruppin strain of RSV or the ts mutant of this strain, NY68 (34). The cells were maintained at the permissive temperature, 35° C. Immunoaffinity chromatography, as described previously (19,24), was used to prepare pp60^{src} from these cells. These preparations were heat-inactivated at 41° C for the indicated times and then phosphotransferase reactions were carried out in the presence of 5 mM Mg^{+2} and 1 μM [γ-^{32}P]ATP (350 Ci/mmol) in the absence of any exogenously added substrates or in the presence of casein (1 mg/ml). After polyacrylamide gel electrophoresis, the phosphorylated proteins were localized by autoradiography, the bands were excised, radioactivity was determined, and percentage activity was calculated from the amount of radioactivity in the bands. o,●, casein; Δ, ▲, pp60^{src}. (We are indebted to Eleanor Erikson and James B. Varner for carrying out this experiment.)

of H. Hanafusa bear on this issue. As mentioned above, newly recovered transforming viruses can be obtained from tumors of chickens infected with partial *src* gene deletion mutants of RSV. With the exception of the carboxy-terminal 20% of the protein, the *src* gene products of these recovered viruses have been derived from normal cellular genetic information (71), and these *src* gene products also show protein kinase activity specific for tyrosine residues. Extensive purification of pp60[c-src] by both ion-exchange or immunoaffinity chromatography has indicated, based on studies to date, that it is indistinguishable from pp60[v-src] in function (50).

The major difference detected to date in the expression of the v-*src* and the c-*src* genes is quantitative. Viral infection results in the synthesis of 50- to 100-fold more pp60[v-src] than the pp60[c-src] normally present in uninfected cells. Consequently, transformation by RSV may result from the overproduction of a protein similar or identical in structure and function to a normal cell protein. Much more detailed study is required before a firm conclusion can be drawn on this issue.

Substrates of the Protein Kinase Activity Associated with pp60[v-src]

The possibility that the protein kinase activity of pp60[src] leads to some properties of the transformed cell prompted a search for evidence of increased protein phosphorylation in RSV-transformed cells. Analyses of phosphotyrosine content revealed a nearly 10-fold increase in RSV-transformed cells, leading to the speculation that tyrosine phosphorylation was essential for cellular transformation by RSV (60). At a more specific level, a transformation-specific phosphoprotein was detected (53) by the techniques described by O'Farrell et al. (46). This 34,000- to 36,000-dalton protein was phosphorylated within 20 min after ts transformation mutant-infected cells were shifted from the nonpermissive to permissive temperature, and this protein was suggested as a possible target of pp60[src] (53). To answer this question directly, the unphosphorylated form of the protein was purified from normal cells and shown to be an *in vitro* substrate of pp60[src] protein kinase activity (18). Moreover, comparative phosphopeptide fingerprints revealed that the site phosphorylated *in vitro* occurs on a tyrosine residue in a tryptic peptide similar or identical to the major phosphopeptide found in the phosphoprotein isolated from transformed cells, thus suggesting that this normal cell protein is phosphorylated directly as a consequence of pp60[src] activity. No data are yet available, however, that show that phosphorylation of this protein is essential for the process of transformation. Nevertheless, these data do show more directly that the protein kinase activity associated with pp60[src] *in vitro* is actually expressed in transformed cells.

Another putative substrate of pp60[v-src] is vinculin (58), a protein that is associated with adhesion plaques and that may have a transmembrane relationship with extracellular proteins (63). The phosphorylation of vinculin is increased in certain transformed cells; however, this protein has not been shown to be a substrate of pp60[v-src] *in vitro*. We believe it is important to have both *in vivo* and *in vitro* data on the phosphorylation of a protein because neither approach used alone is convincing.

FUJINAMI AND PRCII SARCOMA VIRUSES

The Transforming Gene, fps

RSV is no longer the sole representative of ASVs. Two other classes have now been defined based on analyses of their transformation-specific sequences. The first

ASV recognized as distinct from RSV was Fujinami sarcoma virus (FSV) (29,38). Cloned stocks of the virus have biological properties similar to but not identical to RSV since they produce fibromyxosarcomas rather than fibrosarcomas in infected chickens, and fusiform rather than rounded morphology of cells during transformation in culture. In culture, transformed cells could be obtained that were not producing infectious virus or physical particles, although infectious transforming virus could be rescued by superinfection with helper virus. Thus, FSV is a replication-defective virus. The biochemical and biological consequences of replication-defective viruses are discussed in detail by Bister and Duesberg (*this volume*).

When a mixture of FSV and helper virus was used to prepare RNA, two major components were observed, 35S and 28S in size as judged by sucrose gradient sedimentation, corresponding to about 8.5 and 4.5 kb of RNA, respectively. The larger component was derived from the helper virus whereas the smaller was the FSV genome since it contained transformation-specific sequences not found in the helper virus RNA. About 1,000 nucleotides of *gag*-related sequences are present on the 5' end of the genome followed by at least 3,000 nucleotides in the middle of the genome that are transformation specific. These sequences are unrelated to the RSV *src* gene. Sequences at the 3' terminus are related to helper virus RNA.

Although the FSV transformation-specific sequences are unrelated to the *src* gene, they are closely related to those found in another sarcoma virus independently isolated from chickens, PRCII (62). The biological and biochemical properties of this virus are similar to those of FSV (7). It is interesting that these sequences, denoted fps, are also related, in part, to the transformation-specific sequences of the Gardner-Arnstein and Snyder-Theilen feline sarcoma viruses, but discussion of this matter is beyond the scope of this chapter. The structural organization of the PRCII genome is similar to that of the FSV genome.

The Transforming Gene Products, P140$^{gag-fps}$ (FSV) and P105$^{gag-fps}$ (PRCII)

FSV and PRCII have in common a partial *gag* gene fused to RNA sequences that encode transforming information, and produce in transformed cells transformation-specific polypeptides that have *gag*-gene antigenic determinants linked to non-*gag* determinants. The non-*gag* portion of the protein apparently carries the transforming function. Because of the *gag* gene antigenic determinants, the transformation-specific proteins can be immunoprecipitated from transformed cells with the appropriate anti-*gag* serum (4,6,21,29,38,42,44), but not by antiserum against other viral structural proteins. The transformation-specific polypeptides have molecular weights of 140,000 (P140$^{gag-fps}$) and 105,000 (P105$^{gag-fps}$) for FSV and PRCII, respectively. *In vitro* translation of virion RNA confirmed that P140 and P105 are encoded by the 28 S RNA species (16,38). Both P140 and P105 are phosphoproteins, and phosphoamino acid analyses reveal that they contain both phosphoserine and phosphotyrosine. It is possible that the phosphoserine in these polypeptides is present in the p19 sequences encoded by the *gag* gene. Beemon (4) showed by peptide fingerprinting that P140$^{gag-fps}$ and P105$^{gag-fps}$ are structurally related to one another as well as to the feline sarcoma virus transformation-specific protein P85, whereas no homology was observed between these proteins and the transforming proteins of either RSV or Y73 (see below).

When immunoprecipitates containing either P140 or P105 were assayed for protein kinase activity, different results were obtained depending on the antiserum used (21,48). Immunoprecipitates formed with antiserum from RSV-tumor-bearing rabbits, which contains anti-*gag* activity as well as anti-pp60[src] activity, showed protein kinase activity resulting in phosphorylation of the pertinent transformation-specific protein and the heavy chain of IgG, at tyrosine residues. Preadsorption of the serum with purified virion proteins abolished the capacity of the antiserum to immunoprecipitate both the protein and the protein kinase activity, showing that the anti-*gag* activity in TBR serum was responsible for the specific immunoprecipitation and that it was unlikely that antibody against the transformation-specific polypeptide sequences was present. In contrast, when antiserum raised against a purified *gag* protein, such as p19, was used, the immunoprecipitate showed no IgG kinase activity but retained the capacity to phosphorylate the transformation-specific protein at tyrosine residues. One possible explanation for such a result is that TBR IgG is a substrate for the protein kinase activity in the immunoprecipitate but does not have a sufficient affinity for the transformation-specific sequences to permit stable immune complexes to be formed. However, until studies are completed using more conventional assays, the questions raised by these results are likely to remain unanswered.

The results observed with the use of the immune complex assay for protein kinase activity may be interpreted in two ways. Pawson et al. (48) have shown, with one strain of FSV, that the transformed phenotype is ts and that the protein kinase activity and the increased phosphorylation of cellular proteins at tyrosine residues is also ts. These data may indicate that P140 is a protein kinase capable of phosphorylating itself and other cellular proteins. Alternatively, P140 may associate with and activate a cellular protein kinase, but if this were the case, the studies with the FSV ts transformation mutant suggest that the association must also be ts. Studies by Bister et al. (6) support the latter interpretation as they were able to separate the kinase activity from P140 by preincubation of cellular lysates with normal rabbit serum followed by removal of the IgG with *S. aureus* protein A. This issue will be resolved only by study of additional ts mutants in conjunction with conventional biochemical fractionation of the proteins of interest.

Immunoprecipitates of P105[gag-fps] also contain protein kinase activity specific for tyrosine residues (44). Again, strong evidence that the phosphotransferase is encoded by the viral genome is based on the thermolability of the enzymatic activity produced by PRCII mutants defective in their capacity to transform cells at elevated temperatures (P. K. Vogt, *personal communication*) (30).

YAMAGUCHI 73 AND Esh SARCOMA VIRUSES

The Transforming Gene Products, P90[gag-yes] (Y73) and P80[gag-yes] (Esh)

Two recently characterized ASVs, Yamaguchi 73 (Y73) and Esh, produce closely related phosphoproteins (22,23,43). The genomes of these viruses have not been

TABLE 1. *Avian sarcoma viruses*

	Class I	Class II	Class III
Virus and transforming gene product	Rous p60^{src}	Fujinami P140$^{gag\text{-}fps}$ PRCII P104$^{gag\text{-}fps}$	Y73 P90$^{gag\text{-}yes}$ Esh P80$^{gag\text{-}yes}$
Immunoprecipitated by			
Anti-gag	–	+	+
Anti-p60	+	–	–
Phosphotransferase activity for			
Anti-gag IgG	–	–	–
Anti-p60 IgG	+	+	+
"Autophosphorylation"	+	+	+

extensively characterized but it would appear that they are biologically similar to the Class II viruses and have unique transforming genetic information, dubbed *yes*, fused to the *gag* gene (35). The P90 of Y73 and P80 of Esh share all four transformation-specific methionine-containing peptides and seven cysteine-containing peptides, indicating a high degree of homology. However, two nonstructural transformation-specific cysteine-containing peptides were unique for P80 and three were unique for P90. None of these peptides were found in pp60^{src}, PRCII-P105, or FSV-P140. After *in vivo* labeling with ^{32}P, P90 and P80, after trypsin digestion, each yields two major phosphopeptides, one containing phosphoserine and the other phosphotyrosine. *In vitro* phosphorylation using the IgG complex assay results in the phosphorylation of the transformation-specific protein itself, and, if TBR serum is used, IgG heavy chain is phosphorylated as was the case for the Class II ASVs. Thus, although these proteins are antigenically and structurally distinct from those discussed above, they may have functional relatedness since all three protein classes are either protein kinases or strongly associated with protein kinases that readily phosphorylate anti-*src* IgG or tyrosine residues.

The similarity between p60$^{v\text{-}src}$ and P90 and P80 apparently extends to the amino acid sequence around the tyrosine site phosphorylated *in vivo* and *in vitro* because protease degradation yields phosphotyrosine-containing peptides from all three proteins that have a very similar primary structure (45). Thus, as might be expected for proteins of similar functions, there are regions of local homology albeit of a discrete and limited nature. To date, no ts transformation mutants of the Class III viruses have been reported. Should they become available, they will serve to clarify further if *yes*-specific nucleic acid sequences encode the protein kinase activity observed or if *yes* phosphoprotein products are merely substrates for other tyrosine-specific protein kinases.

In Table 1, we summarize the information published to date concerning ASVs, their transforming gene products, and the information available on protein kinase activities.

REFERENCES

1. Ambros, V. R., Chen, L. B., and Buchanan, J. M. (1975):Surface ruffles as markers for studies of cell transformation by Rous sarcoma virus. *Proc. Natl. Acad. Sci. USA*, 72:3144–3148.

2. Ash, J. F., Vogt, P. K., and Singer, S. J. (1976): Reversion from transformed to normal phenotype by inhibition of protein synthesis in rat kidney cells infected with a temperature-sensitive mutant of Rous sarcoma virus. *Proc. Natl. Acad. Sci. USA*, 73:3603–3607.

3. Backman, K., Ptashne, M., and Gilbert, W. (1976): Construction of plasmids carrying the cI gene of bacteriophage λ. *Proc. Natl. Acad. Sci. USA*, 73:4174–4178.

4. Beemon, K. (1981): Transforming proteins of some feline and avian sarcoma viruses are related structurally and functionally. *Cell*, 24:145–153.

5. Bishop, J. M. (1978): Retroviruses. *Annu. Rev. Biochem.*, 47:35–88.

6. Bister, K., Lee, W.-H., and Duesberg, P. H. (1980): Phosphorylation of the nonstructural proteins encoded by three avian acute leukemia viruses and by avian Fujinami sarcoma virus. *J. Virol.*, 36:617–621.

7. Breitman, M. L., Neil, J. C., Moscovici, C., and Vogt, P. K. (1981): The pathogenicity and defectiveness of PRCII: A new type of avian sarcoma virus. *Virology*, 108:1–12.

8. Brugge, J. S., Erikson, E., Collett, M. S., and Erikson, R. L. (1978): Peptide analysis of the transformation-specific antigen from avian sarcoma virus-transformed cells. *J. Virol.*, 26:773–782.

9. Brugge, J. S., and Erikson, R. L. (1977): Identification of a transformation-specific antigen induced by an avian sarcoma virus. *Nature*, 269:346–348.

10. Collett, M. S., Brugge, J. S., and Erikson, R. L. (1978): Characterization of a normal avian cell protein related to the avian sarcoma virus transforming gene product. *Cell*, 15:1363–1369.

11. Collett, M. S., Erikson, E., and Erikson, R. L. (1979): Structural analysis of the avian sarcoma virus transforming protein: Sites of phosphorylation. *J. Virol.*, 29:770–781.

12. Collett, M. S., Erikson, E., Purchio, A. F., Brugge, J. S., and Erikson, R. L. (1979): A normal cell protein similar in structure and function to the avian sarcoma virus transforming gene product. *Proc. Natl. Acad. Sci. USA*, 76:3159–3163.

13. Collett, M. S., and Erikson, R. L. (1978): Protein kinase activity associated with the avian sarcoma virus *src* gene product. *Proc. Natl. Acad. Sci. USA*, 75:2021–2024.

14. Collett, M. S., Purchio, A. F., and Erikson, R. L. (1980): Avian sarcoma virus-transforming protein, pp60src, shows protein kinase activity specific for tyrosine. *Nature*, 285:167–169.

15. Czernilofsky, A. P., Levinson, A. D., Varmus, H. E., Bishop, J. M., Tisher, E., and Goodman, H. M. (1980): Nucleotide sequence of an avian sarcoma virus oncogene *(src)* and proposed amino acid sequence for gene product. *Nature*, 287:198–203.

16. DeLamarter, J. F., Neil, J. C., Ghysdael, J., and Vogt, P. K. (1981): The 28S genomic RNA of avian sarcoma virus PRCII codes for the transformation-specific polyprotein P105. *Virology*, 112:757–761.

17. Erikson, E., Collett, M. S., and Erikson, R. L. (1978): In vitro synthesis of a functional avian sarcoma virus transforming-gene product. *Nature*, 274:919–921.

18. Erikson, E., and Erikson, R. L. (1980): Identification of a cellular protein substrate phosphorylated by the avian sarcoma virus-transforming gene product. *Cell*, 21:829–836.

19. Erikson, R. L., Collett, M. S., Erikson, E., and Purchio, A. F. (1979): Evidence that the avian sarcoma virus transforming gene product is a cyclic AMP-independent protein kinase. *Proc. Natl. Acad. Sci. USA*, 76:6260–6264.

20. Erikson, R. L., Collett, M. S., Erikson, E., Purchio, A. F., and Brugge, J. S. (1979): Protein phosphorylation mediated by partially purified avian sarcoma virus transforming-gene product. *Cold Spring Harbor Symp. Quant. Biol.*, 44:907–917.

21. Feldman, R. A., Hanafusa, T., and Hanafusa, H. (1980): Characterization of protein kinase activity associated with the transforming gene product of Fujinami sarcoma virus. *Cell*, 22:757–765.

22. Ghysdael, J., Neil, J. C., and Vogt, P. K. (1981): A third class of avian sarcoma viruses, defined by related transformation-specific proteins of Yamaguchi 73 and Esh sarcoma viruses. *Proc. Natl. Acad. Sci. USA*, 78:2611–2615.

23. Ghysdael, J., Neil, J. C., Wallbank, A. M., and Vogt, P. K. (1981): Esh sarcoma virus codes for a gag-linked transformation-specific protein with an associated protein kinase activity. *Virology*, 111:386–400.

24. Gilmer, T. M., and Erikson, R. L. (1981): The Rous sarcoma virus transforming protein, p60src, expressed in *Escherichia coli* functions as a protein kinase. *Nature*, 294:771–773.

25. Gilmer, T. M., Parsons, J. T., and Erikson, R. L. (1982): Construction of plasmids for the expression of the Rous sarcoma virus transforming protein, p60src, in *Escherichia coli*. *Proc. Natl. Acad. Sci. USA*, 79:2152–2156.

26. Greengard, P. (1978): Phosphorylated proteins as physiological effectors. *Science*, 199:146–152.
27. Hanafusa, H. (1977): Cell transformation by RNA tumor viruses. In: *Comprehensive Virology*, edited by H. Fraenkel-Conrat and R. P. Wagner, pp. 401–483. Plenum, New York.
28. Hanafusa, H., Halpern, C. C., Buchhagen, D. L., and Kawai, S. (1977): Recovery of avian sarcoma virus from tumors induced by transformation-defective mutants. *J. Exp. Med.*, 146:1735–1747.
29. Hanafusa, T., Wang, L.-H., Anderson, S. M., Karess, R. E., Hayward, W. S., and Hanafusa, H. (1980): Characterization of the transforming gene of Fujinami sarcoma virus. *Proc. Natl. Acad. Sci. USA*, 77:3009–3013.
30. Hirano, A., and Vogt, P. K. (1981): Avian sarcoma virus PRCII: Conditional mutants temperature sensitive in the maintenance of fibroblast transformation. *Virology*, 109:193–197.
31. Hunter, T., and Sefton, B. M. (1980): The transforming gene product of Rous sarcoma virus phosphorylates tyrosine. *Proc. Natl. Acad. Sci. USA*, 77:1311–1315.
32. Karess, R. E., and Hanafusa, H. (1981): Viral and cellular *src* genes contribute to the structure of recovered avian sarcoma virus transforming protein. *Cell*, 24:155–164.
33. Karess, R. E., Hayward, W. S., and Hanafusa, H. (1979): Cellular information in the genome of recovered avian sarcoma virus directs the synthesis of transforming protein. *Proc. Natl. Acad. Sci. USA*, 76:3154–3158.
34. Kawai, S., and Hanafusa, H. (1971): The effects of reciprocal changes in temperature on the transformed state of cells infected with a Rous sarcoma virus mutant. *Virology*, 46:470–479.
35. Kawai, S., Yoshida, M., Segawa, K., Sugiyama, H., Ishizaki, R., and Toyoshima, K. (1980): Characterization of Y73, an avian sarcoma virus: A unique transforming gene and its product, a phosphopolyprotein with protein kinase activity. *Proc. Natl. Acad. Sci. USA*, 77:6199–6203.
36. Krebs, E. G., and Beavo, J. A. (1979): Phosphorylation-dephosphorylation of enzymes. *Annu. Rev. Biochem.*, 48:923–959.
37. Krueger, J. G., Wang, E., and Goldberg, A. R. (1980): Evidence that the *src* gene product of Rous sarcoma virus is membrane associated. *Virology*, 101:25–40.
38. Lee, W-H., Bister, K., Pawson, A., Robins, T., Moscovici, C., and Duesberg, P. H. (1980): Fujinami sarcoma virus: An avian RNA tumor virus with a unique transforming gene. *Proc. Natl. Acad. Sci. USA*, 77:2018–2022.
39. Levinson, A. D., Oppermann, H., Levintow, L., Varmus, H. E., and Bishop, J. M. (1978): Evidence that the transforming gene of avian sarcoma virus encodes a protein kinase associated with a phosphoprotein. *Cell*, 15:561–572.
40. Levinson, A. D., Oppermann, H., Varmus, H. E., and Bishop, J. M. (1980): The purified product of the transforming gene of avian sarcoma virus phosphorylates tyrosine. *J. Biol. Chem.*, 255:11973–11980.
41. Martin, G. S. (1970): Rous sarcoma virus: A function required for the maintenance of the transformed state. *Nature*, 227:1021–1023.
42. Neil, J. C., Breitman, M. L., and Vogt, P. K. (1981): Characterization of a 105,000 molecular weight *gag*-related phosphoprotein from cells transformed by the defective avian sarcoma virus PRCII. *Virology*, 108:98–110.
43. Neil, J. C., DeLamarter, J. F., and Vogt, P. K. (1981): Evidence for three classes of avian sarcoma viruses: Comparison of the transformation-specific proteins of PRCII, Y73, and Fujinami viruses. *Proc. Natl. Acad. Sci. USA*, 78:1906–1910.
44. Neil, J. C., Ghysdael, J., and Vogt, P. K. (1981): Tyrosine-specific protein kinase activity associated with p105 of avian sarcoma virus PRCII. *Virology*, 109:223–228.
45. Neil, J. C., Ghysdael, J., Vogt, P. K., and Smart, J. E. (1981): Homologous tyrosine phosphorylation sites in transformation-specific gene products of distinct avian sarcoma viruses. *Nature*, 291:675–677.
46. O'Farrell, P. Z., Goodman, H. M., and O'Farrell, P. H. (1977): High resolution two-dimensional electrophoresis of basic as well as acidic proteins. *Cell*, 12:1133–1142.
47. Oppermann, H., Levinson, A. D., Varmus, H. E., Levintow, L., and Bishop, J. M. (1979): Uninfected vertebrate cells contain a protein that is closely related to the product of the avian sarcoma virus transforming gene *(src)*. *Proc. Natl. Acad. Sci. USA*, 76:1804–1808.
48. Pawson, T., Guyden, J., Kung, T-H., Radke, K., Gilmore, T., and Martin, G. S. (1980): A strain of Fujinami sarcoma virus which is temperature-sensitive in protein phosphorylation and cellular transformation. *Cell*, 22:767–775.
49. Purchio, A. F., Erikson, E., Brugge, J. S., and Erikson, R. L. (1978): Identification of a polypeptide encoded by the avian sarcoma virus *src* gene. *Proc. Natl. Acad. Sci. USA*, 75:1567–1571.

50. Purchio, A. F., Erikson, E., Collett, M. S., and Erikson, R. L. (1981): Partial purification and characterization of pp60^{c-src}, a normal cellular protein structurally and functionally related to the avian sarcoma virus *src* gene product. In: *Cold Spring Harbor Conferences on Cell Proliferation-Protein Phosphorylation, Vol. 8*, edited by O. M. Rosen and E. G. Krebs, pp. 1203–1215.

51. Purchio, A. F., Erikson, E., and Erikson, R. L. (1977): Translation of 35S and of subgenomic regions of avian sarcoma virus RNA. *Proc. Natl. Acad. Sci. USA*, 74:4661–4665.

52. Purchio, A. F., Jovanovich, S., and Erikson, R. L. (1980): Sites of synthesis of viral proteins in avian sarcoma virus-infected chicken cells. *J. Virol.*, 35:629–636.

53. Radke, K., and Martin, G. S. (1979): Transformation by Rous sarcoma virus: Effects of *src* gene expression on the synthesis and phosphorylation of cellular polypeptides. *Proc. Natl. Acad. Sci. USA*, 76:5212–5216.

54. Rohrschneider, L. R. (1979): Immunofluorescence on avian sarcoma virus-transformed cells: Localization of the *src* gene product. *Cell*, 16:11–24.

55. Rohrschneider, L. R. (1980): Adhesion plaques of Rous sarcoma virus-transformed cells contain the *src* gene product. *Proc. Natl. Acad. Sci. USA*, 77:3514–3518.

56. Rohrschneider, L. R., Eisenman, R. N., and Leitch, C. R. (1979): Identification of a Rous sarcoma virus transformation-related protein in normal avian and mammalian cells. *Proc. Natl. Acad. Sci. USA*, 76:4479–4483.

57. Rübsamen, H., Friis, R. R., and Bauer, H. (1979): *Src* gene product from different strains of avian sarcoma virus: Kinetics and possible mechanism of heat inactivation of protein kinase activity from cells infected by transformation-defective, temperature-sensitive mutant and wild-type virus. *Proc. Natl. Acad. Sci. USA*, 76:967–971.

58. Sefton, B. M., and Hunter, T. (1981): Vinculin: A cytoskeletal target of the transforming protein of Rous sarcoma virus. *Cell*, 24:165–174.

59. Sefton, B. M., Hunter, T., and Beemon, K. (1980): Relationship of polypeptide products of the transforming gene of Rous sarcoma virus and the homologous gene of vertebrates. *Proc. Natl. Acad. Sci. USA*, 77:2059–2063.

60. Sefton, B. M., Hunter, T., Beemon, K., and Eckhart, W. (1980): Evidence that the phosphorylation of tyrosine is essential for cellular transformation by Rous sarcoma virus. *Cell*, 20:807–816.

61. Shalloway, D., Zelenetz, A. D., and Cooper, G. M. (1981): Molecular cloning and characterization of the chicken gene homologous to the transforming gene of Rous sarcoma virus. *Cell*, 24:531–541.

62. Shibuya, M., Hanafusa, T., Hanafusa, H., and Stephenson, J. R. (1980): Homology exists among the transforming sequences of avian and feline sarcoma viruses. *Proc. Natl. Acad. Sci. USA*, 77:6536–6540.

63. Singer, I. I., and Paradiso, P. R. (1981): A transmembrane relationship between fibronectin and Vinculin (130 kd protein): Serum modulation in normal and transformed hamster fibroblasts. *Cell*, 24:481–492.

64. Spector, D. H., Baker, B., Varmus, H. E., and Bishop, J. M. (1978): Characteristics of cellular RNA related to the transforming gene of avian sarcoma viruses. *Cell*, 13:381–386.

65. Spector, D. H., Smith, K., Padgett, T., McCombe, P., Roulland-Dussoix, D., Moscovici, C., Varmus, H. E., and Bishop, J. M. (1978): Uninfected avian cells contain RNA related to the transforming gene of avian sarcoma virus. *Cell*, 13:371–379.

66. Stehelin, D., Varmus, H. E., Bishop, J. M., and Vogt, P. K. (1976): DNA related to the transforming gene(s) of avian sarcoma viruses is present in normal avian DNA. *Nature*, 260:170–173.

67. Takeya, T., Hanafusa, H., Junghans, R., Ju, G., and Skalka, A. M. (1981): Comparison between the viral transforming gene *(src)* of recovered avian sarcoma virus and its cellular homologue. *Mol. Cell. Biol.*, 1:1024–1037.

68. Toyoshima, K., and Vogt, P. K. (1969): Temperature-sensitive mutants of an avian sarcoma virus. *Virology*, 39:930–931.

69. Vogt, P. K. (1977): The genetics of RNA tumor viruses. In: *Comprehensive Virology*, edited by H. Fraenkel-Conrat and R. P. Wagner, pp. 341–455. Plenum, New York.

70. Wang, J. Y. J., and Koshland, D. E., Jr. (1981): The identification of distinct protein kinases and phosphatases in the prokaryote *Salmonella typhimurium*. *J. Biol. Chem.*, 256:4640–4648.

71. Wang, L. H., Halpern, C. C., Nadel, M., and Hanafusa, H. (1978): Recombination between viral and cellular sequences generates transforming sarcoma virus. *Proc. Natl. Acad. Sci. USA*, 75:5812–5816.

72. Wang, S. Y., Hayward, W. S., and Hanafusa, H. (1977): Genetic variation in the RNA transcripts of endogenous virus genes in uninfected chicken cells. *J. Virol.*, 24:64–73.

73. Willingham, M. C., Jay, G., and Paston, I. (1979): Localization of the ASV *src* gene product to the plasma membrane of transformed cells by electron microscopic immunocytochemistry. *Cell*, 18:125–134.

Advances in Viral Oncology, Volume 1,
edited by George Klein. Raven Press,
New York © 1982.

Viral-Encoded Transforming Proteins and Transforming Growth Factors

John R. Stephenson and George J. Todaro

*Laboratory of Viral Carcinogenesis, National Cancer Institute,
National Institutes of Health, Frederick, Maryland 21701*

The initial impetus for studies of the molecular biology of RNA tumor viruses derived from their capacity to transform cells in culture and induce malignant tumors *in vivo*. Such findings raised the possibility that type C viruses might represent significant etiologic agents in naturally occurring cancers of many species, possibly including humans. As a result of these studies, several examples of cancers with a well-established viral etiology have emerged. Among these, viral-induced lymphoid leukemias of avian, murine, and feline species have been examined in greatest detail (89). There is increasing evidence that the role of retroviruses as vectors or for molecular cloning of various cellular genes, including those with transforming potential, may be of even greater significance than their etiologic involvement in spontaneous tumors (28,91). The application of retroviruses to this purpose has led to the identification of a number of transforming genes of cellular origin (oncogenes) and raised the possibility that the representation of such genes within the cellular genome may be relatively limited (28,34,91).

On the basis of functional considerations, type C retroviruses can be classified into two major groups (89). The first consists of the chronic viruses that induce neoplastic transformation, predominantly of hemopoietic cells, *in vivo*. Although viruses of this group are replication-competent, they do not cause morphological transformation of cells in culture and are generally associated with induction of lymphoid tumors *in vivo* only subsequent to prolonged latent periods. In contrast, acute transforming viruses are generally, although not invariably, replication-defective, and they morphologically transform cells in culture and induce tumors *in vivo* within a few weeks of virus inoculation. Isolation of viruses of this second category has been relatively infrequent and, as discussed below, reflects rare recombinational events between type C viral genomic RNAs and cellular genetic sequences with specificity for transforming functions. It is through study of this latter group of viruses that translational products of cellular genes with transforming function are currently being identified and characterized. The availability of well-characterized cellular transforming genes provides a unique opportunity for the analysis of cellular regulatory pathways involved in malignant transformation.

The translational products of many viral transforming genes have been identified and several have been shown to possess associated protein kinase activities with specificity for tyrosine residues (5,14,27,33,38,40,41,52,57,68,105,107). Moreover, several cellular proteins that interact with and/or are specifically phosphorylated by viral-encoded transforming proteins have been identified (24,37,68,69). In other studies, both viral and certain spontaneously transformed *in vitro* propagated cell lines have been shown to exhibit reduced capacity for binding epidermal growth factor (EGF) (94). This, at least in some instances, involves production of low molecular weight (6,000 to 20,000) polypeptide transforming growth factors (TGFs), which morphologically transform cells in culture (93,95,96), compete with radio-labeled EGF for specific membrane binding sites (19), and induce phosphorylation of the EGF cell membrane receptors specifically at tyrosine acceptor sites (64). These interactions between viral- and cellular-gene products and their possible relevance to spontaneously arising cancers represents the major focus of this chapter.

ACQUISITION AND EXPRESSION OF VIRAL-ENCODED TRANSFORMING PROTEINS

Cells nonproductively transformed by several independent isolates of mammalian transforming viruses have been shown to encode virus structural proteins to varying extents. In most instances, these are restricted to *gag* gene-related components and are expressed progressively from the 5' terminus of the viral genome (8,91). This pattern of expression is colinear with the arrangement of *gag* gene-specific components within the helper virus genome, previously established as 5'-p15-p12-p30-p10-3' (8,70). For instance, cells nonproductively transformed by independently derived retrovirus isolates express p15; p15 and p12; or p15, p12 and p30; these are generally in the form of polyproteins that are subject to variable extents of posttranslational cleavage (91). Cells transformed by other viral isolates lack expression of all four *gag* gene-encoded proteins.

Translational products of acquired sequences with transforming function are frequently expressed as a result of their inphase insertion within preexisting type C virus structural genes. In several instances, expression of such sequences has been shown to be in the form of high molecular weight polyproteins consisting of amino terminal *gag* gene structural components covalently linked to acquired sequence-encoded nonstructural components. As summarized in Table 1, such a model has been demonstrated for several mammalian type C viruses, including Abelson murine leukemia virus (Abelson MuLV) (63,71,110), the Rasheed strain of rat sarcoma virus (Rasheed RaSV) (111), and each of three independent feline sarcoma virus (FeSV) isolates (7,41,42,90,101,104). Alternatively, transformation-specific acquired sequences of viruses such as Moloney murine sarcoma virus (MSV) appear to be inserted within, and presumably are under control of, the viral *env* gene (4,53,98). A characteristic of several viruses of this latter group is a variable extent of expression of *gag* gene structural components among independent subclones of the same original transforming isolate (91). The structural and functional properties

TABLE 1. *Mammalian RNA transforming viruses with known polyprotein translational products[a]*

Virus isolate	Polyprotein molecular weight	Structural components	Tyrosine-specific protein kinase	Genetic evidence for transforming function
Mouse				
Abelson MuLV	120,000	p15,p12	+	+
AK-T8 MuLV	110,000	p15,p12	−	NT
3611-MSV	100,000	p15,p12	−	NT
Rat				
Rasheed RaLV	35,000	p15	−	NT
Cat				
Gardner FeSV	110,000	p15,p12	+	+
Snyder-Theilen FeSV	110,000	p15,p12	+	+
MSTF variant	85,000	p15,p12	+	+
McDonough FeSV	170,000	p15,p12,p30	−	+

[a]The identification and characterization of retrovirus polyprotein translational products was performed as described in detail in the text. NT means not tested.

of the gene products of prototype virus isolates of each of these groups are considered below.

TRANSFORMING RETROVIRUSES—MOUSE

Sarcoma Viruses

Two independent type C retroviruses with sarcoma-specific transforming sequences of mouse cell origin have been described. Both transform cells in culture and induce fibrosarcomas *in vivo*. The most thoroughly studied of these, Moloney MSV, represents a genetic recombinant between the Moloney strain of MuLV and transformation-specific sequences of cellular origin (4,36,53,98). By molecular cloning and restriction endonuclease analysis, acquired cellular transforming sequences have been localized within the 3' portion of the Moloney MSV genome (4,53,98). Although initial attempts to demonstrate *in vivo* expression of a translational product corresponding to the Moloney MSV-acquired sequences were unsuccessful, this was primarily due to the lack of an appropriate antiserum. Consistent with this possibility is the demonstration by *in vitro* translation of several related 20,000 to 40,000 molecular weight (M_r) Moloney MSV-acquired sequence-specific proteins (17,54). In other studies, a low (15,000) molecular weight protein with tyrosine-specific protein kinase activity has been identified in Moloney MSV virions (78). This activity is thermolabile when isolated from temperature-sensitive (ts) but not wild type (wt) Moloney MSV pseudotype virions (78), associates with microtubular proteins, and inhibits *in vitro* polymerization of microtubules (77,78). In contrast to many other transforming viruses, transformation by Moloney MSV does not result in an overall elevation of cellular phosphotyrosine levels (76). The Moloney

MSV transforming gene product has recently been identified in transformed cells as a 37,000 M_r phosphoprotein by use of antisera against synthetic peptides corresponding to its predicted C terminus determined based on sequencing of the viral genome (55).

An additional, less well-characterized MSV isolate was originally derived from a naturally occurring sarcoma of a BALB/c mouse (58). This latter virus, designated BALB MSV, represents a genetic recombinant between AKR MuLV and mouse cellular sequences (1,8). Although the position of the acquired sequences within the viral genome has not been established, BALB MSV resembles Moloney MSV in that subclones of the original isolate have been shown to express *gag* gene structural components to variable extents (1,8). Transformation by BALB MSV is associated with the expression of high levels of a 21,000 dalton protein, immunologically related to Harvey MSV p21, discussed below. Additionally, a high degree of sequence homology exists between the BALB MSV and Harvey MSV transforming genes (3).

Acute Leukemia Viruses

Of the mammalian systems studied, the mouse is the only species from which acute transforming viruses have been isolated with *in vivo* specificity for leukemias, rather than sarcomas. The most well-characterized virus of this group, Abelson MuLV, transforms lymphoid cells and embryo fibroblasts in culture and, in the presence of replication-competent helper virus, induces a rapid B-cell lymphoma *in vivo* (2,75). Abelson MuLV genomic RNA is 5.6 kilobases (kb) in length and consists of 1.3 kb and 0.7 kb at its 5' and 3' termini, respectively, derived from the parental Moloney MuLV genome and a central domain of around 3.6 kb corresponding to transformation-specific cellular sequences of mouse origin (31,82).

By competition immunoassay and immunoprecipitation analyses of Abelson MuLV nonproductively transformed cells, a 120,000 dalton polyprotein, P120, consisting of Moloney MuLV amino terminal *gag* gene structural components (p15, p12, and a minor portion of p30), and a less well-defined nonstructural component has been identified (63,110). That P120 represents a direct translational product of the Abelson MuLV genomic RNA has been established by direct *in vitro* translation both in rabbit reticulocyte (110) and *Xenopus oocyte* (71) systems. By tryptic peptide analysis, the nonstructural component of Abelson MuLV P120 has been shown to be encoded by acquired cellular sequences represented within the Abelson MuLV genome (103). The invariable detection of P120 in Abelson MuLV-transformed cell clones and the loss of its expression in morphological revertants of such cells provided initial evidence for its transformation specificity (73). Functional analysis of Abelson MuLV P120 has led to the demonstration of an associated protein kinase activity with specificity for tyrosine acceptor sites both within exogenous substrates and within the polyprotein itself (105,107). Two major *in vitro* phosphorylated acceptor peptides have recently been purified by high performance liquid chromatography and by subsequent amino acid sequence analysis; the phosphorylated tyrosine residues within these sites have been identified six and seven amino acids distal to the trypsin cleavage site (F. H. Reynolds, S. Oroszlan and J. R. Stephenson, *unpublished observations*). In addition to phosphotyrosine, two phosphoserine sites within the p12 structural component of Abelson MuLV P120 and several phosphoserine and phosphothreonine sites in its acquired sequence-encoded component have been identified (67).

A number of independent transformation-defective (td) mutants of Abelson MuLV have been isolated (67,73). Cells nonproductively infected by such viral mutants exhibit a high degree of growth contact inhibition, fail to form colonies in soft agar, and are nontumorigenic *in vivo*. Although the 120,000 M_r polyproteins expressed in td mutant-infected clones are indistinguishable from those in wt Abelson MuLV-transformed cells with respect to level of expression, molecular weight, and [^{35}S]methionine tryptic peptide composition, they lack detectable tyrosine-specific protein kinase activity (67). *In vitro* [γ^{32}P]ATP-mediated phosphorylation of the single Abelson MuLV P120 tyrosine acceptor site is below detectable levels in td mutant-infected cell clones, and Abelson MuLV P120 tyrosine phosphorylation is not observed *in vivo* (67). Moreover, elevated levels of total cellular phosphotyrosine characteristic of wt Abelson MuLV-transformed cells are not observed in td Abelson MuLV-infected clones (Table 2). These findings, in combination with the results of studies by Witte et al. (108) involving analysis of variants of Abelson MuLV-encoding, truncated, kinase-defective polyproteins, establish the involvement of the Abelson MuLV-encoded polyprotein P120 and its associated protein kinase activity in Abelson MuLV tumorigenesis.

Although the normal functions of cellular sequences corresponding to those represented by the acquired sequences of the Abelson MuLV genome are unknown,

TABLE 2. *Phenotypic properties of cells transformed by representative mammalian RNA tumor viruses[a]*

Virus isolate	Growth in soft agar (%)	Phosphotyrosine (% of total cellular phosphoamino acids)	Reduced [^{125}I]-EGF binding	TGF production
Mouse				
Moloney MSV	16	<0.2	+	+
Abelson MuLV				
wild type	21	2.3	+	+
td mutant	<0.01	<0.2	−	−
Rat				
Kirsten MSV	16	<0.2	+	NT
Cat				
Gardner FeSV	16	2.1	+	NT
Snyder-Theilen FeSV				
wild type	21	1.9	+	NT
td mutant	<0.01	<0.2	−	NT
McDonough FeSV	17	<0.2	+	NT

[a]The isolation of cell lines nonproductively transformed by the above retrovirus isolates has been described in detail previously (65–67). NT means not tested.

a 150,000 M_r cellular protein has been identified and shown to share immunologic determinants with the nonstructural component of Abelson MuLV P120 (109). This cellular protein, designated NCP 150, is expressed preferentially in lymphoid organs and, in particular, the thymus.

A second acute murine transforming virus with specificity for lymphoid cells, designated AK-T8, was isolated from a thymic tumor of an AKR mouse and subsequently cloned on mink cells (88). AK-T8 resembles Abelson MuLV in that it encodes as its major translational product a high molecular weight polyprotein. This latter protein, P110, is expressed at readily detectable levels in mink cells nonproductively infected by AK-T8 and consists of AKR MuLV p15 and p12 structural components covalently linked to an acquired sequence component of around 80,000 M_r (74). In contrast to Abelson MuLV P120, AK-T8 P110 lacks detectable protein kinase reactivity and cellular phosphotyrosine concentrations remain at control levels in AK-T8-infected cells (102). Although the carboxy terminal portion of AK-T8 P110 has been shown by tryptic peptide analysis to be encoded by acquired cellular sequences represented within the AK-T8 genome (102), genetic evidence for its involvement in transformation is unavailable. Moreover, on continuous passage, AK-T8 nonproductively infected mink cells lose both their transformed phenotype and rescuable transforming virus, despite the fact that levels of P110 expression remain high.

A third MuLV acute transforming virus, the Friend strain of spleen focus-forming virus (Friend SFFV), differs from the above two isolates in that it is highly tumorigenic, inducing a rapid erythroleukemia *in vivo*, but causes no apparent morphologic alteration of cells in culture (10,72). Cells nonproductively infected with independent variants of Friend SFFV differ in their extent of *gag* gene expression. For instance, cells infected with one Friend SFFV variant associated with polycythemia *in vivo* express only the amino terminal *gag* gene protein, p15 (10), whereas those infected with a second polycythemia-inducing variant express p15 and p12 (46,72). A single isolate of Friend SFFV, which induces a rapid erythroleukemia associated with anemia, rather than polycythemia, encodes p15 and p12 (46). On the basis of genetic evidence, the transforming component of Friend SFFV has been localized within the 3′ region of the viral genome (44,45). In addition to their variable extents of *gag* gene expression, each of the above-described Friend SFFV variants encode envelope glycoproteins of around 52,000 M_r (46,72). Localization of the Friend SFFV-transforming function within the *env* region of the viral genomic RNA implicates this latter gene product in erythroleukemia induction. Such a model is supported by differences in the [^{35}S]methionine tryptic peptide maps of gp52 gene products of the anemia- and polycythemia-inducing variants of Friend SFFV (46).

TRANSFORMING RETROVIRUSES—RAT

Several independent transforming virus isolates with acquired sequences of rat cellular origin have been described (23). These represent genetic recombinants between rat cellular sequences and type C viruses of either mouse origin, as is the case with Harvey and Kirsten MSV (23), or of rat origin, as with Rasheed RaSV (62,111). Of these, the Rasheed strain of RaSV represents a further example of a mammalian type C virus-encoded *gag* gene-related polyprotein translational product; this is in the form of a 29,000 M_r protein consisting of an amino terminal *gag* gene component, p15, covalently linked to an acquired sequence-encoded nonstructural component (111). In contrast, the Harvey and Kirsten strains of MSV encode gene proteins of around 21,000 M_r that are immunologically related both to each other and to Rasheed RaSV p29 but lack *gag* gene-encoded amino terminal p15 immunologic determinants (23). This difference may appear to reflect the relative proximity of the acquired sequences of these independent virus isolates to the 5' terminus of the viral genomes in which they are inserted, the acquired sequences within the Harvey and Kirsten MSV genomes being sufficiently close to the 5' terminus of their respective viral genomes to preclude synthesis of an immunologically detectable *gag* gene product (23).

Functional analysis of the p21 gene products of the Harvey and Kirsten strains of MSV have established their localization in the inner surface of the plasma membrane and led to the demonstration of binding activity for guanine nucleotides (23,85). In addition, both of these viral-encoded transforming proteins possess "autophosphorylating" activities with specificity for threonine rather than tyrosine residues and a preference for GTP or dGTP rather than ATP or dATP as the phosphosyl donor (23,85). Although the expression of immunologically cross-reactive proteins has been demonstrated at low levels in normal cells of many vertebrate species (23,43), their functional significance remains to be determined. Recently, however, transfection of DNA from a human bladder carcinoma cell line has been shown to lead to expression of a cellular protein antigenically related to Harvey MSV p21 (20; L. Parada et al., *personal communication*; M. Barbacid *personal communication*).

TRANSFORMING RETROVIRUSES—FELINE

Three independent replication-defective isolates of FeSV have been obtained from spontaneously arising tumors of cats chronically infected with FeLV (30,49,87). Each transforms embryo fibroblasts in cell culture and induces fibrosarcomas on inoculation *in vivo*. In all three cases, acquired sequences are expressed as high molecular weight polyproteins due to inphase translational readthrough initiated at the 5' terminus of the viral *gag* gene (7,41,42,90,92,101,104). On the basis of structural and functional considerations, these viruses can be separated into two classes: the first consisting of the Gardner and Snyder-Theilen strains of FeSV, and the second of McDonough FeSV (7,26,29,65,101,106).

Gardner and Snyder-Theilen FeSV

The Gardner and Snyder-Theilen strains of FeSV have been shown by competition immunoassay and immunoprecipitation analyses to encode as their major translational products, 110,000 M_r polyproteins (P110), consisting of FeLV structural proteins (p15 and p12) covalently linked to acquired sequence-encoded components (7,41,90). Major posttranslational cleavage products of 72,000 and 80,000 M_r corresponding to the amino terminal portion of the Gardner and Snyder-Theilen FeSV polyproteins, respectively, have also been described (101). A second variant of Snyder-Theilen FeSV encodes an 85,000 protein as its major gene product (5,66), as well as lower levels of an 80,000 M_r cleavage product (F. H. Reynolds and J. R. Stephenson, *unpublished observations*). By immunologic and tryptic peptide analyses, this latter protein corresponds to the 80,000 M_r cleavage product of Snyder-Theilen FeSV P110. Of five methionine-containing tryptic peptides localized within the acquired sequence-encoded components of Gardner FeSV P110, three are present in Snyder-Theilen FeSV P110 and P85, as well as in their 80,000 M_r cleavage products (7,101). These findings argue that the acquired cellular sequences of these independently derived virus isolates have regions in common and that the 85,000 M_r gene product of the variant strain of Snyder-Theilen FeSV represents a truncated form of P110. The relatedness of polyproteins encoded by the Gardner and Snyder-Theilen isolates of FeSV has recently been confirmed by use of monoclonal antibodies directed against their acquired sequence-encoded components (106).

Functional analysis of the Gardner and Snyder-Theilen FeSV-encoded polyproteins has indicated each to possess associated protein kinase activities with specificity for tyrosine acceptor sites (5,68,105). In immunoprecipitate form, these phosphorylate tyrosine residues both in the polyproteins themselves and to a lesser extent in exogenous substrates such as immunoglobulin. Single major tyrosine-containing phosphorylation acceptor sites within the major polyprotein translational products of both Snyder-Theilen FeSV and Gardner FeSV have been identified (12). Tyrosine phosphorylation of these acceptors has been demonstrated both in immunoprecipitates and by direct labeling of unfractionated extracts in the presence of $[\gamma^{32}P]ATP$. By two-dimensional tryptic peptide analysis, tyrosine phosphorylation sites within Snyder-Theilen FeSV P110, P85, and Gardner FeSV P110 closely resemble each other although, unexpectedly, are not identical, possibly reflecting one or more base substitutions occurring subsequent to the recombinational events resulting in the generation of individual FeSV isolates. These acceptor tyrosines each have been localized by sequential Edman degradation at a position seven amino acid residues distal to trypsin cleavage sites (56; F. H. Reynolds, Jr., S. Oroszlan, and J. R. Stephenson, *unpublished observations*).

The involvement of Gardner and Snyder-Theilen FeSV polyprotein-associated protein kinase activities in transformation has been directly established through the isolation and characterization of td mutants (66). Although the major viral polyprotein translational products expressed in td mutant-infected cells are at levels comparable to those of wt transformants, they invariably lack detectable protein kinase activity. Moreover, overall cellular phosphotyrosine levels are not significantly greater in td mutant than in control cells (66). In other studies, each of a number of wt Gardner and Snyder-Theilen FeSV-transformed cell clones were shown to revert to a nontransformed morphology on continuous passage in cell culture. Such nontransformed variants lack detectable polyprotein expression and exhibit overall phosphotyrosine levels similar to those of control cells (66). These findings, in combination with the results of transfection experiments utilizing restriction fragments of Snyder-Theilen FeSV proviral DNA (79), establish the involvement of Gardner and Snyder-Theilen FeSV-encoded polyproteins and their associated tyrosine-specific protein kinase activities in transformation.

In addition to their *in vitro* phosphorylated tyrosine acceptor sites, several *in vivo* phosphorylation sites have been identified in the Gardner and Snyder-Theilen FeSV-encoded polyproteins (105). These include single phosphotyrosine acceptors mapping at positions corresponding to the *in vitro* phosphotyrosine sites and two phosphoserine sites specific to the polyprotein p12 structural components. The similarity in map positions of additional phosphoserine and phosphothreonine peptides further argues for relatedness between the nonstructural components of the independently derived Gardner and Snyder-Theilen isolates of FeSV.

Studies directed toward a determination of metabolic pathways involved in transformation by individual FeSV isolates have led to the identification of a 150,000 M_r cellular substrate specifically recognized by the Gardner and Snyder-Theilen FeSV polyprotein-associated protein kinase activities (68,69). On the basis of immunologic and tryptic peptide analyses, P150 has been shown to be structurally unrelated to polyprotein translational products of either the Gardner, Snyder-Theilen, or McDonough strains of FeSV (68). P150 possesses broadly reactive interspecies antigenic determinants and its expression has been demonstrated in cells of a wide range of mammalian species. Tyrosine residues within P150 are phosphorylated in immunoprecipitates of the Gardner and Snyder-Theilen FeSV-encoded polyproteins as well as in Gardner and Snyder-Theilen FeSV-transformed cells *in vivo*. P150 is highly glycosylated, possesses at least nine major *in vivo*-labeled phosphorylation sites, and exhibits binding affinity for the Gardner and Snyder-Theilen FeSV polyprotein translational products. Although P150 itself possesses an associated protein kinase, this differs from the FeSV P110 enzymatic activities in that it phosphorylates serine and, to a lesser extent, threonine residues rather than tyrosine (68).

McDonough FeSV: An Immunologically and Structurally Distinct Isolate of Feline Origin

In contrast to the Gardner and Snyder-Theilen strains of FeSV, McDonough FeSV encodes as its major gene product a 170,000 M_r polyprotein (P170) containing not only FeLV p15 and p12, but also p30 structural components (7,104). By tryptic peptide analysis, a total of five methionine-containing peptides have been identified within McDonough FeSV P170. Two of these correspond to its p30 structural component; the three remaining peptides are localized in a 120,000 M_r-acquired sequence-encoded component (104). Of three peptides localized within the nonstructural component of McDonough FeSV P170, one is also represented in the polyprotein translational products of the Gardner and Snyder-Theilen strains of

FeSV. As one explanation of this observation, polyproteins encoded by each of these transforming viruses may contain both common and unique components. Alternatively, the similarity in map position of the single methionine-containing peptide apparently shared by these virus isolates may be coincidental.

McDonough FeSV P170 further differs from the Gardner and Snyder-Theilen FeSV-encoded polyproteins in that it is weakly, if at all, phosphorylated *in vivo* and lacks detectable protein kinase activity *in vitro* (65,106). Moreover, overall cellular levels of phosphotyrosine in McDonough FeSV-transformed cells are not significantly elevated over those of nontransformed control cells (Fig. 1). These findings argue for differences in mechanisms of cellular transformation by independently derived FeSV isolates.

Relatedness of Feline and Avian Sarcoma Virus Isolates

Transforming sequences analogous to those represented within the genomic RNAs of Gardner and Snyder-Theilen FeSV have been shown to exhibit sequence homology with Fujinami sarcoma virus (FSV) as well as with the highly related PRCII strain of avian sarcoma virus (ASV) (81). Under conditions of moderate stringency, radioactively labeled DNA complementary to FSV-unique sequences (FSV cDNA) hybridized with PRCII ASV genomic RNA to a final extent of 56%. In addition, FSV cDNA was found to hybridize with RNAs of the Gardner and Snyder-Theilen strains of FeSV to extents of 27 and 19%, respectively, but not to an appreciable degree with McDonough FeSV RNA. On thermal denaturation analysis, melting temperatures (T_m) of the heteroduplexes of the FSV cDNA with RNAs of PRCII ASV and Gardner FeSV were 7 and 12% lower, respectively, than the T_m of the homologous FSV hybrid, suggesting less than 10% mismatching in both heteroduplexes. No detectable cross-hybridization was observed between FSV cDNA and the genomic RNAs of Rous sarcoma virus (RSV), Y73 ASV, representative avian acute leukemia viruses, or Abelson MuLV. Additionally, antigenic cross-reactivity has been demonstrated between the nonstructural components of the polyprotein translational products of the Gardner and Snyder-Theilen strains of FeSV, FSV, and PRCII ASV (6). More recently, the human cellular homologue of transforming sequences common to Gardner and Snyder-Theilen FeSV has been molecularly cloned using a cosmid vector system (32) and shown to exhibit extensive homology with FSV-acquired cellular sequences (J. Groffen et al., *unpublished observations*). Thus, each of two avian and two feline transforming viruses appear to have independently acquired similar cellular sequences that are distinct from those represented within the genomic RNAs of other transforming viruses.

In other studies, the major methionine-containing tryptic peptides common to Gardner and Snyder-Theilen FeSV have been shown to be represented within the nonstructural components of the FSV and PRCII ASV gene products (9). Additionally, PRCII ASV P105 contains unique FSV P140, methionine-containing peptides not present in either of the FeSV-encoded polyproteins. Of interest, the single methionine-containing tryptic peptide common to the Gardner, Snyder-Theilen, and

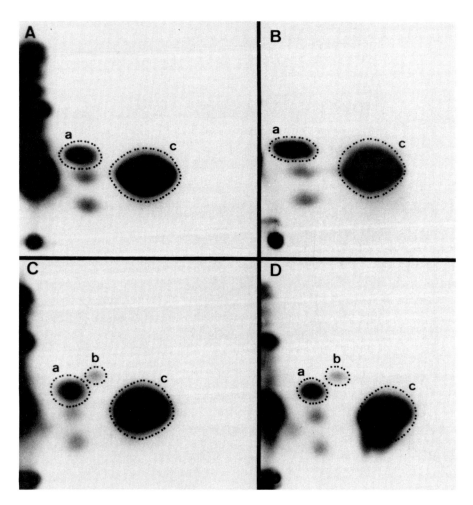

FIG. 1. Identification of major phosphoamino acids in FeSV-transformed cells. Cells were radioactively labeled by overnight incubation in [^{32}P]orthophosphate containing medium, disrupted, hydrolyzed, and subjected to two-dimensional phosphoamino acid analysis as described previously (64). For identification of individual [^{32}P]-labeled phosphoamino acids, unlabeled standards including phosphothreonine *(a)*, phosphotyrosine *(b)*, and phosphoserine *(c)* were mixed at equimolar concentrations with [^{32}P]-labeled hydrolysates of cellular phosphoproteins. Cell lines tested included McDonough FeSV-transformed mink **(A)**, and rat **(B)** cells; Gardner FeSV-transformed mink cells **(C)**; and Snyder-Theilen FeSV-transformed mink cells **(D)**.

McDonough FeSV gene products corresponds to one of the peptides in common with PRCII ASV P105 and FSV P140 (9,104). Thus, despite the lack of detectable sequence homology between McDonough FeSV and FSV genomic RNAs, the possibility that the McDonough FeSV-acquired sequences have one or more minor components in common with those of Gardner and Snyder-Theilen FeSV cannot be excluded.

STRATEGIES FOR IDENTIFICATION OF ADDITIONAL CELLULAR TRANSFORMING GENES

The studies reviewed above establish the potential use of type C viruses for the identification and molecular cloning of cellular genomic sequences with transforming function and indicate that the representation of such genes may be somewhat limited. As an extension of such studies, it will be important to establish more routine and systematic procedures for identification of additional cellular genes, activation of which can lead to expression of the transformed phenotype. Two independent approaches currently being pursued for this purpose in a number of laboratories are described below.

In Vitro Generation of Acute Transforming Retroviruses

Until recently, the frequency of isolation of acute transforming retroviruses has been relatively limited and has, almost exclusively, resulted from *in vivo* passage of nontransforming type C viruses. However, new methods for high frequency generation of mouse sarcoma viruses in cell culture are being developed (60,61). Such acute transforming viruses appear transiently during the spread of rapidly growing ecotropic endogenous mouse viruses in fibroblast cell lines. By isolation of these viruses free of large excesses of nontransforming helper virus, several stable replication-defective isolates have been obtained; these directly transform cells in culture and induce solid tumors *in vivo* (61). To date, virus isolates obtained by this approach have lacked detectable sequence homology to acquired sequence components of previously described mouse transforming viruses and may thus contain unique transformation-specific acquired sequences. The most thoroughly characterized of these viruses to date, 3611-MSV, is replication-defective, transforms embryo fibroblasts in cell culture, and induces a rapid lymphocytic leukemia *in vivo*. The major translational product encoded by the 3611-MSV genome has been identified as a 90,000 M_r polyprotein containing MuLV p15 and p12 covalently linked to a probably acquired sequence-encoded nonstructural component (59). In contrast to the gene products of many of the above-described mammalian transforming viruses, 3611-MSV P90 lacks detectable protein kinase activity and 3611-MSV transformation does not result in an overall elevation of cellular phosphotyrosine levels (59). Further studies involving detection and functional analysis of translational products of additional new isolates are in progress. It will also be important to apply methods successfully utilized for isolation of acute transforming viruses of mouse origin to other mammalian species, possibly including humans.

Detection of Cellular Transforming Genes by Transfection

An alternative approach to the identification of cellular transforming genes has involved DNA transfection techniques. In studies by several groups of investigators, DNAs from a variety of spontaneously and chemically transformed cells have been transfected to, and shown to induce morphologic transformation of, NIH/3T3 mouse cells (15,83,84). The transformed phenotype can be further passaged through a single round of transfection. Evidence that a single or limited number of transforming genes are involved in this process has been obtained by restriction endonuclease analysis of the DNA preparations used for transfection. In these studies, DNAs from methylcholanthrene-transformed mouse fibroblasts were treated with a variety of restriction endonucleases prior to testing their transforming activities by DNA transfer. Identical patterns of sensitivity and resistance to inactivation by different endonucleases were observed in all DNAs studied, suggesting that analogous transforming genes were transferred in each case (86). Induction of transformed foci on mouse cells by transfection of human DNAs from colon and bladder carcinoma cell lines and a promyelocytic leukemia cell line, on the other hand, was shown to involve three different cellular sequences (50). In other studies, Cooper et al. (15) have reported detection of transformed foci using DNAs even from nontransformed cells provided DNA samples are sheared to between 0.5 and 5 kb prior to initial transfection (15). On subsequent transfection cycles, however, transformation efficiencies remain unaltered by shearing (15). As one possibility, it has been hypothesized that the initial shearing may result in separation of the transforming gene from regulatory sequences that normally control its expression.

Recently, transforming sequences of human bladder and lung carcinoma origins have been compared to known retroviral transforming genes. The bladder carcinoma gene corresponds to human cellular homologues of Harvey MSV transforming sequences while the lung carcinoma gene is related to sequences represented in Kirsten MSV (20; L. Parada et al., *personal communication*; M. Barbacid, *personal communication*; M. Goldfarb et al., *personal communication*). These findings suggest that direct transfection of DNAs of human tumor cell origin may provide a means of isolating the cellular homologues of viral oncogenic sequences as functionally active transforming genes.

THE EGF RECEPTOR AND VIRAL TRANSFORMATION

One important objective of studies of RNA tumor viruses has involved the identification of functional pathways involved in expression of transformation. Among several phenotypic changes characteristic of many RNA virus-transformed cells is

TABLE 3. *Properties of growth factors released by viral-transformed rodent fibroblasts and human tumor cells*

Induce phenotypic transformation of cells in culture
Compete with [^{125}I]-labeled EGF for binding the 160,000 M_r EGF membrane receptors
Immunologically and biochemically distinct from EGF
Highly stable to both acid and heat
Induce overall elevation of phosphotyrosine levels in A431 cells and specific tyrosine phosphorylation of the 160,000 M_r EGF membrane receptor
Single chain polypeptides with molecular weight of 7,400 daltons, three disulfide bonds and distant sequence homology to mouse and human EGF
Interact with distinct 60,000 M_r TGF membrane receptors to which EGF does not bind
Conserved amino acid sequence among TGFs of mouse, rat and human origins

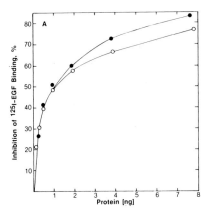
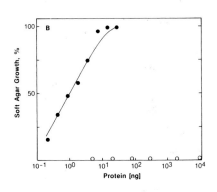

FIG. 2. Comparison of biological properties of highly purified preparations of mouse EGF *(open circles)* and human TGF *(closed circles)*.**A:** Inhibition of specific [^{125}I]-labeled binding to the receptor of formalin-fixed A431 human carcinoma cells. **B:** Soft agar cell colony growth as a function of growth factor concentration. The number of normal rat kidney fibroblasts growing as colonies (> 10 cells) were scored at two weeks and are presented as the maximum percent effect (47).

a reduction in available EGF receptor sites as measured by reduced binding of [^{125}I]-labeled EGF (94). In contrast, the extent of binding of other [^{125}I]-labeled growth factors, such as multiplication-stimulating activity and insulin, remain unaltered following viral transformation (94,95). The reduction in EGF binding is relatively rapid in that it is detectable within a day after infection of a culture with high-titered transforming viruses. The specificity of the reduced EGF binding in Moloney MSV-transformed cells has been established by its rapid reversal following shift of cultures infected with a ts mutant from the permissive to nonpermissive temperature (97).

As summarized in Table 2, levels of EGF binding have also been analyzed in cells morphologically transformed by Abelson MuLV (11), as well as by the Gardner, Snyder-Theilen, and McDonough strains of FeSV (65). The availability of well-characterized morphologic revertants and td mutants in these virus systems provided the necessary genetic controls to establish the transformation specificity of the reduced EGF binding. The extent of EGF binding in each of these transformants is similar to that established by MSV-transformed cell lines. In contrast, in morphologic revertants of Abelson MuLV-, and Gardner and Snyder-Theilen FeSV-transformed cells, levels of EGF binding are restored to levels characteristic of nontransformed control cells (11,65). In fact, the extent of [^{125}I]-labeled EGF binding in partially reverted cultures is inversely proportional to the fraction of the cells that are morphologically transformed. Similarly, in td mutant-infected clones, in which transforming proteins are expressed at levels comparable to those of wt-transformed clones but that lack protein kinase activity, EGF binding is comparable to that of nontransformed control cells (11,66). A functioning protein kinase in these systems appears to be required for the EGF receptor phenotype.

In contrast to RNA tumor virus-transformed cells, cells transformed either by DNA viruses, or by any of a variety of nonviral agents, generally bind EGF efficiently (94). For instance, of several SV40- and polyoma-transformed clones examined, none had diminished numbers of available EGF receptors. Moreover, only around 10% of the chemically transformed cells examined to date have exhibited decreased binding of [^{125}I]-labeled EGF; these have included one clone of benzopyrene-transformed BALB/3T3 cells and a C3H/10T1/2 mouse cell clone transformed by methylcholanthrene. Similarly, of a number of human tumor cell lines examined, only a small percentage were found to exhibit reduced capacity for EGF binding (96) although with some tumor types, such as melanomas and small cell carcinomas of the lung, the frequency is quite high (80). Loss of EGF receptors following transformation, thus, seems to be primarily associated with sarcoma virus transformation, although it does also involve a subset of chemically transformed cells and certain spontaneously arising tumors.

Transforming Growth Factors (TGFs)

As one explanation of the above findings, it was hypothesized that transformation of cells by RNA tumor viruses might result in secondary alteration(s) of the EGF receptors, thereby interfering with their capacity to bind EGF. Alternatively, transformation could be associated with synthesis of low molecular weight growth factors that are able to compete with EGF for binding to its membrane receptor. This latter possibility could lead to noncontrolled proliferative cell growth in that transformed cells would simultaneously produce, and exhibit large numbers of cellular receptors for, growth-stimulating factors. In fact, as discussed below, in several virus model systems and with representative, spontaneously transformed human tumor cells, the involvement of TGFs in sustaining the growth of transformed cells has been established.

Virus-Induced Rodent TGF

Studies designed to resolve these alternative models initially resulted in the demonstration of a family of peptides, designated TGFs, in supernatant culture fluids of Moloney MSV-transformed mouse cells (18). These include three distinct size classes of peptides with molecular weights of 6,000, 10,000, and 20,000 daltons (Table 3). These factors, under appropriate assay conditions, induce morphologic transformation of cultured embryo fibroblasts, are equally as heat- and acid-stable as EGF, and specifically bind to EGF membrane receptors (19,93). The virus specificity of these factors is established by their absence from culture fluids of nontransformed control cell lines. That the 6,000 to 20,000 M_r complex of growth factors released by Moloney MSV-transformed cells is immunologically and functionally distinct from mouse EGF is well-established (18,19). Antisera directed against EGF do not cross-react with TGF as measured either by radioimmunoassay or immunoprecipitation analysis (18,19). A binding protein from mouse serum previously shown to complex to EGF lacks detectable binding affinity for mouse TGF (18,19). An even more critical difference between these growth factors, however, is functional and relates to their effects on susceptible cells. TGF produces a profound phenotypic alteration in cultured cells conferring on them characteristic properties of morphologically transformed cells (18). In response to addition of mouse TGF to culture medium, single cells seeded in agar give rise to large, progressively growing colonies. This phenotypic alteration is dependent on the continued presence of TGF in the culture medium. If cells are recovered from agar and replated in agar in the absence of TGF, they no longer continue to proliferate. EGF, in contrast, has only a minimal effect on monolayer cultures and fails to induce significant growth of cells in soft agar. The growth-stimulatory effects of TGFs on the same cells that produce them (autocrine stimulation) has been shown with viral ts and td mutants (19,99) and with transformed cells and tumor cells plated in agar at low density (96) or in chemically-defined medium (39).

More recently, Abelson MuLV-transformed rat embryo fibroblasts have been found to produce large quantities of TGF (99). Through the analysis of representative td mutants, described in preceding sections, the dependence of the production of these factors on functional activity of the tyrosine-specific protein kinase associated with the major Abelson MuLV gene product, P120, has been established. Following purification from culture fluids of Abelson MuLV-transformed cells, these factors resemble Moloney MSV-induced TGF in that they morphologically transform cells in culture as measured by the soft agar colony assay and compete with [^{125}I]-labeled EGF for binding cell receptors. Amino acid sequence analysis shows no differences in the first 19 residues between mouse TGF and Abelson MuLV- induced rat TGF, and only two amino acid substitutions when compared to human melanoma-derived TGF (see below) (H. Marquardt et al., *unpublished observations*).

These distinct molecular weight species of TGF synthesized by both Moloney MSV- and Abelson MuLV-transformed cells resemble each other, but can be distinguished from EGF on the basis of their high performance liquid chromatography elution profiles. Whether these represent distinct factors, or, as would seem more probable, multiple forms of a single factor is not known. The similarities in growth factors detected in cells transformed by retroviruses containing genetically distinct acquired cellular sequences strongly argues that these represent cellular rather than viral gene products.

Human Tumor Cell TGF

Although the above studies involved only viral-transformed cells, they raised the possibility that at least some human tumor cells, in particular those that lack detectable EGF receptors as measured by binding affinity for [^{125}I]-labeled EGF, may release growth-stimulating factors. To test this possibility, culture fluids of several human tumor cell lines were tested for growth factor activity. Of these, three cell lines—including 9812, a bronchogenic carcinoma; A673, a rhabdomyosarcoma; and A2058, a metastatic melanoma—all of which lack functional EGF receptors and readily form colonies in soft agar, were found to produce such factors (96). These factors are analogous to the Moloney MSV and Abelson MuLV TGFs with respect to interference with EGF binding and stimulation of colony growth in soft agar. In contrast, under similar assay conditions, culture fluids of normal embryonal lung fibroblasts, which lack capacity for growth in soft agar, and the A431 epidermoid carcinoma cell line, which has a very high number of EGF receptors and grows poorly in soft agar, lack detectable growth-stimulating activity.

By molecular size analysis, preparations of human TGFs have been shown to resemble the viral-associated TGFs in that they consist of several distinguishable 6,000 to 20,000 M_r components (96). The 7,400 M_r form of human TGF has been extensively purified by sequential carboxy methyl cellulose and reverse-phase high performance liquid chromatography. Soft agar growth-stimulating activity and the EGF-competing activity co-elute in a single fraction, corresponding to a well-resolved protein peak (97). This inability to separate physically EGF receptor binding activity from the transforming activity further argues that these two activities are attributable to the same protein moiety. Highly purified human TGF competes as well as EGF on a molar basis for binding to the EGF receptor; it also stimulates cells to grow in agar at 0.1 to 1.0 ng/ml whereas EGF, even at 1 to 10 μg/ml, does not produce soft agar colonies (Fig. 2).

GROWTH FACTOR INDUCTION OF TYROSINE PHOSPHORYLATION

In an effort to elucidate the mechanisms of cellular transformation by viral-induced TGFs, and relate these to RNA tumor virus transformation, phosphotyrosine levels have been examined in various growth factor-stimulated rodent and human cell lines (64). The human tumor line with the greatest concentration of available EGF receptors, A431, exhibited a pronounced increase in total phosphotyrosine in response either to EGF or TGFs isolated from culture fluids of Moloney MSV-transformed mouse cells, Abelson MuLV-transformed rat cells, or human tumor cells. The overall extent of tyrosine phosphorylation in these growth factor-treated cells was comparable to that characteristic of cells transformed by RNA tumor viruses encoding tyrosine-specific protein kinases. Concentrations of phosphotyrosine in other human cell lines, including two lines, A673 and A2058, which themselves are high level producers of TGF, were relatively low and remained unaltered following exposure to growth factors (64).

An *in vitro* extract labeling procedure shown previously to result in preferential phosphorylation of tyrosine acceptor sites (12) was utilized in an effort to identify the major cellular substrate labeled in response to the above growth factors. By this approach, a major 160,000 M_r A431 cell substrate(s) phosphorylated in response to EGF (13,64,100) and TGFs from each of the above-described sources (64) was identified. By two-dimensional phosphoamino acid analysis, tyrosine has been shown in each case to represent the predominant P160 acceptor phosphorylated under these conditions. Although low levels of serine phosphorylation were also observed, these are highly variable, and their significance is as yet not determined. On the basis both of molecular weight and immunoprecipitation analysis, this substrate was indistinguishable from the previously described 160,000 M_r EGF membrane receptor. Both A673 human tumor-derived TGF and growth factors from supernatant fluids of Moloney MSV- and Abelson MuLV-transformed cells, induced P160 phosphorylation to an extent comparable to that observed with relatively high concentrations of mouse EGF.

By tryptic peptide analysis of the 160,000 M_r EGF receptor in A431 cells following either EGF- or TGF-induced phosphorylation, one major and six minor phosphorylated peptides have been identified (64). The predominant phosphorylated acceptor, in each of these peptides, is tyrosine. The map positions and relative intensities of phosphorylation of acceptor sites are analogous in response to activation by EGF and TGFs of various sources. The similar receptor phosphorylation responses of A431 cells observed in response to TGFs as compared to EGF must be reconciled with differences in the phenotypic response of cells to these two classes of growth factors. As one possibility, in addition to their binding to, and phosphorylation of, the 160,000 M_r major EGF membrane receptor, TGFs may specifically interact with another cell receptor. Alternatively, interaction of growth factors with, and subsequent tyrosine phosphorylation of, the 160,000 M_r EGF receptor could be on a pathway resulting directly in expression of the transformed phenotype, or this interaction may simply provide a means of transporting the factors into the cell. Studies using [^{125}I]-labeled mouse TGF have identified a 60,000 M_r receptor on the membranes of NRK cells that does not interact with EGF but does bind either mouse or rat TGF and thus may be the receptor which mediates some or most of the effects that lead to phenotypic transformation (48).

At least two cellular substrates, in addition to P160, are phosphorylated in tyrosine residues in response to EGF. These include 39,000 and 80,000 M_r proteins, both of which are also phosphorylated in cells transformed by retroviruses of the Gardner/Snyder-Theilen FeSV and Fujinami ASV group. Additionally, the 39,000 M_r cellular substrate is tyrosine phosphorylated in response to transformation by several other retroviruses, encoding tyrosine-specific protein kinases, such as Abelson MuLV, Rous sarcoma virus and avian transforming viruses of the Y73 class (16,25; J. A. Cooper and T. Hunter, *personal communications*). In contrast, platelet-derived growth factor (PDGF) induces phosphorylation of tyrosine residues of membrane proteins with apparent molecular weights of 175,000 and 130,000 (22), and a 46,000 M_r cellular substrate which is phosphorylated in cells transformed by each of the above-described retroviruses, but not in response to EGF (J. A. Cooper and T. Hunter, *personal communications*). Of the three classes of growth factors known to induce tyrosine phosphorylation of these various cellular substrates (EGF, TGF and PDGF) it is only the TGF family that is commonly expressed by a variety of RNA tumor virus-transformed cells and tumors of various morphological types and which induces phenotypic transformation of cells in culture.

CONCLUSIONS

The developments reviewed above establish the potential value of retroviruses as unique vectors for the identification, molecular cloning, and characterization of cellular genes involved in expression of the transformed phenotype. Presumably because recombination between viral and cellular genes occurs at the RNA, rather than DNA level, preexisting introns within transformation-specific cellular sequences are removed in the generation of recombinant transforming viruses, thus eliminating the requirement for a spliced mRNA in their expression. In view of their highly conserved nature, cellular sequences acquired by this means have probable functional significance to the species from which they were isolated. One possibility is that these genes are involved in differentiation and are transiently expressed at various stages of embryogenesis. Genetic recombination of such cellular genes with viral sequences could result in their separation from cellular control elements and result in the generation of acute transforming viruses. Similarly, perturbation of cellular regulatory controls influencing expression of such sequences by chemical carcinogens or other factors could lead to unregulated proliferative growth and resulting tumor development.

The frequency of occurrence within the cellular genome of genetic loci with transforming potential that are subject to acquisition by retroviruses appears quite limited. This is indicated by the relatedness of acquired sequences of Gardner and Snyder-Theilen FeSV to those of the independently derived Fujinami and PRCII strains of ASV (81). Similarly, several independent avian acute leukemia virus isolates have been shown to have represented, within their genomic RNAs, highly related, cellular-derived, transformation-specific sequences (21,34). Activation of analogous cellular sequences has been demonstrated in a high percentage of chronic retrovirus-induced lymphoid tumors of chickens (35,51). This is apparently due to downstream promotion as a result of integration of a nontransforming viral genome adjacent to an existing cellular gene with transforming function. In other studies, transforming sequences represented within the Harvey and Kirsten MSV and Rasheed RaSV genomic RNAs have been reported to encode immunologically cross-reactive products (23) and appear to be related to transforming sequences isolated from certain human tumor cells. Finally, as discussed above, recent data derived by restriction endonuclease analysis of cellular DNAs with transforming activity, as measured by transfection, also argue for a limited occurrence of sequences with capacity for transformation (15,86). This apparent, relatively limited number of cellular genes with transforming potential should facilitate a determination of the role of such sequences in spontaneous and chemically-induced tumors of their natural hosts.

As a consequence of recent advances reviewed above, many promising avenues of investigation pertaining to the molecular basis of malignant transformation are being opened. The identification and molecular cloning of cellular genetic sequences involved in transformation is progressing rapidly. Functional analysis of transformation-specific proteins encoded by such genes, both in normal and transformed human cells, should provide insight into the etiology of spontaneously developing tumors of humans. Although translational products of many of the cellular genes initially identified and molecularly cloned by use of type C viruses are tyrosine-specific protein kinases, further study will presumably lead to the demonstration of additional functional activities relevant to transformation. This approach, in combination with studies of the interaction of TGFs, both with these and functionally related cellular proteins, should significantly further our understanding of cellular metabolic pathways involved in malignant transformation.

REFERENCES

1. Aaronson, S. A., and Barbacid, M. (1978): Origin and biological properties of a new BALB/c mouse sarcoma virus. *J. Virol.*, 27:366–373.
2. Abelson, H. T., and Rabstein, L. S. (1970): Lymphosarcoma virus-induced thymic independent disease in mice. *Cancer Res.*, 30:2213–2222.
3. Andersen, P. R., Devare, S. G., Tronick, S. R., Ellis, R. W., Aaronson, S. A., and Scolnick, E. M. (1981): Generation of BALB-MSV and Ha-MSV by type C virus transduction of homologous transforming genes from different species. *Cell*, 26:129–134.
4. Andersson, P., Goldfarb, M. P., and Weinberg, R. A. (1979): A defined subgenomic fragment of in vitro synthesized Moloney sarcoma virus DNA can induce cell transformation upon transfection. *Cell*, 16:63–75.
5. Barbacid, M., Beemon, K., and Devare, S. G. (1980): Origin and functional properties of the major gene product of the Snyder-Theilen strain of feline sarcoma virus. *Proc. Natl. Acad. Sci. USA*, 77:5158–5162.
6. Barbacid, M., Breitman, M. L., Lauver, A. V., Long, L. K., and Vogt, P. K. (1981): The transformation-specific proteins of avian (Fujinami and PRC-II) and feline (Snyder-Theilen and Gardner-Arnstein) sarcoma viruses are immunologically related. *Virology*, 110:411–419.
7. Barbacid, M., Lauver, A. V., and Devare, S. G. (1980): Biochemical and immunological characterization of polyproteins coded for by McDonough, Gardner-Arnstein, and Snyder-Theilen strains of feline sarcoma virus. *J. Virol.*, 33:196–207.
8. Barbacid, M., Stephenson, J. R., and Aaronson, S. A. (1976): *gag* Gene of mammalian type-C RNA tumour viruses. *Nature*, 262:554–559.
9. Beemon, K. (1981): Transforming proteins of some feline and avian sarcoma viruses are related structurally and functionally. *Cell*, 24:145–153.
10. Bernstein, A., Mak, T. W., and Stephenson, J. R. (1977): The Friend virus genome: Evidence for the stable association of MuLV sequences and sequences involved in erythroleukemic transformation. *Cell*, 12:287–294.
11. Blomberg, J., Reynolds, F. H., Jr., Van de Ven, W. J. M., and Stephenson, J. R. (1980): Abelson murine leukemia virus transformation involves loss of epidermal growth factor binding sites. *Nature*, 286:504–507.
12. Blomberg, J., Van de Ven, W. J. M., Reynolds, F. H., Jr., Nalewaik, R. P., and Stephenson, J. R. (1981): Snyder-Theilen FeSV P85 contains a single phosphotyrosine acceptor site recognized by its associated protein kinase. *J. Virol.*, 38:886–894
13. Cohen, S., Ushiro, H., Stoscheck, C., and Chinkers, M. (1982): A native 170,000 epidermal growth factor receptor-kinase complex from shed plasma membrane vesicles. *J. Biol. Chem.*, 257:1523–1531.
14. Collett, M. S., Purchio, A. F., and Erikson, R. L. (1980): Avian sarcoma virus-transforming protein pp60^{src} shows kinase activity specific for tyrosine. *Nature*, 285:167–169.
15. Cooper, G. M., Okenquist, S., and Silverman, L. (1980): Transforming activity of DNA of chemically transformed and normal cells. *Nature*, 284:418–421.
16. Cooper, J. A., and Hunter, T. (1981): Changes in protein phosphorylation in Rous sarcoma virus-transformed chicken embryo cells. *Mol. Cell. Biol.*, 1:165–178.
17. Cremer, K., Reddy, E. P., and Aaronson, S. A. (1981): Translational products of Moloney murine sarcoma virus RNA: Identification of proteins encoded by the murine sarcoma virus *src* gene. *J. Virol.*, 38:704–711.
18. De Larco, J. E., and Todaro, G. J. (1978): Growth factors from murine sarcoma virus-transformed cells. *Proc. Natl. Acad. Sci. USA*, 75:4001–4005.
19. De Larco, J. E., and Todaro, G. J. (1980): Sarcoma growth factor (SGF): Specific binding to epidermal growth factor (EGF) membrane receptors. *J. Cell. Physiol.*, 102:267–277.
20. Der, C. J., Krontiris, T. G., and Cooper, G. M. (1982): Transforming genes of human bladder and lung carcinoma cell lines are homologous to the *ras* genes of Harvey and Kirsten sarcoma viruses. *Proc. Natl. Acad. Sci. USA*, *(in press)*.
21. Duesberg, P. H., and Vogt, P. K. (1979): Avian acute leukemia viruses MC29 and MH2 share specific RNA sequences: Evidence for a second class of transforming genes. *Proc. Natl. Acad. Sci. USA*, 76:1633–1637.
22. Ek, B., Westermark, B., Wasteson, A., and Heldin, C.-H. (1982): Stimulation of tyrosine-specific phosphorylation by platelet-derived growth factor. *Nature*, 295:419–420.

23. Ellis, R. W., DeFeo, D., Shih, T. Y., Gonda, M. A., Young, H. A., Tsuchido, N., Lowy, D., and Scolnick, E. M. (1981): The p21 src genes of the Harvey and Kirsten sarcoma viruses originate from divergent members of a family of normal vertebrate genes. *Nature*, 292:506–511.

24. Erikson, E., and Erikson, R. L. (1980): Identification of a cellular protein substrate phosphorylated by the avian sarcoma virus transforming gene product. *Cell*, 21:829–836.

25. Erikson, E., Shealy, D. J., and Erikson, R. L. (1981): Evidence that viral transforming gene products and epidermal growth factor stimulate phosphorylation of the same cellular protein with similar specificity. *J. Biol. Chem.*, 256:11381–11384.

26. Fedele, L. A., Even, J., Garon, C. F., Donner, L., and Sherr, C. J. (1981): Recombinant bacteriophages containing the integrated transforming provirus of Gardner-Arnstein feline sarcoma virus. *Proc. Natl. Acad. Sci. USA*, 78:4036–4040.

27. Feldman, R. A., Hanafusa, T., and Hanafusa, H. (1980): Characterization of protein kinase activity associated with the transforming gene product of Fujinami sarcoma virus. *Cell*, 22:757–765.

28. Fischinger, P. J. (1980): Type C RNA transforming viruses. In: *Molecular Biology of RNA Tumor Viruses*, edited by J. R. Stephenson. Academic Press, New York. pp. 163–198.

29. Frankel, A. E., Gilbert, J. H., Porzig, K. J., Scolnick, E. M., and Aaronson, S. A. (1979): Nature and distribution of feline sarcoma virus nucleotide sequences. *J. Virol.*, 30:821–827.

30. Gardner, M. B., Rongey, R. W., Arnstein, P., Estes, J. D., Sarma, P., Huebner, R. J., and Richard, C. G. (1970): Experimental transmission of feline fibrosarcoma of cats and dogs. *Nature*, 226:807–809.

31. Goff, S. P., Gilboa, E., Witte, O. N., and Baltimore, D. (1980): Structure of the Abelson murine leukemia virus genome and the homologous cellular gene: Studies with cloned viral DNA. *Cell*, 22:777–785.

32. Groffen, J., Heisterkamp, N., Grosveld, F., Van de Ven, W. J. M., and Stephenson, J. R. (1982): Isolation of human oncogene sequences (v-*fes* homolog) from a cosmid library. *Science*, 216:1136–1138.

33. Hanafusa, T., Wang, L. H., Anderson, S. M., Karess, R. E., Hayward, W. S., and Hanafusa, H. (1980): Characterization of the transforming gene of Fujinami sarcoma virus. *Proc. Natl. Acad. Sci. USA*, 77:3009–3013.

34. Hayman, M. J. (1981): Transforming proteins of avian retroviruses. *J. Gen. Virol.*, 52:1–14.

35. Hayward, W. S., Neel, B. G., and Astrin, S. M. (1981): Activation of a cellular *onc* gene by promoter insertion in ALV-induced lymphoid leukosis. *Nature*, 290:475–480.

36. Hu, S., Davidson, N., and Verma, I. M. (1977): A heteroduplex study of the sequence relationships between the RNAs of M-MSV and M-MLV. *Cell*, 10:469–477.

37. Hunter, T. (1980): Protein phosphorylated by the RSV transforming function. *Cell*, 22:647–648.

38. Hunter, T., and Sefton, B. M. (1980): Transforming gene product of Rous sarcoma virus phosphorylates tyrosine. *Proc. Natl. Acad. Sci. USA*, 77:1311–1315.

39. Kaplan, P. L., Anderson, M., and Ozanne, B. (1982): Transforming growth factor(s) production enables cells to grow in the absence of serum. *Proc. Natl. Acad. Sci. U.S.A.*, 79:485–489.

40. Kawai, S., Yoshida, M., Segawa, K., Sugiyama, H., Ishizaki, R., and Toyoshima, K. (1980): Characterization of Y73, an avian sarcoma virus: A unique transforming gene and its product, a phosphopolyprotein with protein kinase activity. *Proc. Natl. Acad. Sci. USA*, 77:6199–6203.

41. Khan, A. S., Deobagkar, D. N., and Stephenson, J. R. (1978): Isolation and characterization of a feline sarcoma virus-coded precursor polyprotein: Competition immunoassay for nonstructural component(s). *J. Biol. Chem.*, 253:8894–8901.

42. Khan, A. S., and Stephenson, J. R. (1977): Feline leukemia virus: Biochemical and immunological characterization of *gag* gene-coded structural proteins. *J. Virol.*, 23:599–607.

43. Langbeheim, H., Shih, T. Y., and Scolnick, E. M. (1980): Identification of a normal vertebrate cell protein related to the p21 *src* of Harvey murine sarcoma virus. *Virology*, 106:292–300.

44. Linemeyer, D. L., Ruscetti, S. K., Menke, J. G., and Scolnick, E. M. (1980): Recovery of biologically active spleen focus-forming virus from molecularly cloned spleen focus-forming virus-pBR322 circular DNA by cotransfection with infectious type C retroviral DNA. *J. Virol.*, 35:710–721.

45. Linemeyer, D. L., Ruscetti, S. K., Scolnick, E. M., Evans, L. H., and Duesberg, P. H. (1981): Biological activity of the spleen focus-forming virus is encoded by a molecularly cloned subgenomic fragment of spleen focus-forming virus DNA. *Proc. Natl. Acad. Sci. USA*, 78:1401–1405.

46. MacDonald, M. E., Reynolds, F. H., Jr., Van de Ven, W. J. M., Stephenson, J. R., Mak, T. W., and Bernstein, A. (1980): Anemia- and polycythemia-inducing isolates of Friend spleen focus-

forming virus: Biological and molecular evidence for two distinct viral genomes. *J. Exp. Med.*, 151:1477–1492.

47. Marquardt, H., and Todaro, G. J. (1982): Human transforming growth factor: Production by a melanoma cell line, purification, and initial characterization. *J. Biol. Chem.*, 257:5220–5225.

48. Massague, J., Czech, M. P., Iwata, K., De Larco, J. E. and Todaro, G. J.: Affinity-labeling of a transforming growth factor (TGF) receptor that does not interact with epidermal growth factor (EGF). *(in preparation)*.

49. McDonough, S. K., Larsen, S., Brodey, R. S., Stock, N. D., and Hardy, W. D., Jr. (1971): A transmissible feline fibrosarcoma of viral origin. *Cancer Res.*, 31:953–956.

50. Murray, M. J., Shilo, B-Z., Shih, C., Cowing, D., Hsu, H. W., and Weinberg, R. A. (1981): Three different human tumor cell lines contain different oncogenes. *Cell*, 25:355–361.

51. Neel, B. G., Hayward, W. S., Robinson, H. L., Fang, J., and Astrin, S. (1981): Avian leukosis virus-induced tumors have common proviral integration sites and synthesize discrete new RNAs: Oncogenesis by promoter insertion. *Cell*, 23:323–334.

52. Neil, J. C., Delamarter, J. F., and Vogt, P. K. (1981): Evidence for three classes of avian sarcoma viruses: Comparison of the transformation-specific proteins of PRCII, Y73, and Fujinami viruses. *Proc. Natl. Acad. Sci. USA*, 78:1906–1910.

53. Oskarsson, M., McClements, W. L., Blair, D. G., Maizel, J. V., and Vande Woude, G. F. (1980): Properties of a normal mouse cell DNA sequence (sarc) homologous to the src sequence of Moloney sarcoma virus. *Science*, 207:1222–1224.

54. Papkoff, J., Hunter, T., and Beemon, K. (1980): *In vitro* translation of virion RNA from Moloney murine sarcoma virus. *Virology*, 101:91–103.

55. Papkoff, J., Verma, I. M., and Hunter, T. (1982): Detection of a transforming gene product in Moloney murine sarcoma virus transformed cells. *Cell, (in press)*.

56. Patschinsky, T., Hunter, T., Esch, F. S. and Cooper, J. A. (1982): Analysis of amino acids surrounding sites of tyrosine phosphorylation. *Proc. Natl. Acad. Sci. USA*, 79:973–977.

57. Pawson, T., Guyden, J., Kung, T-H., Radke, K., Gilmore, T., and Martin, G. S. (1980): A strain of Fujinami sarcoma virus which is temperature-sensitive in protein phosphorylation and cellular transformation. *Cell*, 22:767–775.

58. Peters, R. L., Rabstein, L. S., VanVleck, R., Kelloff, G. J., and Huebner, R. J. (1974): Naturally occurring sarcoma virus of the BALB/cCr mouse. *J. Natl. Cancer Inst.*, 53:1725–1729.

59. Rapp, U. R., Reynolds, F. H., Jr., and Stephenson, J. R.: New mammalian transforming retrovirus: Demonstration of a polyprotein gene product. *(in preparation)*.

60. Rapp, U. R., and Todaro, G. J. (1978): Generation of new mouse sarcoma viruses in cell culture. *Science*, 201:821–824.

61. Rapp, U. R., and Todaro, G. J. (1980): Generation of oncogenic mouse type C viruses: In vitro selection of carcinoma-inducing variants. *Proc. Natl. Acad. Sci. USA*, 77:624–628.

62. Rasheed, S., Gardner, M. B., and Huebner, R. J. (1978): *In vitro* isolation of stable rat sarcoma viruses. *Proc. Natl. Acad. Sci. USA*, 75:2972–2976.

63. Reynolds, F. H., Jr., Sacks, T. L., Deobagkar, D. N., and Stephenson, J. R. (1978): Cells non-productively transformed by Abelson murine leukemia virus express a high molecular weight polyprotein containing structural and nonstructural components. *Proc. Natl. Acad. Sci. USA*, 75:3974–3978.

64. Reynolds, F. H., Jr., Todaro, G. J., Fryling, C., and Stephenson, J. R. (1981): Human growth factors (TGFs) specifically induce phosphorylation of tyrosine residues in epidermal growth factor (EGF) membrane receptors. *Nature*, 292:259–262.

65. Reynolds, F. H., Jr., Van de Ven, W. J. M., Blomberg, J., and Stephenson, J. R. (1981): Differences in mechanisms of transformation by independent feline sarcoma virus isolates. *J. Virol.*, 38:1084–1089.

66. Reynolds, F. H., Jr., Van de Ven, W. J. M., Blomberg, J., and Stephenson, J. R. (1981): Involvement of a high molecular weight polyprotein translational product of Snyder-Theilen FeSV in malignant transformation. *J. Virol.*, 37:643–653.

67. Reynolds, F. H., Jr., Van de Ven, W. J. M., and Stephenson, J. R. (1980): Abelson murine leukemia virus transformation defective mutants with impaired P120 associated protein kinase activity. *J. Virol.*, 36:374–386.

68. Reynolds, F. H., Jr., Van de Ven, W. J. M., and Stephenson, J. R. (1980): Feline sarcoma P115-associated protein kinase phosphorylates tyrosine: Identification of a cellular substrate conserved during evolution. *J. Biol. Chem.*, 255:11040–11047.

69. Reynolds, F. H., Jr., Van de Ven, W. J. M., and Stephenson, J. R. (1980): Feline sarcoma virus polyprotein P115 binds a host phosphoprotein in transformed cells. *Nature*, 286:409–412.
70. Reynolds, R. K., and Stephenson, J. R. (1977): Intracistronic mapping of the murine type C viral *gag* gene by use of conditional lethal replication mutants. *Virology*, 81:328–340.
71. Reynolds, R. K., Van de Ven, W. J. M., and Stephenson, J. R. (1978): Translation of type C viral RNAs in *Xenopus laevis* oocytes: Evidence that the 120,000-molecular-weight polyprotein expressed in Abelson leukemia virus-transformed cells is virus coded. *J. Virol.*, 28:665–670.
72. Ruscetti, S., Troxler, D., Linemeyer, D., and Scolnick, E. (1980): Three laboratory strains of spleen focus-forming virus: Comparison of their genomes and translational products. *J. Virol.*, 33:140–151.
73. Sacks, T. L., Hershey, E. J., and Stephenson, J. R. (1979): Abelson murine leukemia virus-infected cell lines defective in transformation. *Virology*, 97:231–240.
74. Sacks, T. L., Reynolds, F. H., Jr., Deobagkar, D. N., and Stephenson, J. R. (1978): Murine leukemia virus (T-8)-transformed cells: Identification of a precursor polyprotein containing *gag* gene-coded (p15 and p12) and a nonstructural component. *J. Virol.*, 27:809–814.
75. Scher, C. D., and Siegler, R. (1975): Direct transformation of 3T3 cells by Abelson murine leukemia virus. *Nature*, 253:739–741.
76. Sefton, B. M., Hunter, T., Beemon, K., and Eckart, W. (1980): Evidence that the phosphorylation of tyrosine is essential for cellular transformation by Rous sarcoma virus. *Cell*, 20:807–816.
77. Sen, A., and Todaro, G. J. (1979): A murine sarcoma virus-associated protein kinase: Interaction with actin and microtubular protein. *Cell*, 17:347–356.
78. Sen, A., Todaro, G. J., Blair, D. G., and Robey, W. G. (1979): Thermolabile protein kinase molecules in a temperature sensitive murine sarcoma virus pseudotype. *Proc. Natl. Acad. Sci. USA*, 76:3617–3621.
79. Sherr, C. J., Fedele, L. A., Donner, L., and Turek, L. P. (1979): Restriction endonuclease mapping of unintegrated proviral DNA of Snyder-Theilen feline sarcoma virus: Localization of sarcoma-specific sequences. *J. Virol.*, 32:860–875.
80. Sherwin, S. A., Minna, J. D., Gazdar, A. F., and Todaro, G. J. (1981): Expression of epidermal and nerve growth factor receptors and soft agar growth factor production by human lung cancer cells. *Cancer Res.*, 41:3538–3542.
81. Shibuya, M., Hanafusa, T., Hanafusa, H., and Stephenson, J. R. (1980): Homology exists among the transforming sequences of avian and feline sarcoma viruses. *Proc. Natl. Acad. Sci. USA*, 787:6536–6540.
82. Shields, A., Goff, S., Pasking, M., Otto, G., and Baltimore, D. (1979): Structure of the Abelson murine leukemia virus genome. *Cell*, 18:955–962.
83. Shih, C., Padhy, L. C., Murray, M., and Weinberg, R. A. (1981): Transforming genes of carcinomas and neuroblastomas introduced into mouse fibroblasts. *Nature*, 290:261–264.
84. Shih, C., Shilo, B-Z., Goldfarb, M. P., Dannenberg, A., and Weinberg, R. A. (1979): Passage of phenotypes of chemically transformed cells via transfection of DNA and chromatin. *Proc. Natl. Acad. Sci. USA*, 76:5714–5718.
85. Shih, T. Y., Papageorge, A. G., Stokes, P. E., Weeks, M. O., and Scolnick, E. M. (1980): Guanine nucleotide-binding and autophosphorylating activities associated with the p21[src] protein of Harvey murine sarcoma virus. *Nature*, 287:686–691.
86. Shilo, B. Z., and Weinberg, R. A. (1981): Unique transforming gene in carcinogen-transformed mouse cells. *Nature*, 289:607–609.
87. Snyder, S. P., and Theilen, G. H. (1969): Transmissible feline fibrosarcoma. *Nature*, 221:1074–1075.
88. Staal, S. P., Hartley, J. W., and Rowe, W. P. (1977): Isolation of transforming murine leukemia viruses from mice with a high incidence of spontaneous lymphoma. *Proc. Natl. Acad. Sci. USA*, 74:3065–3067.
89. Stephenson, J. R., ed. (1980): *Molecular Biology of RNA Tumor Viruses*. Academic Press, New York.
90. Stephenson, J. R., Khan, A. S., Sliski, A. H., and Essex, M. (1977): Feline oncornavirus-associated cell membrane antigen: Evidence for an immunologically crossreactive feline sarcoma virus-coded protein. *Proc. Natl. Acad. Sci. USA*, 74:5608–5612.
91. Stephenson, J. R., Khan, A. S., Van de Ven, W. J. M., and Reynolds, F. H., Jr. (1979): Guest Editorial: Type C retroviruses as vectors for cloning cellular genes with probable transforming function. *J. Natl. Cancer Inst.*, 63:1111–1119.

92. Stephenson, J. R., Van de Ven, W. J. M., Khan, A. S., and Reynolds, F. H., Jr. (1980): Mammalian RNA type C transforming viruses: Characterization of virus-coded polyproteins containing phosphorylated components with possible transforming function. *Cold Spring Harbor Symp. Viral Oncogenes*, 44:865–874.
93. Todaro, G. J., and De Larco, J. E. (1978): Growth factors produced by sarcoma virus transformed cells. *Cancer Res.*, 38:4147–4154.
94. Todaro, G. J., De Larco, J. E., and Cohen, S. (1976): Transformation by murine and feline sarcoma viruses specifically blocks binding of epidermal growth factor (EGF) to cells. *Nature*, 264:26–31.
95. Todaro, G. J., De Larco, J. E., Fryling, C., Johnson, P. A., and Sporn, M. B. (1981): Transforming growth factors (TGFs): Properties and possible mechanisms of action. *J. Supramol. Struct.*, 15:287–301.
96. Todaro, G. J., Fryling, C., and De Larco, J. E. (1980): Transforming growth factors produced by certain human tumor cells: Polypeptides that interact with epidermal growth factor receptors. *Proc. Natl. Acad. Sci. USA*, 77:5258–5262.
97. Todaro, G. J., Marquardt, H., De Larco, J. E., Reynolds, F. H., Jr., and Stephenson, J. R. (1981): Transforming growth factors produced by human tumor cells: Interactions with epidermal growth factor (EGF) membrane receptors. In: *Cellular Responses to Molecular Modulators*, edited by W. Scott, R. Werner, and J. Schultz. Academic Press, New York. pp. 183–204.
98. Tronick, S. R., Robbins, K. C., Canaani, E., Devare, S. G., Andersen, P. R., and Aaronson, S. A. (1979): Molecular cloning of Moloney murine sarcoma virus: Arrangement of virus-related sequences within the normal mouse genome. *Proc. Natl. Acad. Sci. USA*, 76:6314–6318.
99. Twardzik, D. R., Todaro, G. J., Marquardt, H., Reynolds, F. H., Jr., and Stephenson, J. R. (1982): Transformation induced by Abelson murine leukemia virus involves production of a polypeptide growth factor. *Science*, 216:894–897.
100. Ushiro, H., and Cohen, S. (1980): Identification of phosphotyrosine as a product of epidermal growth factor-activated protein kinase in A-431 cell membranes. *J. Biol. Chem.*, 255:8363–8365.
101. Van de Ven, W. J. M., Khan, A. S., Reynolds, F. H., Jr., Mason, K. T., and Stephenson, J. R. (1980): Translational products encoded by newly acquired sequences of independently derived feline sarcoma virus isolates are structurally related. *J. Virol.*, 33:1034–1045.
102. Van de Ven, W. J. M., Reynolds, F. H., Jr., Blomberg, J., and Stephenson, J. R. (1980): Identification of tryptic peptides unique to a 110,000 molecular weight polyprotein encoded by the T-8 isolate of murine leukemia virus. *J. Exp. Med.*, 152:589–612.
103. Van de Ven, W. J. M., Reynolds, F. H., Jr., Nalewaik, R. P., and Stephenson, J. R. (1979): The nonstructural component of the Abelson murine leukemia virus polyprotein P120 is encoded by newly acquired genetic sequences. *J. Virol.*, 32:1041–1045.
104. Van de Ven, W. J. M., Reynolds, F. H., Jr., Nalewaik, R. P., and Stephenson, J. R. (1980): Characterization of a 170,000-dalton polyprotein encoded by the McDonough strain of feline sarcoma virus. *J. Virol.*, 35:165–175.
105. Van de Ven, W. J. M., Reynolds, F. H., Jr., and Stephenson, J. R. (1980): The nonstructural components of polyproteins encoded by replication-defective mammalian transforming retroviruses are phosphorylated and have associated protein kinase activity. *Virology*, 101:185–197.
106. Veronese, F., Kelloff, G. J., Reynolds, F. H., Jr., Hill, R., and Stephenson, J. R. (1982): Monoclonal antibodies specific to transforming polyproteins encoded by independent isolates of feline sarcoma virus. *J. Virol. (in press)*.
107. Witte, O. N., Dasgupta, A., and Baltimore, D. (1980): Abelson murine leukemia virus protein is phosphorylated *in vitro* to form phosphotyrosine. *Nature*, 283:826–831.
108. Witte, O. N., Goff, S., Rosenberg, N., and Baltimore, D. (1980): A transformation-defective mutant of Abelson murine leukemia virus lacks protein kinase activity. *Proc. Natl. Acad. Sci. USA*, 77:4993–4997.
109. Witte, O. N., Rosenberg, N., and Baltimore, D. (1979): A normal cell protein cross-reactive to the major Abelson murine leukaemia virus gene product. *Nature*, 281:396–398.
110. Witte, O. N., Rosenberg, N., Paskind, M., Shields, A., and Baltimore, D. (1978): Identification of an Abelson murine leukemia virus-encoded protein present in transformed fibroblasts and lymphoid cells. *Proc. Natl. Acad. Sci. USA*, 75:2488–2492.
111. Young, H. A., Rasheed, S., Sowder, R., Benton, C. V., and Henderson, L. E. (1981): Rat sarcoma virus: Further analysis of individual viral isolates and the gene product. *J. Virol.*, 38:286–293.

Advances in Viral Oncology, Volume 1
edited by George Klein. Raven Press,
New York © 1982.

Transformation of Hemopoietic Cells with Avian Leukemia Viruses

*Carlo Moscovici and **Louis Gazzolo

*Tumor Virology Laboratory, Veterans Administration Medical Center, and
Department of Pathology, College of Medicine, University of Florida, Gainesville,
Florida 32602; and **Virology Unit, INSERM, U. 51, Groupe de Recherche CNRS 33,
69371 Lyon Cedex 2, France*

Few comprehensive studies on the biology of avian retroviruses are now available in the literature (3,4,44,53,75). The purpose of this chapter is to assemble the data derived from the *in vivo* experiments together with those obtained from *in vitro* studies, with emphasis on the interaction of retroviruses with cells of hemopoietic origin.

Avian leukemia viruses (ALV) are recognized as the etiological agents for causing a large spectrum of diseases mainly in chickens. The hemopoietic system is most affected by some viral strains, although a wide variety of solid tumors can also be obtained. The ALV have been divided into two groups: acute leukemia viruses and lymphoid leukosis viruses (LLV).

These two classes of ALV differ in two main parameters in terms of their ability to transform cells *in vitro* and in terms of their genetic complexity. All acute leukemia viruses so far are defective for replication and can produce infectious progeny only when one or more lymphoid leukosis helper viruses are present in the viral stock. Moreover, acute leukemia viruses do cause a variety of morphological changes in hemopoietic and nonhemopoietic cells cultured *in vitro*.

In contrast, the LLV are competent and hence replicate independently. They are unable to induce transformation of cells in culture, but some do cause a cytopathic effect mainly in cultured chicken fibroblasts.

HEMOPOIESIS IN CHICKENS

Hemopoiesis embraces the different successive steps leading to the formation of blood cells circulating in the peripheral blood or localized in tissues. These cells, which have finite life spans, derive from the proliferation and differentiation of immature cells. The different populations of immature cells (stem and progenitor cells) that home in the blood-forming organs have been analyzed intensively as new cloning techniques have been introduced (73), thus providing new insights into the development of the three main lineages of hemopoietic differentiation: erythropoiesis, granulopoiesis, and lymphopoiesis. The analysis of the *in vitro* transforming ability of ALV has greatly benefited from a better understanding of the properties of hemopoietic stem and progenitor cells. Therefore, it seems of interest to summarize briefly the recent observations obtained in the field of chicken hemopoiesis.

Blood-Forming Organs

In chickens, the ontogenetic development of hemopoietic tissue has been studied mainly by histological means; for a review, see Romanoff (91) and Le Douarin (67). These studies revealed that hemopoiesis occurs at different successive sites in the embryonic stage than in the adult life. The first blood cells appear after 18 hr of incubation in the blood islands (Wolff islands) disseminated in the blastoderm. Then, the yolk sac represents the main site of blood formation in the developing embryo until 15 days; thereafter, the bone marrow becomes increasingly important until hatching time and remains the principal hemopoietic tissue through the adult life. Spleen, bursa, liver, and thymus are other hemopoietic organs. Lymphopoiesis occurs mainly in thymus and in spleen during adult life, whereas the bursa, from which precursors of B lymphocytes originate, is also a transient granulopoietic organ.

Finally, recent observations have shown that, in the developing embryo, intraembryonic sites may be the source of the hemopoietic stem cells during the adult life. These sites are found in the aortic endothelium, close to the lungs and spleen. They are also observed in the endothelium of the heart and aortic arches and are disseminated in the intraembryonic mesoderm. Experiments with quail/chick chimeras have suggested the role of these intraembryonic sites in the definitive hemopoiesis (24,25). Quail embryos severed from their own yolk sac are grafted at an early stage of development onto the yolk sac of chick embryos. The recognition of chick and quail erythrocytes is made possible thanks to differences in the structure of the interphase nucleus between these two species. The proportion of quail and chick erythrocytes is also assayed through a differential immunohemolysis technique. It was then demonstrated that yolk sac stem cells were capable of colonizing intraembryonic organs, mainly the spleen, but were unable to seed a permanent intraembryonic erythropoiesis. Therefore, stem cells from the intraembryonic sites might be at the origin of hemopoiesis by colonizing the bone marrow after the involution of yolk sac.

Hemopoietic Cell Differentiation

Analysis of stem and progenitor cells in the different hemopoietic tissues has also been useful in clarifying the origin of medullar hemopoiesis as well as exploring the regulatory mechanisms of blood cell production (Table 1).

Stem Cells

As in the mouse system, hemopoietic stem cells are characterized by an extensive ability of self-replication in order to maintain the stem cell compartment itself while

TABLE 1. *Hemopoietic colony-forming cells in chickens*

Hemopoietic precursor	Abbreviation (characterization)	Frequency[a]	Progeny	Differentiation markers of cells in colony
In vivo				
Colony-forming unit in marrow	CFU-M (stem cell) (or early progenitor)	3–4 (95,100)	$>10^5$	Erythroblasts, hemoglobin synthesis
In vitro				
Burst forming unit erythroid	BFU-E (early progenitor)	110–160 (97) 300–600 (97)	1–2×10^3	Normoblasts-hemoglobin synthesis
Colony-forming unit erythroid	CFU-E (late progenitor)	500–2,000 (97) 1,500–1,800 (97)	8–150	Normoblasts-hemoglobin synthesis
Colony-forming cell granulocyte-macrophage	CFC (early progenitor)	250–400 (27,37) 100–200 (27)	50–1,000	Fc receptors, C3 receptors, phagocytosis
Cluster-forming cell granulocyte-macrophage	— (late progenitor)	1,000–1,300 (37) 100–200 (39)	3–50	Fc receptors, C3 receptors phagocytosis

[a]Expressed as per 10^5 cells. First line indicates frequency in bone marrow, the second line that in yolk sac. Numbers in parentheses refer to the literature cited.

generating the various progenitor cells committed to the different lineages. These cells, after a limited proliferation, give rise to the formation of more differentiated cells that can be morphologically identified (70). Further differentiation of these cells leads to the production of mature cells (granulocytes, macrophages, erythrocytes, and lymphocytes), most of which are incapable of further proliferation.

Attempts to identify hemopoietic chicken stem cells have been performed according to transplantation experiments by Till and McCulloch (113) to identify the mouse hemopoietic stem cell. Samarut and Nigon and associates (96,101) transplanted normal chicken bone marrow or yolk sac cells into irradiated chickens. Six days later, macroscopic colonies of an erythrocytic nature were observed only on the surface of the tibial marrow. Each colony was shown to originate from a single cell, hence the name of "colony-forming unit in marrow" (CFU-M). The CFU-M might not be considered as bona fide stem cells. Even if they are capable of self-renewal, they are not fulfilling another important condition of stem cells, i.e., that of differentiation into the various types of mature blood cells. In fact, neither macrophage-granulocytic colonies nor mixed types of colonies were observed in the marrow of the irradiated chickens. The medullar environment probably does not favor the development of such colonies. Alternatively, these CFU-M might represent stem cells at the earliest step of commitment in the erythroid lineage. Contrary to those of medullar origin, vitelline CFU-M are not self-replicating (100). This observation is another indication that the yolk sac membrane is not a site of production of stem cells during embryonic life.

Myeloid Progenitor Cells

Chicken progenitor cells belonging to the erythrocyte or granulocyte-macrophage lineage have been grown *in vitro*, in plasma clots, methylcellulose, or soft agar cultures. Granulocyte macrophage progenitor cells from bone marrow cells cultured in soft agar or methylcellulose form colonies composed of granulocytes or macrophages or both in the presence of a colony stimulating factor (CSF). The progenitor cells that originated these colonies are designated as "granulocyte-macrophage colony-forming cells" (GM-CFC). The wide variations in the colony size indicate that these progenitor cells display various degrees of maturity. The more immature CFC give rise to colonies containing 50 to more than 2,000 cells (27,28). The more mature CFC give rise to clusters containing 3 to 50 cells (37). These CFC were found in the various chicken hemopoietic tissues of embryonic and adult life (27,28,111). The observation (111) that CFC can be detected in yolk sac only at 6 days of incubation is surprising because macrophages have been observed in 2-day-old embryos (91). It might be that the frequency of CFC in yolk sac before the sixth day of incubation is under detectable levels. However, we were able to enumerate CFC in blastoderms incubated for 24 hr (C. Moscovici et al., *unpublished observations*). A higher percentage of CFC was also found in embryonic spleen and bone marrow. After chicks hatched, the frequency dropped rapidly. Interestingly, in the bursa, a peak of CFC occurred on days 14 and 15 of incubation, indicating that stem cells colonizing the bursal anlagen differentiate first toward granulopoiesis and then toward lymphopoiesis (111).

The source of CSF used to grow the CFC varies from one study to another. In some experiments, an underlayer of macrophages was used (51). Others were performed by adding to the semi-solid medium either egg albumin (111) or serum from chickens injected with endotoxin (26) or a culture medium conditioned by chicken fibroblasts (27,28,37). Leukemic AMV-transformed (avian myeloblastosis virus) cells were shown also to produce CSF (107).

Erythroid Progenitor Cells

Two classes of erythroid progenitor cells have been identified in cultures of hemopoietic cells. With the use of plasma clot or methylcellulose milieu, immature erythrocytic burst forming units (BFU-E) may give rise, after six days of culture, to large aggregates made of several benzidine-positive clusters containing 1,000 erythrocytes (21,98). These BFU-E are highly sensitive to factor(s) present in pokeweed-mitogen spleen-cell-conditioned medium, burst promoting activity (BPA) (98), and depend on high concentrations of erythropoietin, contained in anemic chicken serum or partially purified from the same source (95).

After three days of incubation, the more mature erythroid colony-forming unit-erythrocyte (CFU-E) proliferates to form one compact colony of 8 to 150 benzidine-positive erythrocytes (20,97–100). The development of CFU-E does require lower concentrations of erythropoietin than those required by BFU-E. BFU-E and CFU-E were detected in yolk sac and embryonic and adult marrows, and BFU-E may be found in the blastoderm at the primitive streak stage (18 hr of incubation), when CFU-E were not yet detectable (98).

In the mouse, by varying culture conditions, subpopulations of BFU-E at different steps of maturation have been observed (52). The presence of similar subpopulations of BFU-E in the chicken has not yet been demonstrated. Besides their different requirements of erythropoietin and BPA, CFU-E and BFU-E have recently been distinguished by different antigenic membrane properties (38,97). An antigen specific to immature red cells is present on CFU-E and not detectable on BFU-E. Conversely, a chicken brain-related antigen is expressed on BFU-E and less expressed on CFU-E. Committed lymphoid progenitors have not yet been cultured from chicken hemopoietic tissues.

PATHOGENESIS OF ALV

Defective Leukemia Viruses

As documented by the broad spectrum of neoplasms observed, one of the main characteristics of the pathogenesis of defective leukemia viruses (DLV) is the pleiotropic response of chickens to infection (3,4). In view of the previously well-detailed description of these tumors (4,89) we believe that it is sufficient in this chapter to recapitulate the most salient pathogenic features of DLV by summarizing the response of the chicken after exposure to the myeloid and erythroid groups of viruses. *In vivo* oncogenesis will also be complemented by considering the transforming alteration observed with the respective target cell *in vitro*.

Myeloid Group

AMV Strain

Only one strain of virus is known to be able exclusively to induce an acute myeloblastic leukemia in the chicken. Pseudotypes containing either subgroup A, B, or C can all induce the same type of disease. Infection of embryonated eggs of very young birds injected by the intravenous route results in a fatal disease that can be diagnosed by the characteristic myeloblasts circulating in the peripheral blood a few days after viral infection.

Histopathological examination of dead birds reveals massive infiltration of leukemic cells in liver, spleen, and bone marrow. Nephroblastomas and osteopetrosis, which were described in an earlier report, are essentially produced by either of the two helpers associated with AMV, namely MAV1 and MAV2 (108).

MC29 Strain

The oncogenic response induced in the chicken by this virus has been extensively studied by Beard and associates (4,74). Injection of birds 1 day old or older results in a disease that is essentially aleukemic, with occasional onset of a stem cell leukemia not yet clearly defined. However, when 12-day-old embryonated eggs were injected intravenously, a typical myelocytic leukemia resulted in the hatched birds (C. Moscovici, *unpublished observations*). This leukemia is often accompanied by a number of different types of tumors, as have been described in the literature. These tumors include liver and kidney carcinomas, hemangiomas, myelocytomas, and sarcomas. Sarcomas have been observed only when young chicks or baby Japanese quail were injected subcutaneously into the wing web (C. Moscovici, *unpublished observations*). Unlike Rous-induced sarcomas (fibrosarcomas), the MC29 sarcomas were predominantly of the round cell type and produced very little extracellular matrix.

MH2 Strain

This virus is another agent in the myeloid group that induces a wide spectrum of oncogenic response in the chicken. Originally the tumors were described only as endotheliomas (6), but a recent reexamination of the disease (1,76) showed that several different types of tumors similar to the ones described for MC29 were obtained. The major difference was that none of the MH2-infected birds ever developed myeloblastosis or myelocytomatosis. Moreover, no hemorrhagic hepatocarcinomas were obtained with MH2 or MC29. Adenocarcinomas were similar in both cases.

E26 Strain

This strain was isolated in Bulgaria and was found to induce in quail a leukemia involving erythroid and myeloid cells (61,83). In chickens, the same virus can induce only an erythroblastic leukemia. These findings were recently confirmed (81) by examining buffy coats derived from leukemic chickens. When surface markers were assayed on these cells grown *in vitro*, about half of them expressed erythroid antigens and the other half showed Fc receptors. Such findings indicate that E26 in chickens induces both an erythroblastic and a myeloid leukemia. These results are in variance with those obtained by *in vitro* transformation studies, which show that E26 transforms cells of the myeloid lineage. No solid tumors have so far been obtained in E26-infected chickens.

CMII and OK10 Strains

Except for the original reports, no further pathological studies have been described. CMII was described by Löliger (68), who showed that CMII is probably very similar to MC29, since it causes myelocytomas accompanied by other types of tumors, including nephroblastomas (69). The OK10 strain was isolated from a liver carcinoma in a chicken that had previously been injected with a field isolate of a leukosis virus (85). The pathology of the virus infection in chickens has many features in common with that described for MH2 virus. It also causes a not-well-defined leukemoid disease accompanied by visceral tumors.

Erythroid Group

AEV (Avian Erythroblastosis Virus) Strain

Inoculation of embryonated eggs or of young chickens with AEV strain ES4 or strain R leads to an acute erythroleukemia within a few days after infection (33,46). The incubation period is influenced by the virus source, the dose and route of inoculation, and the age and genetic constitution of the host (89). Both strains can also cause anemia likely due to the associated helper viruses present in the viral stocks (50,60). When birds were injected intramuscularly or subcutaneously, fibrosarcomas did develop.

In view of the complexity of the response of the host to various avian retrovirus, it would be worthwhile, in some cases, to reevaluate their oncogenic potential *in vivo* in relation to their transforming ability *in vitro*. In fact, the tumor specificity does not always reflect the target cell specificity. A recent study (81) showed that the response of Japanese quail and chickens to AEV or E26 depends on the host species. The results suggest that classification of DLV (8,45,48) based only on *in vitro* studies may not be definitive.

Nondefective Leukosis Viruses (LLV)

Viruses of this category are found in almost all chicken flocks and belong to the replication-competent members of the exogenous leukosis virus group (89). Infection with LLV usually leads to a B-cell lymphoma after a relatively long period of latency. Although LLV viruses multiply in most organs of the body, the cells of the bursa of Fabricius are the principal target cells for neoplastic transformation (35). The LLVs are multipotent viruses, and a broad oncogenic spectrum has been observed in addition to lymphomas (36). The most common neoplasm associated with LLV in experimental inoculation and transmission of these viruses is erythroblastosis (14,15).

It is well established that the frequency of occurrence of lymphoma and other tumors, including erythroblastosis fibrosarcoma, hemangioma, nephroblastoma, and osteopetrosis, is correlated with the high doses of virus injected into the susceptible host. A detailed description of the histopathological characteristics caused by these viruses in the chicken is now available (89).

CELL-DERIVED ONCOGENES: THEIR ROLE IN THE TRANSFORMING EVENTS

DLV

As it is shown in Table 2, with the exception of AMV, most of the avian acute leukemia viruses display a broad oncogenic spectrum. This broad oncogenic spectrum is paralleled by the ability of these viruses to transform fibroblasts and epithelial and hemopoietic cells *in vitro*. However, the predominant neoplasm induced by these viruses *in vivo* is an acute leukemia. *In vitro* studies of transformation of hemopoietic cells by these viruses have led in recent years to a better understanding of the oncobiology of DLV.

Moreover, molecular studies have shown that the *onc* genes of DLV are defined by internal specific sequences (2,9,10,12,17,18,29,30,72,102–106) unrelated to the *src* gene (18,109). Complementary DNA (cDNA) specific for the internal sequences of each virus was prepared. Hybridization studies have shown that these cDNA probes are related to sequences present in the DNA of uninfected chicken cells (92,105,110). Therefore, the viral specific sequences represent transduced

TABLE 2. In vivo *and* in vitro *transforming abilities of defective leukemia viruses in chickens[a]*

Virus strain	Neoplasms	Transforming ability	
		Hemopoietic cells	Fibroblasts
AEV	Erythroblastosis, sarcoma (33,46)	+ (51) (erythroid)	+ (93)
AMV	Myeloblastosis (3,75)	+ (5,78) (myeloid)	− (75)
E26	Erythroblastosis (61,83)	+ (8,47) (myeloid)	− (47)
MC29	Myelocytomatosis, carcinoma, hemangioma, sarcoma (4,74)	+ (66,79) (myeloid)	+ (93,115)
MH2	Carcinoma, sarcoma, leukemia (rare) (6,76)	+ (37,58) (myeloid)	+ (59)
OK10	Carcinoma (85)	+ (8,47) (myeloid)	+ (47)
CMII	Myelocytomatosis, carcinoma (68,69)	+ (8) (myeloid)	+ (49)

[a]Numbers in parentheses refer to literature cited.

cellular nucleotide sequences, designated as proto-oncogenes. Moreover, the same studies have indicated that the viral genes of viruses with similar oncogenic potential are closely related. These *onc* genes derived from cellular sequences were named after the name of the *in vitro* transformed hemopoietic cells. Hence they were designated *erb* (erythroblasts) for AEV, *myb* (myeloblasts) for AMV, and *myc* (macrophages) for MC29 and related viruses. In most viruses, the acquired cellular sequences are expressed as a fusion protein comprising part of the *gag* gene product together with the cellular sequence product (11,54–56,59,63,65,86,114). These nonstructural proteins are found in transformed cells of hemopoietic and nonhemopoietic origin. They represent the best candidates for transforming proteins.

In fact, recent genetic experiments have implicated the cell-derived oncogenes in the transformation process. One nonconditional mutant of AEV, td359, can transform fibroblasts, but cannot transform erythroid progenitors (94). The mutation has been assigned to a deletion in the region of *erb* coding for p75 (7). Three nonconditional mutants of MC29 have been shown to transform hemopoietic cells with reduced efficiency but have retained the ability to transform fibroblasts. Deletions have been found in the *myc* sequences of these three mutants (90).

Insights into the mechanism(s) by which these *onc* genes are able to mediate the transformation of hemopoietic cells were provided by two main groups of studies. The first considered the characterization and identification of the target cells for neoplastic transformation of DLV. The second concerned the phenotype of the cells transformed by these viruses. Both studies benefited from the development of techniques permitting the culture of DLV-transformed cells and the assay *in vitro* of the transforming capability of these viruses.

Characterization and Identification of the Target Cells of DLV

The studies carried out in this field have established: first, lineage-specific transformation of the hemopoietic cells by these viruses, and second, their target cell specificity inside the respective lineage.

Assays

Methods for assaying *in vitro* the oncogenic capability of these viruses were a prerequisite for characterizing their target cells. As noted, these assays benefited from the ameliorations introduced in the clonal cultures of hemopoietic progenitor cells. Two types of assay for transformation of hemopoietic cells have been developed: a focus assay based on the transformation of adherent secondary cultures overlaid with agar (58,78–80) and a colony assay using cells obtained directly from hemopoietic tissues and seeded in soft agar or in methylcellulose medium (37,41,42).

The observation that the number of transformed colonies or foci is directly proportional to the dilution of virus indicates that a single virus particle is capable of inducing transformation. The colony assay has shown: first, that the ability of DLV to induce transformation *in vitro* correlates with the hemopoietic activity of the various organs at the time of infection, and second, that the frequency of target cells in hemopoietic tissues for the three types of DLV is very low. The number of target cells per one million of bone marrow cells was found to range from 2,000 to 3,500 for MC29, 700 to 2,000 for AMV, and 50 to 200 for AEV (37,38,51). These values might represent minimum estimates, since they may be affected by many unknowns, such as plating efficiency and loss of viability during handling as well as by the physiological state of the infected population (cell cycle status). Further, variations in the number of target cells from several experiments are wide, perhaps reflecting other unknown physiological factors. The addition of CSF in the colony assay of AMV and MC29 was found to increase the cloning efficiency of the transformed cells (79). Recently, BPA and serum from anemic chickens were observed to increase the frequency of AEV target cells (J. Samarut and L. Gazzolo, *unpublished observations*).

Lineage-Specific Transformation

Results recently obtained after complement-dependent immune cytolysis demonstrate that AEV target cells are recruited exclusively among erythroid cells, since in the presence of complement they are killed by an antierythrocyte serum and an antierythroblast serum. AMV and MC29 target cells are not sensitive to the effects of these sera. Conversely, AMV and MC29 target cells are equally susceptible to an antimyeloblast serum, which suggests that the target cells of these viruses are recruited among the myeloid cells. Finally, an antimacrophage serum lyses a higher percentage of target cells for MC29 than it does for AMV (51). These last results may suggest that MC29 transforms bone marrow cells of different degrees of maturation (immature cells and macrophages), whereas AMV transforms cells only at an immature stage.

However, our observations (37) do not support the last conclusion, nor do more recent observations by Durban and Boettiger (31), which confirm that macrophages are target cells for AMV.

Target Cell Specificity

Attempts have been made to characterize these cells by their density, velocity sedimentation, adherence, and phagocytic ability. The results of these experiments summarized in Table 3 have shown that AEV on the one hand, and AMV and MC29 on the other, transform cells already committed in their maturation (37,38,51). These target cells for AEV have been precisely identified recently. Cell fractionations and immune cytolysis experiments indicate that the target cells for AEV are essentially recruited among BFU-E (38). Indeed, these target cells, like BFU-E, were found to be cells of light density and were expressing an immature erythroid antigen at a low level and a brain-related antigen at a high level. The other erythroid progenitors, CFU-E, display antigenic properties just the opposite of those of BFU-E. They could support viral replication, but were not transformed by AEV. In the case of AMV, cell fractionations have shown that these target cells are recruited among cells located just beyond the stage of the myeloid progenitors, i.e., CFC (37), and already committed toward the macrophage lineage. MC29 seems to share

TABLE 3. *Physical, antigenic, and functional properties of target cells transformed by AMV, MC29, and AEV*

Target cells	Density (g/cm³)	Sedimentation velocity (mm/hr)	Cell surface antigens[a]					Phagocytosis[b]	Adhesiveness[b]
			Myeloblast	Macrophage	Erythroblast	Brain	Immature		
AMV	1.060–1.065[c]	4.5[d] (3.6–6.2)	+++	+	–	ND	ND	0	4–15
MC29	1.060–1.070	4.1 (3.6–4.9)	+++	+++	–	ND	ND	50	50–65
AEV	1.060–1.065	5.1 (4.2–5.8)	ND	–	+	+++	+	0	0

[a] + = slightly positive, +++ = strongly positive, ND = not done.
[b] Percentage of positive cells.
[c] Range of values.
[d] Peak sedimentation velocity (the two values in parentheses indicate the distribution of the majority of cells). Data from Gazzolo et al. (37,38) and Graf et al. (51).

the same target cells with AMV and also can transform cells that are more mature, as judged by their greater adherence and phagocytosis (51).

Finally, experiments have confirmed previous observations concluding that AMV and MC29 could transform macrophages obtained from cultured yolk sac or from the peripheral blood (37,78). However, the efficiency of transformation was proportional to the proliferative capacity of these cells. When these cells stopped dividing, no transformation was occurring. AMV-transformed cells expressed differentiation markers of macrophages, indicating that target cells might be recruited among cells committed to macrophages. In fact, if target cells for AMV are recruited among mononuclear phagocytes, the leukemia induced by this virus should be classified as a monocytic leukemia. In contrast, another report claims that target cells for AMV are recruited among myeloblasts, which were considered in this study as the immediate precursors of granulocytes (44). However, no correlation has been found between the granulocyte-lineage cells and the number of AMV-transformed cells observed in yolk sac cultures infected with this virus (13,31; E. H. Durban and D. Boettiger, *personal communication*). This result indicates that granulocytic cells do not serve as potential targets for AMV transformation.

Phenotype of the DLV-Transformed Cells

The first indications that hemopoietic cells are transformed by DLV are their ability to proliferate and their diminished adhesiveness. In recent years, attempts have been aimed to characterize the phenotype of these cells, and a synopsis of their properties follows.

Differentiation Parameters

Along the differentiation pathway toward the mature functional cells, in an orderly programmed fashion, progenitor cells acquire functional characteristics and surface markers through a series of cell divisions. The expression of these differentiation parameters is closely correlated with the acquisition of mature cell functions and is independent of standard morphologic criteria. Therefore, these differentiation parameters were found to be essential in analyzing the phenotype of hemopoietic cells transformed by DLV.

The myeloid parameters that were analyzed in cells transformed by AMV, MC29, and other related viruses are fully expressed in normal macrophages. The main functional property of macrophages is their ability to phagocytize particles. This phagocytosis is mediated either by nonspecific receptors (phagocytosis of latex particles or killed bacteria) or by specific receptors, which are the receptors for the Fc portion of the immunoglobulin G (immune-phagocytosis of antibody-coated erythrocytes). In addition, macrophages possess receptors for the C3 component of complement. Acid phosphatase and adenosine triphosphatase (ATPase) were also checked in the cytoplasm and at the membrane level of the transformed cells. Finally, antibodies directed against myeloblasts or macrophages allowed the detection of antigens related to these cells belonging to two different compartments of the myeloid lineage. Unfortunately, lysozyme synthesis was not assayed in the avian-transformed cells in the same manner as it was done in the murine myeloid leukemic cells.

Hemoglobin synthesis was assayed either by benzidine staining or by radioimmune assay. Histone H5, which is present in erythroid cells of avian and other nonmammalian species, was detected by indirect immunofluorescence. In addition, carbonic anhydrase was found to be fully expressed in erythrocytes. Finally, the presence of cell surface antigens (of erythroblastic and erythrocytic nature) was detected by immunofluorescence or immunocytolysis techniques.

AMV-Transformed Cells

The AMV-transformed cells can be maintained in culture for long periods of time (82). They were obtained either from colonies of transformed bone marrow or yolk sac cells, from foci of macrophage cultures, or from the peripheral blood of moribund leukemic chickens. Regardless of their origin, they are morphologically the same and have the same functional and surface properties (Table 4).

These cells are mostly nonadherent, round, and have a diameter of about 10 μm. Their large and eccentric nucleus is surrounded by a rim of cytoplasm containing small granules. The presence of surface marker characteristics of macrophages was investigated on the membrane of AMV-transformed cells (8,32,37,45). It was found that receptors for the Fc part of immunoglobulins are expressed on the surface of these cells, whereas receptors for the C3 component of complement are not expressed. Both receptors were present on normal avian macrophages. Moreover, AMV-transformed cells were shown to be able to engulf latex particles (phagocytosis mediated by nonspecific receptors). However, phagocytosis mediated by Fc receptors did not occur, which indicated that these receptors are not functional. The search for enzymatic and antigenic surface markers has shown the presence of ATPase, the expression at a high level of a myeloblast-related antigen, and the expression of a macrophage-related antigen. Finally, when treated with phorbol myristate acetate, AMV-transformed cells adhere to the surface of the culture flask, and differentiate into macrophages (88).

MC29-Transformed Cells

Hemopoietic cells transformed *in vitro* differ greatly from those observed in the peripheral blood of diseased chickens injected either during their embryonic life or when newly hatched. Although the blood shows the typical morphology of myelocytes, recognizable by the presence of large azurophilic granules, the cells transformed *in vitro* do not share the same phenotype as seen *in vivo*. Moreover, cells of buffy coats from myelocytic birds, when cultured *in vitro*, display the same characteristics as those transformed by MC29 *in vitro*. These cells are slightly adherent, are 15 to 20 μm in diameter, and have an irregular shape with pseudopodia. The nucleus is eccentrically located, and their cytoplasm contains numerous vacuoles. Fc and C3 receptors were present on the surface of MC29-transformed cells, which are able to phagocytize latex particles (37). Immune phagocytosis was also

TABLE 4. *Expression of myeloid differentiation parameters by hemopoietic cells transformed by myeloid defective leukemia viruses*

Cell type	Adhesiveness	Surface receptors[a]		Phagocytosis[a]		Enzyme activities[b]		Cell surface antigens[b]		
		Fc	C3	Nonspecific	Immune	Acid F'tase	ATPase	Myeloblast	Macrophage	Erythrocyte
Normal macrophages	+++	95–98	75	97	95	+++	++++	+	+++	–
AMV transformed	–	9–73	1	35–85	0	+	++++	+++	+	–
E26 transformed	–	15	ND	39	ND	ND	++++	+++	+	–
MC29 transformed	+	80–95	15	77–85	90	+++	+	+	+++	–
MH2 transformed	+	47–96	13	91–95	90	ND	+	+	+++	–
CMII transformed	+	85	ND	81	ND	ND	+	+	+++	–
OK10 transformed	+	82	ND	92	ND	ND	+	+	+++	–

[a]Percentage of positive cells.
[b]+ = slightly positive, +++ = strongly positive, – = not detectable, ND = not done.
Data from Beug et al. (8), Durban and Boettiger (32), and Gazzolo et al. (37).

observed, indicating that Fc receptors are functional (8,37). ATPase was not demonstrated on their surface, which strongly expresses a macrophage-related surface antigen, while weakly expressing a myeloblast-related surface antigen. Hemopoietic cells transformed with CMII, OK10, or MH2 were found to display the same phenotype of differentiation as MC29-transformed cells (8,45).

AEV-Transformed Cells

AEV-transformed cells *in vitro* or *in vivo* have morphologically similar phenotypes. These cells of a diameter of 10 μm are nonadherent and have a centrally located nucleus and a cytoplasm devoid of any granulation. They strongly express the histone H5. They weakly react with an immune serum directed against normal erythrocytes. The hemoglobin content was very low and varied considerably among different clones. It was estimated as 0.3 to 1.0% of the amount of hemoglobin in mature erythrocytes. Carbonic anhydrase is present in AEV-transformed cells, although 5 to 10 times less than in erythrocytes (8,45). Finally, in cells transformed by a thermosensitive mutant of AEV (ts 34), an increase of hemoglobin and carbonic anhydrase activity was observed when these cells were shifted to the nonpermissive temperature (43).

In conclusion, assays for the detection of erythroid and myeloid differentiation parameters confirm that AEV transforms cells of erythroid nature and AMV and MC29 transform cells of myeloid origin. Moreover, AEV- and AMV-transformed cells do not fully express differentiation-marker characteristics of the mature cells inside the respective lineage. These observations indicate that these viruses interfere with the maturation of the transformed cells. The MC29-transformed cells and normal macrophages have an identical phenotype. Their proliferating ability and their loose adherence distinguish them from their normal counterparts. Moreover, ATPase is not detected on the surface of these cells, whereas it is found on the membrane of normal macrophages (32). Therefore, MC29 prevents either the expression of this enzyme or its activity at the cell surface. A previous study had indicated that ATPase was not present on normal macrophages (8), but this observation was not valid, since the ATPase was assayed after trypsinization of the macrophages.

Target Cells of LLV

As noted above, lymphoid tumor induction by these viruses depends on the presence of bursa during the 12 weeks after injection of 1-day-old birds (35). In fact, surgical or chemical bursectomy up to 12 weeks reduced drastically the incidence of LLV and did not affect the incidence of erythroblastosis, but bursectomy did result in an increase of the incidence of osteopetrosis. These experiments indicate that the target cells of LLV are in the bursa. These cells are at a very immature stage during lymphocyte development because it was shown that LLV-transformed cells produce IgM, but not IgG and IgA (22). Therefore, the target cells of LLV are recruited among early precursors in the lymphoid lineage, and LLV interfere with the intraclonal switch from IgM to IgG and IgA production. An *in vitro* transformation assay might be useful to get a better characterization of the target cell of LLV. Finally, some LLV can induce cytopathic alterations in fibroblasts, leading to the formation of plaques under appropriate conditions (40,62,77).

Several hypotheses have been proposed to explain the transformation event induced by LLV (23). Among them, the most promising was in favor of the transcription of proto-oncogenes initiated at viral promoters. Recently, this hypothesis has been supported by experimental data (57,84,87), which show that the rare event leading to the proliferation of tumor cells, in at least some cases, is the integration of the LLV provirus, in a position adjacent to the proto-oncogene *myc*. Then, transcription of this proto-oncogene initiating from a viral promoter causes enhanced expression of the cellular *myc*, leading to neoplastic transformation.

Mechanisms of Cell Transformation

Studies on the characterization of target cells and on the expression of hemopoietic phenotypic differentiation provide insights on the mechanism by which oncogenes transform hemopoietic cells. Two main conclusions may be drawn from these studies.

First, the specific requirements of ALV for one lineage and for definite target cells suggest that the transformation event depends on the expression of specific differentiation functions. This conclusion is drawn from the observation that target cells for neoplastic transformation are recruited among cells already committed in their respective lineage of differentiation. AEV transform early erythroid progenitors (i.e., BFU-E). AEV may infect cells located within a compartment situated beyond the target cells (i.e., CFU-E), but these cells are not transformed. Therefore, the oncogenes of AEV will be efficient only at the BFU-E stage and active at the CFU-E stage.

However, AMV, MC29, or other members related to the myeloid group transform cells at late stages of the myeloid lineage and, in order to be transformed, they must express some or all of the differentiation parameters of mature macrophages. Nevertheless, infection could occur in immature cells, but transformation will be triggered when these immature cells will acquire some of the differentiation markers. Therefore, for AMV or MC29, expression of the transforming ability of their *onc* genes may depend on events closely related to terminal maturation of macrophages.

Second, transformation of hemopoietic target cells by DLV or LLV leads to the proliferation of cells that display distinct phenotypes of differentiation. AEV-transformed cells do not synthesize hemoglobin (8,112); AMV-transformed cells do not express immune phagocytosis (37); and LLV-transformed cells are unable to produce IgG or IgA (22). It was first postulated that these viruses transform their target cells by blocking maturation (44). However, the expression of several differentiation parameters by the transformed cells may be distinct from the expression of the same parameters by normal hemopoietic cells. This abnormal pattern is well documented for AMV- or MC29-transformed cells and speaks in favor of a model of neodifferentiation that was recently proposed (E. M. Durban and D. Boettiger, *personal communication*). This model implies that derangement of the normal pathway of differentiation is the main effect of the transforming ability of these two viruses.

The two models, block or derangement of differentiation, may not be exclusive with each other. Moreover, they do not leave out the possibility of limited dedifferentiation (as proposed in Fig. 1) when AMV or MC29 transform macrophages (37).

Finally, if one considers that nondividing macrophages are transformed by AMV or MC29, the main effect of the transforming ability of these two viruses may be to induce these cells to proliferate. Alternatively, the proliferation of the AEV-transformed cells may not be under the direct control of the transforming gene, since the target cells are early progenitors that already have a high mitotic activity before infection.

Perspectives

From these conclusions, the transformation event of hemopoietic cells may be defined as a specific event involving the transforming sequences of these viruses and the phenotypic program of the target cells. The insertion promoter model (57) implies that neoplastic transformation by DLV or LLV is initiated from the enhanced expression of a normal cellular gene. In the case of LLV, the viral promoters are inserted adjacent to these proto-oncogenes. Moreover, since LLV infection induces not only lymphoid lymphomatosis but also other neoplasms, such as erythroblastosis, it is feasible that activation of other proto-oncogenes (*erb*-related, in this case) might also occur in target tissues.

In the case of DLV, the proto-oncogenes have been inserted into the viral genome and are then controlled by viral promoters. The promoter insertion model may explain how a DLV has originated from the recombination between the specific proto-oncogene and LLV-replicative genes, with a subsequent partial or complete deletion of some replicative genes (19,29,34). The transforming sequences of DLV represent transduced normal cellular genes. The extensive homology between the viral transforming genes and the homologous cellular genes (92), the conservation of these proto-oncogenes during the evolution of vertebrates (92), and the expression of these proto-oncogenes in normal uninfected cells (16,92) raise the possibility that viral and cellular genes encode similar or identical functions and participate in normal regulatory processes of differentiation. Moreover, recent observations indicate that proto-oncogenes for AMV were expressed more efficiently in hemopoietic organs than in other tissues (16). Therefore, these proto-oncogenes may be considered as essential in the regulation of normal hemopoiesis. Target cell specificity of ALV could be explained, if one considers that proto-oncogenes are expressed at different levels in the compartments of hemopoietic lineages. Indeed, DLV would transform cells in which the proto-oncogenes are fully expressed and efficient, by overloading these cells with normal gene products. This permanent overload will prevent them from maturing further. If this hypothesis is correct, it

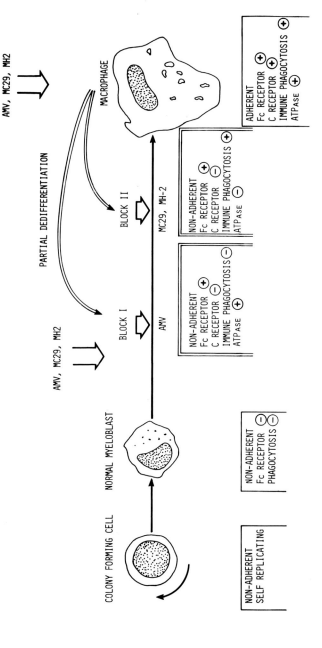

FIG. 1. Avian myeloid differentiation after leukemia viruses infection *in vitro*: A proposed model.

implies that *erb*-related proteins might be very efficient only at the BFU-E stage of the erythroid differentiation. By the same rationale, *myb*- and *myc*-related proteins will be efficient throughout late stages of macrophage differentiation. To test this hypothesis, it will be necessary to demonstrate at the cytological level that target cells are expressing cellular sequences related to the *onc* genes at a higher level than those of nontarget cells. This analysis might be performed by using cDNA probes of *onc* genes or antibodies against the specific proteins coded for by the *onc* genes or both. A prerequisite for this analysis is the preparation of cell fractions enriched in target cells for one DLV. In this regard, physical and immunological cell separations seem the best available methods for reaching this goal.

The knowledge of the mechanisms by which cell-derived oncogenes induce neoplastic transformation in hemopoietic tissues may allow us to define their role in cellular growth, differentiation, and development. From the data presented in this chapter, it might be postulated that *myc*-related proto-oncogenes are genes controlling cell multiplication, whereas *erb*-related proto-oncogenes are more involved in the control of erythroid differentiation.

In conclusion, studies of the oncobiology of ALV underline that an understanding of neoplastic phenomena may stem from the knowledge of the regulatory and developmental parameters that characterize normal populations at each stage of differentiation. Furthermore, these viruses should provide useful tools to the oncodevelopmental biologist for unraveling the mechanisms governing development and differentiation (71).

ACKNOWLEDGMENTS

We would like to thank Drs. M. G. Moscovici, M. Duc Dodon, G. A. Quash, and J. Samarut for providing helpful comments on the manuscript, and Drs. E. Durban and D. Boettiger for permission to include unpublished data. The first author was supported by National Cancer Institute grant 10697 and the Medical Research Service of the Veterans Administration. The second author was supported by research grants from Institut National Santé et Recherche Médicale, and "Vaincre le cancer," and by contracts within the Virus-Cancer program of the National Cancer Institute and INSERM.

REFERENCES

1. Alexander, R. W., Moscovici, C., and Vogt, P. K. (1979): Avian oncovirus Mill Hill no. 2: Pathogenicity in chickens. *J. Natl. Cancer Inst.*, 62:359–366.
2. Anderson, S. M., Hayward, W. S., Neel, B. G., and Hanafusa, H. (1980): Avian erythroblastosis virus produces two mRNA's. *J. Virol.*, 36:676–683.
3. Beard, J. W. (1963): Avian virus growths and their etiologic agents. *Adv. Cancer Res.*, 7:1–127.
4. Beard, J. W. (1980): Biology of avian oncornaviruses. In: *Viral Oncology*, edited by G. Klein, pp. 55–87. Raven Press, New York.
5. Beaudreau, G. S., Becker, C., Bonar, R. A., Wallbank, A. M., Beard, D., and Beard, J. W. (1960): Virus of avian myeloblastosis. XIV. Neoplastic response of normal chicken bone marrow treated with the virus in tissue culture. *J. Natl. Cancer Inst.*, 24:395–415.
6. Begg, A. M. (1927): A filterable endothelioma of the fowl. *Lancet*, 1:912–915.

7. Beug, H., Kitchener, G., Doederlein, G., Graf, T., and Hayman, M. J. (1980): Mutant of avian erythroblastosis virus defective for erythroblast transformation: Deletion in the *erb* portion of p75 suggests function of the protein in leukemogenesis. *Proc. Natl. Acad. Sci. USA*, 77:6683–6686.

8. Beug, H., von Kirchbach, A., Doederlein, G., Conscience, J.-F., and Graf, T. (1979): Chicken hematopoietic cells transformed by seven strains of defective avian leukemia viruses display three distinct phenotypes of differentiation. *Cell*, 18:375–390.

9. Bister, K., and Duesberg, P. H. (1979): Structure and specific sequences of avian erythroblastosis virus RNA: Evidence for multiple classes of transforming genes among avian tumor viruses. *Proc. Natl. Acad. Sci. USA*, 76:5023–5027.

10. Bister, K., and Duesberg, P. H. (1980): Genetic structure of avian acute leukemia viruses. *Cold Spring Harbor Symp. Quant. Biol.*, 44:801–822.

11. Bister, K., Hayman, M. J., and Vogt, P. K. (1977): Defectiveness of avian myelocytomatosis virus MC29: Isolation of long-term nonproducer cultures and analysis of virus-specific polypeptide synthesis. *Virology*, 82:431–448.

12. Bister, K., Ramsay, G., Hayman, M. J., and Duesberg, P. H. (1980): OK10, an avian acute leukemia virus of the MC29 subgroup with a unique genetic structure. *Proc. Natl. Acad. Sci. USA*, 77:7142–7146.

13. Boettiger, D., and Durban, E. M. (1980): Progenitor-cell populations can be infected by RNA tumor viruses, but transformation is dependent on the expression of specific differentiated functions. *Cold Spring Harbor Symp. Quant. Biol.*, 44:1249–1254.

14. Burmester, B. R., Fontes, A. K., and Walter, W. G. (1960): Pathogenicity of a viral strain (RPL12) causing avian visceral lymphomatosis and related neoplasms. III. Influence of host age and route of inoculation. *J. Natl. Cancer Inst.*, 24:1423–1442.

15. Burmester, B. R., Gross, M. A., Walter, W. G., and Fontes, A. K. (1959): Pathogenicity of a viral strain (RPL12) causing avian visceral lymphomatosis and related neoplasms. II. Host-virus interrelations affecting response. *J. Natl. Cancer Inst.*, 22:103–127.

16. Chen, J. H. (1980): Expression of endogenous avian myeloblastosis virus information in different chicken cells. *J. Virol.*, 36:162–170.

17. Chen, J. H., Hayward, W. S., and Moscovici, C. (1981): Size and content of virus-specific RNA in myeloblasts transformed by avian myeloblastosis virus (AMV). *Virology*, 110:128–136.

18. Chen, J. H., Moscovici, M. G., and Moscovici, C. (1980): Isolation of complementary DNA unique to the genome of avian myeloblastosis virus (AMV). *Virology*, 103:112–122.

19. Coffin, J. M. (1979): Structure, replication, and recombination of retrovirus genomes: Some unifying hypotheses. *J. Gen. Virol.*, 42:1–26.

20. Coll, J., and Ingram, V. M. (1978): Stimulation of heme accumulation and erythroid colony formation in cultures of chick bone marrow cells by chicken plasma. *J. Cell Biol.*, 76:184–190.

21. Coll, J., and Ingram, V. M. (1981): Identification of ovotransferrin as a heme-, colony- and burst-stimulating factor in chick erythroid cell cultures. *Exp. Cell Res.*, 131:173–184.

22. Cooper, M. D., Purchase, H. G., Brockman, D. E., and Gathings, W. E. (1974): Studies on the nature of the abnormality of B cell differentiation in avian lymphoid leukosis: Production of heterogeneous IgM by tumor cells. *J. Immunol.*, 113:1210–1222.

23. Crittenden, L. B. (1980): New hypotheses for viral induction of lymphoid leukosis in chickens. *Cold Spring Harbor Conf. Cell Prolif.*, 7:529–541.

24. Dieterlen-Lievre, F. (1975): On the origin of haemopoietic stem cells in the avian embryo: An experimental approach. *J. Embryol. Exp. Morphol.*, 33:607–619.

25. Dieterlen-Lievre, F., Beaupain, D., and Martin, C. (1976): Origin of erythropoietic stem cells in avian development: Shift from yolk sac to an intraembryonic site. *Ann. Immunol.*, 127C:857–863.

26. Dodge, W. H., and Hansell, C. C. (1978): The marrow colony forming cell and serum colony stimulating factor of the chicken. *Exp. Hematol.*, 6:661–672.

27. Dodge, W. H., and Moscovici, C. (1973): Colony formation by chicken hematopoietic cells and virus induced myeloblasts. *J. Cell Physiol.*, 81:371–386.

28. Dodge, W. H., Silva, R. F., and Moscovici, C. (1975): The origin of chicken hematopoietic colonies as assayed in semi solid agar. *J. Cell Physiol.*, 85:25–30.

29. Duesberg, P. H. (1980): Transforming genes of retroviruses. *Cold Spring Harbor Symp. Quant. Biol.*, 44:13–29.

30. Duesberg, P. H., and Vogt, P. K. (1978): Avian acute leukemia viruses MC29 and MH2 share specific RNA sequences: Evidence for a second class of transforming genes. *Proc. Natl. Acad. Sci. USA*, 76:1633–1637.

31. Durban, E. M., and Boettiger, D. (1981): Replicating, differentiated macrophages can serve as in vitro targets for transformation by avian myeloblastosis virus. *J. Virol.*, 37:488–492.
32. Durban, E. M., and Boettiger, D. (1981): Differential effects of transforming avian RNA tumor viruses on avian macrophages. *Proc. Natl. Acad. Sci. USA*, 78:3600–3604.
33. Engelbreth-Holm, J., and Rathe-Meyer, A. (1935): On the connection between erythroblastosis (haemocytoblastosis), myelosis, and sarcoma in chicken. *Arch. Pathol. Microbiol. Scand.*, 12:352–365.
34. Eisenman, R. N., Linial, M., Groudine, M., Shaikh, R., Brown, S., and Neiman, P. E. (1980): Recombination in the avian oncoviruses as a model for the generation of defective transforming viruses. *Cold Spring Harbor Symp. Quant. Biol.*, 44:1235–1247.
35. Fadly, A. M., Purchase, H. G., and Gilmour, D. G. (1981): Tumor latency in avian lymphoid leukosis. *J. Natl. Cancer Inst.*, 66:549–552.
36. Fredrickson, T. N., Purchase, H. G., and Burmester, B. R. (1964): Transmission of virus from field cases of avian lymphomatosis. III. Variation in the oncogenic spectra of passaged virus isolates. *Natl. Cancer Inst. Monogr.*, 17:1–27.
37. Gazzolo, L., Moscovici, C., Moscovici, M. G., and Samarut, J. (1979): Response of hemopoietic cells to avian acute leukemia viruses: Effects on the differentiation of the target cells. *Cell*, 16:627–638.
38. Gazzolo, L., Samarut, J., Bouabdelli, M., and Blanchet, J. P. (1980): Early precursors in the erythroid lineage are the specific target cells of avian erythroblastosis virus in vitro. *Cell*, 22:683–691.
39. Gazzolo, L., Samarut, J., Moscovici, C., Moscovici, M. G., and Quash, G. (1978): Identification of chicken hemopoietic cells and their response to avian myeloblastosis virus. In: *Avian RNA Tumor Viruses*, edited by S. Barlati and C. De Giuli, pp. 35–44, Piccin Medical Books, Padua, Italy.
40. Graf, T. (1972): A plaque assay for avian RNA tumor viruses. *Virology*, 50:567–578.
41. Graf, T. (1973): Two types of target cells for transformation with avian myelocytomatosis virus. *Virology*, 54:398–413.
42. Graf, T. (1975): In vitro transformation of chicken bone-marrow cells with avian erythroblastosis virus. *Z. Naturforsch. [C.]*, 30:847–851.
43. Graf, T., Ade, N., and Beug, H. (1978): Temperature-sensitive mutant of avian erythroblastosis virus suggests a block of differentiation as mechanism of leukemogenesis. *Nature*, 275:496–501.
44. Graf, T., and Beug, H. (1978): Avian leukemia viruses: Interaction with their target cells in vivo and in vitro. *Biochim. Biophys. Acta*, 516:269–299.
45. Graf, T., Beug, H., von Kirchbach, A., and Hayman, M. J. (1980): Three new types of viral oncogenes in defective avian leukemia viruses. II. Biological, genetic, and immunochemical evidence. *Cold Spring Harbor Symp. Quant. Biol.*, 44:1225–1234.
46. Graf, T., Fink, D., Beug, H., and Royer-Pokora, B. (1977): Oncornavirus-induced sarcoma formation obscured by rapid development of lethal leukemia. *Cancer Res.*, 37:59–63.
47. Graf, T., Okerblom, N., Todorov, T. G., and Beug, H. (1979): Transforming capacities and defectiveness of avian leukemia viruses OK10 and E26. *Virology*, 99:431–436.
48. Graf, T., Royer-Pokora, B., Meyer-Glauner, W., and Beug, H. (1977): Tumor specificity of acute avian leukemia viruses reflected by their transformation target cell specificity in vitro. *Med. Microbiol. Immunol. (Berl.)*, 164:139–153.
49. Graf, T., Royer-Pokora, B., Meyer-Glauner, W., Claviez, M., Gotz, E., and Beug, H. (1977): In vitro transformation with avian myelocytomatosis virus strain CMII: Characterization of the virus and its target cell. *Virology*, 83:96–109.
50. Graf, T., Royer-Pokora, B., Schubert, G. E., and Beug, H. (1976): Evidence for the multiple oncogenic potential of cloned leukemia virus: In vitro and in vivo studies with avian erythroblastosis virus. *Virology*, 71:423–433.
51. Graf, T., von Kirchbach, A., and Beug, H. (1981): Characterization of the hematopoietic target cells of AEV, MC29 and AMV avian leukemia viruses. *Exp. Cell Res.*, 131:331–343.
52. Gregory, C. J., and Eaves, A. C. (1978): Three stages of erythropoietic progenitor cell differentiation distinguished by a number of physical and biological properties. *Blood*, 51:527–537.
53. Hanafusa, H. (1977): Cell transformation by RNA tumor viruses. In: *Comprehensive Virology*, edited by H. Fraenkel-Conrat and R. R. Wagner, pp. 401–488. Plenum, New York.
54. Hayman, M. J. (1981): Transforming proteins of avian retroviruses. *J. Gen. Virol.*, 52:1–14.
55. Hayman, M. J., Kitchener, G., and Graf, T. (1979): Cells transformed by avian myelocytomatosis virus strain CMII contain a 90K *gag*-related protein. *Virology*, 98:191–199.

56. Hayman, M. J., Royer-Pokora, B., and Graf, T. (1979): Defectiveness of avian erythroblastosis virus: Synthesis of a 75K *gag*-related protein. *Virology*, 92:31–45.
57. Hayward, W. S., Neel, B. G., and Astrin, S. M. (1981): Activation of a cellular *onc* gene by promoter insertion of ALV-induced lymphoid leukosis. *Nature*, 290:475–480.
58. Hu, S. S. F., Duesberg, P. H., Lai, M. M. C., and Vogt, P. K. (1979): Avian oncovirus MH2: Preferential growth in marcophages and exact size of the genome. *Virology*, 96:302–306.
59. Hu, S. S. F., Moscovici, C., and Vogt, P. K. (1978). The defectiveness of Mill Hill 2, a carcinoma-inducing avian oncovirus. *Virology*, 89:162–178.
60. Ishizaki, R., and Shimizu, T. (1970): Heterogeneity of strain R avian (erythroblastosis) virus. *Cancer Res.*, 30:2827–2831.
61. Ivanov, X., Mladenov, Z., Nedyalkov, S., Todorov, T. G., and Yakimov, M. (1964): Experimental investigations into avian leukosis. V. Transmission, haematology and morphology of avian myelocytomatosis. *Bull. Inst. Pathol. Comp. Animaux Domest. (Sofia)*, 10:5–38.
62. Kawai, S., and Hanafusa, H. (1972): Plaque assay for some strains of avian leukosis virus. *Virology*, 48:126–135.
63. Kitchener, G., and Hayman, M. J. (1980): Comparative tryptic peptide mapping studies suggest a role in cell transformation for the *gag*-related protein of avian erythroblastosis virus and avian myelocytomatosis virus strains CMII and MC29. *Proc. Natl. Acad. Sci. USA*, 77:1637–1641.
64. Lai, M. M. C., Hu, S. S. F., and Vogt, P. K. (1979): Avian erythroblastosis virus: Transformation-specific sequences form a contiguous segment of 3.25 kb located in the middle of the 6 kb genome. *Virology*, 97:366–377.
65. Lai, M. M. C., Neil, J. C., and Vogt, P. K. (1980): Cell-free translation of avian erythroblastosis virus RNA yields two specific and distinct proteins with molecular weights of 75,000 and 40,000. *Virology*, 100:475–483.
66. Langlois, A. J., Fritz, R. B., Heine, U., Beard, D., Bolognesi, D. P., and Beard, J. W. (1969): Response of bone marrow to MC29 avian leukosis virus. *Cancer Res.*, 29:2056–2063.
67. Le Douarin, N. (1966): L'hematopoièse dans les formes embryonnaires et jeunes des vertébrés. *Ann. Biol.*, 5:105–171.
68. Löliger, H.-C. (1964): Histogenetic correlations between the reticular tissue and the different types of avian leukosis and related neoplasms. *J. Natl. Cancer Inst.*, 17:37–61.
69. Löliger, H.-C., and Schubert, H. J. (1966): Übertragungsversuche mit aviaren Myelozytomen (tumorförmige Chloroleukose, s. Chlorome). *Pathol. Vet.*, 3:492–505.
70. Lucas, A. B., and Jamroz, C. (1961): *Atlas of Avian Hematology*. Agriculture monograph 25, United States Department of Agriculture, Washington, D.C.
71. Maltzman, W., and Levine, A. J. (1981): Viruses as probes for development and differentiation. *Adv. Virus Res.*, 26:65–116.
72. Mellon, P., Pawson, A., Bister, K., Martin, G. S., and Duesberg, P. H. (1978): Specific RNA sequences and gene products of MC29 avian acute leukemia virus. *Proc. Natl. Acad. Sci. USA*, 75:5874–5878.
73. Metcalf, D. (1977): Hemopoietic colonies. In vitro cloning of normal and leukemic cells. *Recent Results Cancer Res.*, 61:1–227.
74. Mladenov, Z., Heine, U., Beard, D., and Beard, J. W. (1967): Strain MC29 avian leukosis virus. Myelocytoma, endothelioma, and renal growths: Pathomorphological and ultrastructural aspects. *J. Natl. Cancer Inst.*, 38:251–285.
75. Moscovici, C. (1975): Leukemia transformation with avian myeloblastosis virus: Present status. *Curr. Top. Microbiol. Immunol.*, 71:79–101.
76. Moscovici, C., Alexander, R. W., Moscovici, M. G., and Vogt, P. K. (1978): Transforming and oncogenic effects of MH2 virus. In: *Avian RNA Tumor Viruses*, edited by S. Barlati and C. De Giuli, pp. 45–56, Piccin Medical Books, Padua, Italy.
77. Moscovici, C., Chi, D., Gazzolo, L., and Moscovici, M. G. (1976): A study of plaque formation with avian RNA tumor viruses. *Virology*, 73:181–189.
78. Moscovici, C., Gazzolo, L., and Moscovici, M. G. (1975): Focus assay and defectiveness of avian myeloblastosis virus. *Virology*, 68:173–181.
79. Moscovici, C., Gazzolo, L., and Moscovici, M. G. (1978): Avian acute leukemia viruses: Transforming ability in vitro. *Microbiologica*, 1:1–13.
80. Moscovici, C., and Moscovici, M. G. (1973): Tissue culture of avian hematopoietic cells. *Methods Cell Biol.*, 7:313–328.
81. Moscovici, C., Samarut, J., Gazzolo, L., and Moscovici, M. G. (1981): Myeloid and erythroid neoplastic responses to avian defective leukemia viruses in chickens and in quail. *Virology*, 113:765–768.

82. Moscovici, M. G., and Moscovici, C. (1980): AMV-induced transformation of hemopoietic cells: Growth patterns of producers and nonproducers. In: *In Vivo and In Vitro Erythropoiesis: The Friend System*, edited by G. B. Rossi, pp. 503–514. Elsevier/North-Holland Biomedical Press, Amsterdam.

83. Nedyalkov, S. T., Bozhkov, S. P., and Todorov, G. (1975): Experimental erythroblastosis in the Japanese quail *(Coturnix coturnix japonica)* induced by E26 leukosis strain. *Acta Vet. (Brno.)*, 44:75–78.

84. Neel, B. G., Hayward, W. S., Robinson, H. L., Fang, J. F., and Astrin, S. M. (1981): Avian leukosis virus-induced tumors have common proviral integration sites and synthesize discrete new RNAs: Oncogenesis by promoter insertion. *Cell*, 23:323–334.

85. Oker-Blom, N., Hortling, L., Kallio, A., Nurmiaho, E.-L., and Westermarck, H. (1978): OK 10 virus, an avian retrovirus resembling the acute leukaemia viruses. *J. Gen. Virol.*, 40:623–633.

86. Pawson, T., and Martin, G. (1980): Cell-free translation of avian erythroblastosis virus RNA. *J. Virol.*, 34:280–284.

87. Payne, G. S., Courtneidge, S. A., Crittenden, L. B., Fadly, A. M., Bishop, J. M., and Varmus, H. E. (1981): Analysis of avian leukosis virus DNA and RNA in bursal tumors: Viral gene expression is not required for maintenance of the tumor state. *Cell*, 23:311–322.

88. Pessano, S., Gazzolo, L., and Moscovici, C. (1979): The effect of a tumor promoter on avian leukemic cells. *Microbiologica*, 2:379–392.

89. Purchase, H. G., and Burmester, B. R. (1978): Neoplastic diseases: Leukosis/sarcoma group. In: *Diseases of Poultry, 7th ed.*, edited by M. S. Hofstad, B. W. Calnek, C. F. Helmboldt, W. M. Reid, and H. W. Yoder, Jr., pp. 418–468, Iowa State University Press, Ames.

90. Ramsay, G., Graf, T., and Hayman, M. H. (1981): Mutants of avian myelocytomatosis virus with smaller *gag* gene-related proteins have an altered transforming ability. *Nature*, 288:170–172.

91. Romanoff, A. L. (1960): *The Avian Embryo. Structural and Functional Development*. Macmillan, New York.

92. Roussel, M., Saule, C., Lagrou, C., Rommens, H., Beug, H., Graf, T., and Stehelin, D. (1979): Three new types of viral oncogene of cellular origin specific for hematopoietic cell transformation. *Nature*, 281:452–455.

93. Royer-Pokora, B., Beug, H., Claviez, M., Winkhardt, H. J., Friis, R. R., and Graf, T. (1978): Transformation parameters in chicken fibroblasts transformed by AEV and MC29 avian leukemia viruses. *Cell*, 13:751–760.

94. Royer-Pokora, B., Grieser, S., Beug, H., and Graf, T. (1979): Mutant avian erythroblastosis virus with restricted target cell specificity. *Nature*, 282:750–752.

95. Samarut, J. (1978): Isolation of an erythropoietic stimulating factor from the serum of anemic chicks. *Exp. Cell Res.*, 115:123–126.

96. Samarut, J., Blanchet, J. P., Godet, J., and Nigon, V. (1976): Kinetics and biochemical properties of haemopoietic stem cells during chicken development. *Ann. Inst. Pasteur (Paris)*, 127C:873–880.

97. Samarut, J., Blanchet, J. P., and Nigon, V. (1979): Antigenic characterization of chick erythrocytes and erythropoietic precursors: Identification of several definitive populations during embryogenesis. *Dev. Biol.*, 72:155–166.

98. Samarut, J., and Bouabdelli, M. (1980): In vitro development of CFU-E and BFU-E in cultures of embryonic and post-embryonic chicken hematopoietic cells. *J. Cell Physiol.*, 105:553–563.

99. Samarut, J., Jurdic, P., and Nigon, V. (1979): Production of erythropoietic colony-forming units and erythrocytes during chick embryo development: An attempt at modelization of chick embryo erythropoiesis. *J. Embryol. Exp. Morphol.*, 50:1–20.

100. Samarut, J., and Nigon, V. (1976): In vitro development of chicken erythropoietin sensitive cells. *Exp. Cell Res.*, 100:245–248.

101. Samarut, J., and Nigon, V. (1976): Properties and development of erythropoietic stem cells in the chick embryo. *J. Embryol. Exp. Morphol.*, 36:247–260.

102. Sheiness, D., and Bishop, J. M. (1979): DNA and RNA from uninfected vertebrate cells contain nucleotide sequences related to the putative transforming gene of avian myelocytomatosis virus. *J. Virol.*, 31:514–521.

103. Sheiness, D., Bister, K., Moscovici, C., Fanshier, L., Gonda, T., and Bishop, J. M. (1980): Avian retroviruses that cause carcinoma and leukemia: Identification of nucleotide sequences associated with pathogenicity. *J. Virol.*, 33:962–968.

104. Sheiness, D., Fanshier, L., and Bishop, J. M. (1978): Identification of nucleotide sequences which may encode the oncogenic capacity of avian retrovirus MC29. *J. Virol.*, 28:600–610.

105. Sheiness, D., Hughes, S. H., Varmus, H. E., Stubblefield, E., and Bishop, J. M. (1980): The vertebrate homolog of the putative transforming gene of avian myelocytomatosis virus: Characteristics of the DNA locus and its RNA transcript. *Virology*, 195:415–424.
106. Sheiness, D., Vennstrom, B., and Bishop, J. M. (1981): Virus-specific RNAs in cells infected by avian myelocytomatosis virus and avian erythroblastosis virus: Modes of oncogene expression. *Cell*, 23:291–300.
107. Silva, R. F., Dodge, W. H., and Moscovici, C. (1974): The role of humoral factors in the regression of leukemia in chickens as measured by in vitro colony formation. *J. Cell Physiol.*, 83:187–192.
108. Smith, R. E., and Moscovici, C. (1969): The oncogenic effects of nontransforming viruses from avian myeloblastosis virus. *Cancer Res.*, 29:1356–1366.
109. Stehelin, D., and Graf, T. (1978): Avian myelocytomatosis and erythroblastosis viruses lack the transforming gene *src* of avian sarcoma viruses. *Cell*, 13:745–750.
110. Stehelin, D., Saule, S., Roussel, M., Sergeant, A., Lagrou, C., Rommens, C., and Raes, M. B. (1980): Three new types of viral oncogenes in defective leukemia viruses. I. Specific nucleotide sequences of cellular origin correlate with specific transformation. *Cold Spring Harbor Symp. Quant. Biol.*, 44:1215–1223.
111. Szenberg, A. (1977): Ontogeny of myelopoietic precursor cells in the chicken embryo. *Adv. Exp. Med. Biol.*, 88:3–11.
112. Therwath, A., and Scherrer, K. (1978): Post-transcriptional gene expression in cells transformed by avian erythroblastosis virus. *Proc. Natl. Acad. Sci. USA*, 75:3776–3780.
113. Till, J. E., and McCulloch, E. A. (1961): A direct measurement of the radiation sensitivity of normal bone marrow cells. *Radiat. Res.*, 14:213–222.
114. Yoshida, M., and Toyoshima, K. (1980): In vitro translation of avian erythroblastosis virus RNA: Identification of two major polypeptides. *Virology*, 100:484–487.
115. Zeller, N. K., Gazzolo, L., and Moscovici, C. (1980): A study of the epithelioid transformation of MC29-infected chicken embryo cells. *Virology*, 104:239–242.

Advances in Viral Oncology, Volume 1,
edited by George Klein. Raven Press,
New York © 1982.

The Viral and Cellular p21 (ras) Gene Family

*Ronald W. Ellis, **Douglas R. Lowy, and *Edward M. Scolnick

*Virus and Cell Biology Research, Merck Sharp & Dohme Research Laboratories,
West Point, Pennsylvania 19486, **Dermatology Branch, National Cancer Institute,
National Institutes of Health, Bethesda, Maryland 20205

Retroviruses can be grouped into two broad classes based on their biological activities: the nontransforming leukemia or leukosis viruses and the transforming sarcoma or acute leukemia viruses (reviewed in 7,26,48,57). The molecular biology of the transforming viruses has been of special interest because viruses of this class enable cellular transformation related to a defined genetic sequence and its gene product(s) to be studied in great detail and under a high degree of experimental control. Many of these viruses exercise their biological action by means of a single, transformation-specific protein encoded by the viral genome (6,8,49,56,62). In light of the fact that many of these proteins are expressed at low levels in normal cells from a variety of species (5,14,32,63), the mechanism of action of these transforming proteins is a particularly salient question in the field of oncology.

In this chapter, we shall discuss several mammalian transforming retroviruses whose transforming protein is a 21,000 dalton phosphoprotein called p21 ras. The p21 proteins encoded by these genes are immunologically related to one another and to the cellular p21 found in low levels in normal cells. The discussion will focus principally on Harvey and Kirsten murine sarcoma viruses (Ha-MuSV, Ki-MuSV) and the cellular homologs of their p21 coding sequences. Our emphasis here will be on the origin and biology of the viruses, genetic studies of the viral transforming sequences, analysis of two ras-encoding rat cellular genes, and biochemical studies of the viral and cellular ras polypeptides. The designation of the p21 coding genes follows the recently proposed nomenclature for the transforming (onc) genes of retroviruses (13).

ORIGIN AND PATHOLOGY OF p21-ENCODING SARCOMA VIRUSES

As is true of other mammalian sarcoma viruses, the sarcoma viruses that encode ras are helper-dependent because they lack genetic sequences that encode virion structural proteins (reviewed in 7,26,48,57). Therefore, sarcoma virus virions are always a pseudotype of the sarcoma virus RNA genome, which is surrounded by virion proteins encoded by a helper-independent virus. Conversely, all sarcoma virus virion preparations are a mixture of the sarcoma virus and the helper-independent virus, and all mammalian sarcoma viruses originally have been detected as mixed preparations.

Initially, the biological activity of a sarcoma virus genome was deduced from the fact that the biological properties of these virus preparations differed from those observed with the helper-independent virus alone. Subsequently, the finding that a single sarcoma virus particle could induce transformation of cells in tissue culture made it possible, by using appropriate dilutions of virus stocks that contained a favorable ratio of sarcoma virus to helper-independent virus, to isolate cells that had been transformed by the sarcoma virus genome but had not been co-infected with the helper-independent virus (1). Since the transformed cells did not release infectious virus, these results established both that the cellular transformation was induced by the sarcoma virus virions and that these genomes were defective for making progeny virus. This separation of the sarcoma virus from the helper-independent virus also provided cells in which expression of the sarcoma virus genome could be studied independently of the helper-independent virus. Moreover, when these "nonproducer" cells were superinfected with any one of a variety of helper-independent C-type viruses, the transforming activity of the sarcoma virus could be "rescued" from the cells by making a new pseudotype (23,28). The effect (or lack thereof) of different helper-independent viruses on the biologic activity of the sarcoma viruses then could be used to define further the biological potential encoded by the sarcoma viral genome.

The Ha-MuSV strain was the first sarcoma virus isolated from mammals. It was discovered by Harvey in 1964 when a preparation of Moloney murine leukemia virus (Mo-MuLV, which is of mouse origin) was found to induce sarcomas and splenomegaly in newborn BALB/c mice (27). This preparation of Mo-MuLV had been taken from the plasma of a leukemic Chester-Beatty rat, the strain in which Harvey had passaged the virus routinely. Following a short latent period (usually two to three weeks), Ha-MuSV induced pleomorphic sarcomas near the site of injection and elsewhere in many newborn mice, rats, and hamsters. In mice, splenomegaly was even more common than sarcomas. In newborn mice and rats, but not in hamsters, abdominal distention and splenomegaly usually were present by two weeks after inoculation and were an almost universal feature of this disease. Splenomegaly also was induced regularly in adult mice, but not in adult rats. Histologically, erythroblastosis similar to that induced by the Friend virus complex was found in the spleen and peripheral blood (11). Although the early studies were carried out with Mo-MuLV pseudotypes of Ha-MuSV, similar results in mice were obtained with other MuLV pseudotypes of Ha-MuSV (39). The finding that different pseudotypes of the same sarcoma virus possessed similar novel biological activity strengthened the inference that these properties were encoded by the sarcoma virus genome.

The Ki-MuSV strain was isolated by Kirsten and Mayer in 1967 (30,31). Following Harvey's observation, they repeatedly passaged Kirsten murine leukemia virus (Ki-MuLV, a helper-independent virus of mouse origin similar to Mo-MuLV) through Wistar-Furth rats. As was found with Ha-MuSV, Ki-MuSV preparations induced pleomorphic sarcomas and hepatosplenomegaly in newborn mice and rats. The erythroblastosis induced by Ki-MuSV apparently was less malignant than that induced by Ha-MuSV; splenic rupture was not observed with Ki-MuSV, even though it was a common cause of death with Ha-MuSV.

Whereas Ha-MuSV and Ki-MuSV had been isolated by *in vivo* passage of MuLV in rats, Rasheed et al. recently have isolated a rat "sarcoma" virus (RaSV) by *in vitro* cocultivation of a Sprague-Dawley (SD-1) rat embryo cell line with any of several chemically transformed rat cell lines (38). The SD-1 cell line releases an endogenous nontransforming helper-independent type-C virus that is infectious for rat cells. The virus preparations derived from the cocultivations can transform rat cells in culture; recently they have been shown to be pathogenic for animals (Rasheed et al., *unpublished data*).

A fourth *ras*-encoding sarcoma virus was isolated by Peters et al. from a BALB/c mouse (37). This BALB/c mouse sarcoma virus (B-MuSV) was isolated by passage of plasma filtrate from a BALB/c mouse with a spontaneous chloroleukemia. By the fourth *in vivo* passage, it induced hemangiosarcomas with a latent period of less than one month.

STRUCTURE OF THE VIRAL GENOMES

Ha-MuSV and Ki-MuSV were isolated earlier than RaSV or B-MuSV, and they have been studied more intensely than have the latter two viruses. The RNA genome length of Ha-MuSV is about 5.5 kb, whereas that of Ki-MuSV is about 6.5 kb. As is true of other murine retroviruses, the unintegrated or integrated linear viral DNA genomes of each virus is 0.6 kb longer than its RNA genomes, since 0.5 kb of sequences from the 3′ end of the viral RNA are duplicated at the 5′ end of the viral DNA and 0.1 kb of sequences from the 5′ end of the viral RNA are duplicated at the 3′ end of the viral DNA (22,25). In the viral DNA, these 0.6 kbp of duplicated sequences form the long terminal repeat (LTR), which is a characteristic structural feature of all retroviral DNAs.

The isolation of Ha-MuSV and Ki-MuSV from mouse MuLVs passaged in rats had suggested that these viruses either were entirely of rat origin or were interspecies recombinants between rat and mouse genetic information. Nucleic acid hybridization studies demonstrated that Ha- and Ki-MuSV contained both MuLV and rat-derived sequences (42,43), indicating that both viruses are interspecies recombinants.

Oligonucleotide fingerprinting and viral RNA heteroduplexing elucidated many structural features of the Ha- and Ki-MuSV genomes (12,51). Most of the sequences of both viruses are derived from rat cellular information (4.5 kb for Ha- and 5.5 kb for Ki-MuSV). The MuLV sequences are limited to the 5′ and 3′ ends of the viral genome: approximately 0.1 kb at the 5′ end and 0.9 kb at the 3′ end of these RNAs are derived from MuLV sequences. In the viral DNA, the LTR of both viruses, therefore, is composed of Mo-MuLV sequences.

Most of the rat cellular information is derived from sequences that express themselves in some rat cells as 30S RNA (3,40,46,54). Some uninfected rat cell lines express high constitutive levels of RNA homologous to rat sequences of Ha- and Ki-MuSV, and the predominant molecular RNA species in these cells sediment at 30S in sucrose density gradients (40,54). These rat "30S" sequences are retrovirus-like in several respects. Namely, they are present as multiple copies in rat cellular DNA, are poorly conserved evolutionarily, are inducible by halogenated pyrimidines, can be pseudotyped by helper-independent type C viruses, can be reverse transcribed, and are transmissible to heterologous cells (3,20,44,46). Since 30S are replication-defective and nontransforming, it is difficult to assign these sequences a specific genetic function. However, their presence in both viruses suggests that they may have been essential to the formation of these interspecies recombinants.

The development of recombinant DNA clones for Ha-MuSV, Ki-MuSV, and 30S has enabled us to characterize further the rat genetic sequences of Ha- and Ki-MuSV by means of heteroduplexing and Southern blot hybridization analysis (20,64). Both 1.0 kb in the 5′ half of the Ha-MuSV genome and at least 1 kb in the 5′ half of the Ki-MuSV genome are nonhomologous to 30S. Therefore, the RNA genomes of Ha-MuSV and Ki-MuSV are each tripartite, consisting of MuLV sequences, 30S sequences highly reiterated in rats, and a third set of unrelated sequences (Fig. 1). The relationship between the two kinds of rat-derived sequences in normal cell DNA will be discussed in subsequent sections.

GENETIC LOCALIZATION OF THE VIRAL TRANSFORMING FUNCTION

In the avian sarcoma virus system, the viral *src* gene was mapped by the development of deletion mutants and temperature-sensitive mutants of the Rous sarcoma virus (RSV) (7,26,57,58). These studies were facilitated greatly by virtue of the helper-independent nature of RSV. Consequently, it was possible to isolate transformation-defective viruses that were still helper-independent. The lack of a second selectable marker among the mammalian sarcoma viruses complicated this genetic approach for these viruses. Molecular cloning of sarcoma viral DNA circumvented this problem; this technique made available unlimited amounts of genomic viral DNA from which could be derived rigidly defined subgenomic fragments whose infectivity could be assessed in mammalian cells.

Two technical observations were of considerable importance in making these experiments possible. First, the calcium phosphate precipitation technique of Graham and van der Eb (24), originally developed for adenovirus DNA, greatly enhanced the sensitivity of DNA-mediated transfection of retroviral DNA. The second observation was that NIH3T3 cells were very sensitive for infectivity by helper-independent viral DNA (Mo-MuLV) (52), for nonproductive transformation by helper-dependent viral DNA (Ha-MuSV) (34), and finally for subgenomic viral DNA fragments (Mo-MuSV) (4). Indeed, a transfected NIH3T3 cell could be transformed directly by avian sarcoma virus DNA, although these same viral DNAs failed to transform certain other mouse cells or chick embryo cells directly (17).

Among the *ras*-encoding sarcoma viruses, the functional organization of the Ha-MuSV genome has been studied more completely than has that of the other viruses

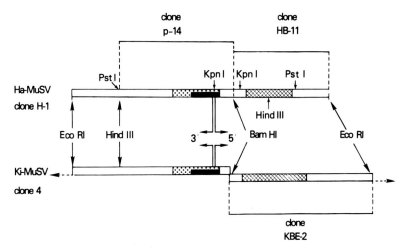

FIG. 1. Structural relationship among the viral clones. The molecular clonings of the full-genome-length DNA molecules Ha-MuSV clone H-1 and Ki-MuSV clone 4 have been described (10,55). The 5'- and 3'-halves of these circularly permuted genomes are indicated on the DNA maps. The subgenomic fragments p-14, HB-11, and KBE-2 were derived from their respective parental clones by means of double digestion with the indicated restriction endonucleases, preparative gel electrophoresis, and molecular cloning at the appropriate sites in pBR322 (18,21). Clone p-14 contains the LTR sequences *(solid box)* which have a promoter-like sequence of the same 5'-3' polarity as the viral genome (19) and which significantly enhance the transformation efficiency of viral transforming genes. Clones HB-11 and KBE-2 contain the viral *ras* genes *(cross-hatched box)*. *Open box*, 30S-derived; *dotted box*, MuLV-derived. (Reproduced with slight modifications from Ellis et al., ref. 21.)

because it was the first of these viral DNAs to be molecularly cloned (25). Most of the studies of Ha-MuSV DNA were carried out on viral DNA that had been cloned from circular genomic DNA isolated from a Hirt supernatant extract of permissive cells that had been acutely infected with a Mo-MuLV pseudotype of Ha-MuSV. The ability of Ha-MuSV to induce high p21-*ras* levels (as described below) provided an important biochemical assay for the viral specificity of DNA-induced focal transformation of the NIH3T3 cells.

The Ha-MuSV circular genomic DNA was chosen to be cloned principally for technical reasons. Most cloning vectors had been designed around the *Eco*RI restriction endonuclease site, and preliminary restriction mapping of the viral DNA revealed that it contained a unique *Eco*RI site near the middle of the viral DNA (25). This meant that a linear genomic Ha-MuSV DNA molecule would be cleaved into two *Eco*RI fragments, whereas *Eco*RI digestion of the circular viral DNA would yield a full-length viral molecule that would be circularly permuted with respect to the linear viral DNA. Therefore, the Ha-MuSV DNA was cloned from the *in vivo* circular DNA at its *Eco*RI site in λ-phage (25). Viral DNA clones containing one, two, and three tandem copies of the viral LTR were obtained. Except for the number of LTRs, the viral DNAs were identical to each other and had the expected permuted order of sequences: *Eco*RI—3' half—LTR(1, 2, or 3)—5' half—*Eco*RI.

When transfected onto NIH3T3 cells, molecules with one, two, or three LTRs induced foci of transformed cells (25). For each viral DNA, its specific infectivity followed single-hit kinetics, it possessed similar efficiencies of transformation, and infectivity was unaffected by digestion with *Eco*RI, which separated the viral DNA insert from its λ vector. However, the infectivity of the permuted DNA was one to two orders of magnitude less efficient than that of uncloned unintegrated linear viral DNA, in agreement with studies using noncloned viral DNAs. Because the infectivity of the three sizes of cloned Ha-MuSV DNA was similar, it was chosen to focus further infectivity studies on a clone with only one LTR. This viral DNA was recloned at the *Eco*RI site of pBR322 as a 5.5 kbp insert designated clone H-1 (10).

The transforming region of Rous sarcoma virus and Mo-MuSV previously had been localized at the 3′ end of the viral RNA (57,58) to acquire nonviral (i.e., not essential for virus replication) sequences. Since the principal region of nonhomology between retroviral sequences and those of Ha- and Ki-MuSV lay near the 5′ end of the viral genome, it seemed possible that the transforming function of both viruses might reside at this end, and this turned out to be the case.

The first approach to defining biologically the transforming region of Ha-MuSV DNA involved the transfection of subgenomic fragments (10,20). A 3.8 kbp clone, spanning the segment between *Pst*I sites 1.5 kbp to the left of the LTR and 1.6 kbp to the right of the LTR (Fig. 1), still transformed with an efficiency about one-fifth that of the full-length clone. A second clone, which contained only the 5′ half of the linear viral DNA (LTR and 5′ end down to the *Eco*RI site), also induced foci. Transformants induced by each type of viral DNA produced levels of p21 *ras* as high as those in Ha-MuSV transformed cells. These results localized the transforming (and v-Ha-*ras*) region to the 2.3 kbp spanning the LTR and the 5′ portion of the viral DNA. This localization of the transforming region was confirmed by studies of viral RNA expression in the transformed cells (10). Although many clones transformed by the cloned genomic viral DNA did not express sequences from the 3′ half of the viral genome, they all expressed high levels of RNA from the 5′ half of the viral genome. Further confirmation was obtained through the abrogation of transformation by digestion at the *Hin*dIII site in this segment (Fig. 1); ligation restored transformation and p21 coding (20).

A second approach, the creation of insertion and deletion mutants of the viral DNA (59), yielded similar results. In this method, circularized Ha-MuSV DNA was partially digested with *Hae*III under conditions favoring restriction at only one or two of the many genomic *Hae*III sites. *Sal*I linkers were ligated to the blunt ends (Ha-MuSV DNA does not contain a *Sal*I site), and the viral DNAs were inserted to a *Sal*I λ vector. The lesions of 14 mutant clones were mapped and their transforming activity assessed on NIH3T3 cells (59). In 10 of the clones, the mutations involved the region previously determined to be nonessential for transformation, and their infectivity was similar to that of the parental clone. The mutations in the other 4 clones were located in the non-LTR sequences near the 5′ end of the viral DNA; their infectivity was greatly reduced or totally absent. These results therefore, complemented those obtained with the subgenomic fragments.

The experiments noted above localized the transforming region to the viral LTR and the 1.8 kb immediately downstream from the LTR. With respect to the role of the LTR, it had been observed that digestion with a restriction endonuclease, which digested within the LTR, almost totally abolished the infectivity of the viral DNA (9). However, it was possible to introduce a deletion between the *Kpn*I site in the LTR located to the right of the start site of viral RNA synthesis and a *Kpn*I site 0.4 kb downstream while retaining considerable transforming activity of the viral DNA (9). These deleted molecules specified the synthesis of high levels of normal v-Ha-*ras* p21. These genetic results localized the p21 coding region to the 1.3 kbp segment between the *Kpn*I NS *Pst*I sites, the segment that contained all the non-30S rat sequences of Ha-MuSV. One *Sal*I mutant of Ha-MuSV DNA had its 0.5 kb deletion in this segment, and this mutant was devoid of transforming activity. These observations also indicated that, in the transfection system, two components of the viral DNA were necessary for efficient viral-induced transformation—the v-Ha-*ras* coding region and the viral LTR. Neither region by itself induced transformation efficiently. It also appeared that for Ha-MuSV DNA, the LTR must be placed upstream from the v-Ha-*ras* coding sequences for the induction, since attempts to induce transformation by ligating the LTR downstream from the v-Ha-*ras* coding region have been unsuccessful (Ellis, Lowy, and Scolnick, *unpublished data*).

The transforming region of Ki-MuSV has been studied less completely than has that of Ha-MuSV. However, its v-Ki-*ras* coding region also has been localized to sequences located in the 5′ half of the viral genome. Ki-MuSV DNA has an *Eco*RI site located near the middle of the linear viral DNA and a *Bam*HI site located 3.1 kbp to the left of the *Eco*RI site and 0.2 kbp to the right of the viral LTR (21,55). These two sites correspond to homologous sites in the Ha-MuSV clone H-1. When this cloned 3.1 kb *Bam*HI/*Eco*RI fragment of Ki-MuSV DNA (clone KBE-2, Fig. 1) was ligated downstream from a nontransforming DNA fragment that contained the LTR of Ha-MuSV (clone p-14, Fig. 1), it transformed NIH3T3 cells and synthesized high levels of v-Ki-*ras* p21 (21). Without the viral LTR, this *Bam*HI/*Eco*RI fragment, which contains the sequences of nonhomology to rat 30S, is almost completely devoid of transforming activity, as was also true of the v-Ha-*ras* p21 coding region (clone HB-11, Fig. 1).

In summary, the biological and structural studies of Ha-MuSV and Ki-MuSV strongly suggested that the 5′ sequences unrelated to 30S encode p21 and the transforming function. Our ability to clone from rat DNA two transforming, p21-encoding genes homologous to the non-30S sequences provided direct support for this hypothesis.

DETECTION OF CELLULAR SEQUENCES HOMOLOGOUS TO v-Ha-*ras* AND v-Ki-*ras* CODING SEQUENCES

As described above, the use of recombinant DNA clones from Ha-MuSV, Ki-MuSV, and 30S enabled us to define the location of the Ha-MuSV and Ki-MuSV *ras* sequences in the 5′ halves of the respective viral genomes. To achieve a finer comparison between the viral *ras* sequences (21), we performed heteroduplex, hybridization, and restriction enzyme analyses on clones derived from the 5' half of both viral genomes (Ha-MuSV clone HB-11 and Ki-MuSV clone KBE-2, Fig. 2). The restriction maps of these clones reveal a complete site mismatch in the respective v-*ras* sequences, whereas virtually every site in the adjacent 30S sequences is present in each clone. When the two v-*ras* regions were compared by heteroduplex analysis under nonstringent hybridization conditions, two domains were recognized with each v-*ras* region. One domain represents v-*ras* sequences unique to each of the viral genes. The second domain, a 0.3 kb segment, is shared

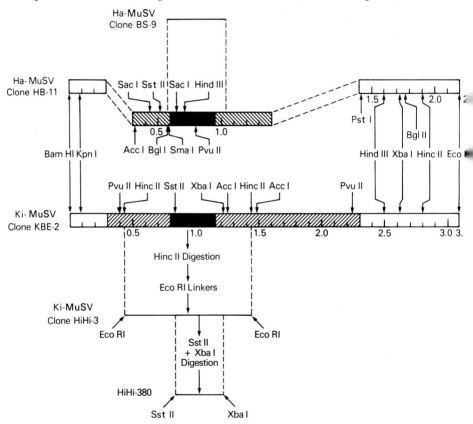

FIG. 2. Detailed structure of Ha-MuSV and Ki-MuSV v-*ras* genes. Detailed restriction endonuclease maps, on scales demarcated in kbp, were developed for Ha-MuSV clone HB-11 (18) and Ki-MuSV clone KBE-2 (21). Superimposed on these maps are heteroduplex data (21), where *the open box* represents common rat 30S RNA sequences, *the solid box* represents v-*ras* sequences shared by Ha-MuSV and Ki-MuSV, and *the hatched boxes* represent v-*ras* sequences unique to either Ha-MuSV *(left-hatched)* or Ki-MuSV *(right-hatched)*. Note the discontinuity of scale on clone HB-11 *(dotted lines)*, drawn to compensate for the size differential between v-Ha-*ras* and v-Ki-*ras*; the substantially larger size of v-Ki-*ras* diagnosed by heteroduplexing may result from the presence of non-*ras* sequences (e.g., 30S) in the region 1.5 to 2.3 kbp on the clone KBE-2 map. The derivations of HiHi-380 and clones BS-9 and HiHi-3 have been described (20,21). (From Ellis et al., ref. 21.)

by the two *ras* genes. Under stringent hybridization conditions, Southern blot analysis between the two genes demonstrated no homology. These results suggest that this shared domain is approximately 10 to 15% divergent between the two viruses. Comparison of the Ki-MuSV and Ha-MuSV p21 tryptic peptides showed that only about two-thirds of the peptide spots of one viral p21 was shared by the other p21 (21). These results therefore were consistent with the partial homology noted between the Ki- and Ha-v-*ras* genes.

When the v-*ras* sequences of Ha-MuSV and Ki-MuSV were compared with those of the other two v-*ras* encoding sarcoma viruses, v-Ha-*ras* region hybridized strongly, under stringent conditions, to RaSV and B-MuSV, whereas the v-Ki-*ras* region did not hybridize with these viruses (2,18). These findings suggest that the v-*ras* coding regions of RaSV and B-MuSV are related more closely to the v-Ha-*ras* than to the v-Ki-*ras* coding regions.

Although Ha-MuSV and Ki-MuSV *ras* genes encode structurally, serologically, and enzymatically related p21 *ras* proteins (41,47,50), the nonreactivity between the v-*ras* genes under stringent hybridization conditions suggested that these two viral p21 coding genes might be derived from distinct cellular *ras* genes. To test this hypothesis, *ras*-specific DNA probes free of 30S sequences were cloned from the respective v-*ras* regions (20,21), denoted Ha-MuSV clone BS-9 and Ki-MuSV HiHi-380 (Fig. 2).

When these two probes were hybridized to *Eco*RI-digested genomic DNA from rat, chicken, human, and mouse, each probe hybridized to at least one *Eco*RI fragment in each DNA (Fig. 3). For each species, the fragments detected by the Ha-specific probe were clearly different in size from the corresponding Ki-specific fragments. These results demonstrated that sequences in each probe were conserved evolutionarily, as is true of other transforming genes, and that the Ha- and Ki-specific probes recognized different gene sequences in genomic DNA. As controls for the specificity of the Ha- and Ki-specific *ras* probes, the Ki-specific probe, but not the Ha-specific probe, detected an extra band in *Eco*RI-digested DNA from mouse cells nonproductively transformed by Ki-MuSV. Conversely, when *Eco*RI-digested DNA from RaSV-transformed mouse cells were hybridized with the Ha- and Ki-*ras* probes, an extra band relative to control cells was detected only with the Ha-specific probe, not the Ki-specific probe. The weak hybridization of the Ki-specific probe to the chicken DNA fragments sized 2.1 and 4.2 kbp raises the possibility that the normal c-*ras* sequences related to Ki-MuSV, having diverged more rapidly in chickens, are not as broadly conserved evolutionarily as are the c-Ha-*ras* sequences. Nevertheless, these data clearly demonstrate that the *ras* sequences of Ha- and Ki-MuSV are derived from distinct c-*ras* genes and suggest that genomic DNA may contain more than one gene that encodes a p21 *ras*.

CLONING AND ANALYSIS OF HARVEY c-*ras* SEQUENCES FROM RAT DNA

Consistent with the evolutionarily conserved nature of the Ha- and Ki-MuSV *ras* genes is the expression of a related, but distinguishable, p21 *ras* in normal cells

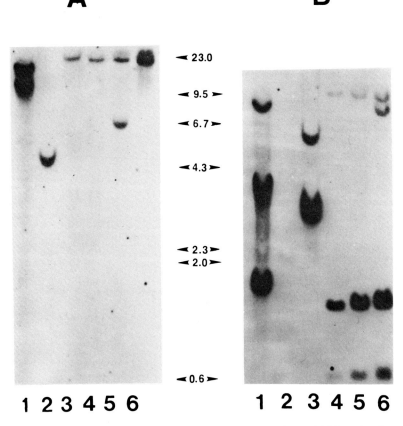

FIG. 3. Southern blot analysis of restriction endonuclease-digested high molecular-weight cellular DNA. Fifty micrograms of cellular DNA were digested 16 hr with 100 units *Eco*RI, electrophoresed, blotted, and hybridized to either of two ^{32}P-labeled DNA probes (1.5 × 10^7 cpm): **(A)** ^{32}P-labeled BS-9 (v-Ha-*ras* specific) DNA or **(B)** ^{32}P-labeled HiHi-380 (v-Ki-*ras* specific) DNA.

Sources of high molecular-weight DNA were: *1*, FRE rat cells; *2*, chicken cells; *3*, human cells; *4*, uninfected NIH3T3 cells; *5*, NIH3T3 cells transformed by RaSV; *6*, NIH3T3 cells transformed by Ki-MuSV. The *arrows* indicate the positions of ^{32}P-labeled λ/*Hind*III DNA markers (length in kbp). Panel **A** lane *1* portrays the two c-*ras* genes, c-Ha-*ras*1 (13 kbp) and c-Ha-*ras*2 (20 kpb). (From Ellis et al., ref. 21.)

from a wide variety of species (32). To understand better any differences in the structure, biology, and regulation of expression between viral p21 (v-*ras*) and cellular p21 (c-*ras*) proteins, studies were initiated into the structure and function of rat c-*ras* genes. Two genes, c-Ha-*ras*2 and c-Ha-*ras*1, have been cloned from rat cellular DNA (18), being derived respectively from the 13 and 20 kbp bands present in *Eco*RI-digested rat DNA hybridized by the v-Ha-*ras* probe (Fig. 3A, lane 1). For surveying the gross structural relationship between v-Ha-*ras* and c-Ha-*ras* sequences, heteroduplex mapping was performed among these DNA mol-

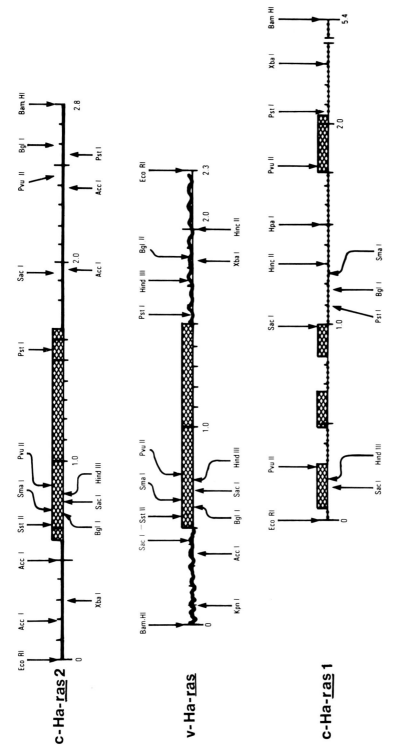

FIG. 4. Restriction endonuclease maps of *v-Ha-ras* and *c-Ha-ras* genes. Restriction maps have been constructed on scales demarcated in kbp (18). As deduced from both heteroduplex analysis and Southern blot hybridization, the homologous *v-ras* and *c-ras* sequences in the three fragments are highlighted by *cross-hatches*. Sequences in each molecule that are nonhomologous to sequences in other molecules are denoted by *solid (top), wavy (middle)*, and *dotted (bottom)* lines. (From DeFeo et al., ref. 18.)

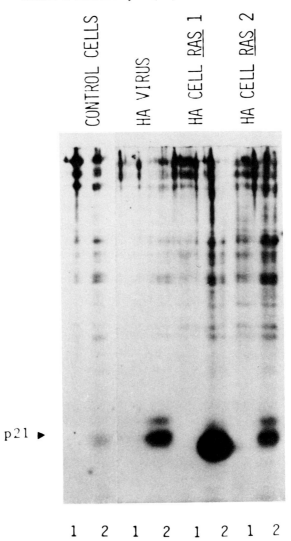

CONTROL CELLS   HA VIRUS   HA CELL RAS 1   HA CELL RAS 2

p21 ▶

1   2   1   2   1   2   1   2

FIG. 5. Immunoprecipitation of p21-*ras* from extracts of NIH3T3 cells transformed by v-Ha-*ras*, c-Ha-*ras*1, and c-Ha-*ras*2. Cells were labeled for 24 hr at 37° with ^{35}S met, cell extracts were prepared, and immunoprecipitations were performed as detailed previously (49,50). NIH3T3 cells either untransformed or transformed by v-*ras* (Ha virus), c-Ha-*ras*2 (Ha cell *ras*2), or c-Ha-*ras*1 (Ha cell *ras*1), and extracts were immunoprecipitated by either control (1) or immune (2) rat antisera.

ecules (Fig. 4). A comparison of c-Ha-*ras*1 with v-Ha-*ras* revealed 0.9 kbp of homology interrupted in c-Ha-*ras*1 by three intervening sequences sized 0.2, 0.2, and 0.8 kbp. In contrast, c-Ha-*ras*2 and v-Ha-*ras* hybridized to an uninterrupted 0.9 kbp segment. The heteroduplex formed between the two c-Ha-*ras* clones was consistent with these results: 0.9 kbp of homology interrupted in the c-Ha-*ras*1 clone by three intervening sequences. These results indicate that Ha-*ras* genes may contain several or no introns and may be present in more than one copy per haploid genome. It is also noteworthy that c-Ha-*ras*1 and c-Ha-*ras*2 contained no homology beyond the 0.9 kb of sequences related to the viral *src*, meaning that c-Ha-*ras* contained no 30S sequences. Since Ha-MuSV is composed of three components, these data would suggest that Ha-MuSV arose after at least two recombinational events.

The juxtaposition of an evolutionarily conserved *onc* gene with an evolutionarily nonconserved sequence (30S) in these viruses constitutes a heretofore novel structural arrangement among transforming retroviruses. To the extent that other transforming retroviruses have been analyzed, the entire genomes have been shown to be composed exclusively of leukemia/helper viral sequences and *onc* genes derived from the host species. Since the 30S component is unrelated to transformation and encodes no known gene products, its biological role in these viruses remains to be elucidated. Nevertheless, it is important to consider whether 30S did play a role in the genesis of these viruses, which were derived following interspecies infections. Our analysis of the c-*ras* genes has shown that these genes are not flanked by 30S sequences, implying that Ha-MuSV and Ki-MuSV are double recombinants among Mo-MuLV, 30S, and c-*ras*. It is possible that 30S functions as an "adapter" or transposable genetic element to facilitate the incorporation of c-Ha-*ras* sequences into these interspecies viruses. Consistent with this role for 30S is the apparent absence of 30S sequences in RaSV, an exclusively rat-derived transforming virus that encodes a protein (p29 *gag-ras*) that is closely related serologically and biochemically to v-Ha-*ras* (66), and in the B-MuSV (2), an exclusively mouse-derived transforming virus that also encodes p21 (v-Ha-*ras*-mouse).

When restriction endonuclease maps of the pBR322 subclones of both c-Ha-*ras* sequences were constructed and compared with the v-Ha-*ras* map (Fig. 4), the colinearity of the c-Ha-*ras*2/v-Ha-*ras* heteroduplex was complemented by the total correspondence of a series of sites (top and middle, *Sst*II, *Bgl*I, *Sma*I, *Sac*I, *Hind*III, *Pvu*II) (18). In contrast, c-Ha-*ras*1 (bottom) has only three of these six sites (*Sac*I, *Hind*III, *Pvu*II), which are clustered in v-Ha-*ras* (middle); in addition, c-Ha-*ras*1 contains a second *Pvu*II site. The close similarity between c-Ha-*ras*2 and v-Ha-*ras* suggests that v-Ha-*ras* was derived from c-Ha-*ras*2. In this regard, the origin of the v-Ha-*ras* sequences would be analogous to that of Mo-MuSV, whose *onc* gene (v-*mos*) also is derived from a colinear cellular *onc* gene (c-*mos*) (35).

In contrast to c-Ha-*ras*2, the structure of c-Ha-*ras*1 is divergent significantly from v-Ha-*ras*. Therefore, we sought biological evidence for its relationship to the Ha-MuSV transforming sequences. Unlike Ha-MuSV DNA, c-Ha-*ras*1 failed by itself to induce foci of transformed NIH3T3 cells in the DNA transfection assay. As noted previously, the viral LTR, which contains a promoter-like sequence of the same 5'–3' polarity as the viral genome (19), significantly enhances the transformation efficiency of v-*ras* genes (9). Accordingly, we ligated the Ha-MuSV LTR with synthetic *Eco*RI termini to the *Eco*RI-*Bam*HI subclone of c-Ha-*ras*1 (Fig. 4). Transfection of this preparation resulted in a low but significant level of focus formation (18). To confirm the specificity of the focus induction, we tested cell extracts for the presence of the transformation-specific p21 *ras*. Immunoprecipitation of cell extracts with p21 *ras*-specific antiserum detected high levels of p21 *ras* in each of three independent foci. Therefore, despite the structural differences between c-Ha-*ras*1 and v-Ha-*ras*, the ability of this cellular DNA clone to transform cells and to induce p21 *ras* expression unambiguously demonstrates its close relationship to the v-Ha-*ras* gene.

By means of a molecular construction similar in principle to that used for c-Ha-*ras*2, the c-Ha-*ras*2 gene is also capable of inducing cellular transformation and high level p21 *ras* expression. By SDS-gel electrophoresis, the ^{35}S-methionine labeled p21 of c-Ha-*ras*2 contains the double band characteristic of cells transformed by v-Ha-*ras*, whereas the p21 of c-Ha-*ras*1 is closer in mobility and appearance to the endogenous p21 of normal cells (Fig. 5). These results strongly support the hypothesis that v-Ha-*ras* is derived from c-Ha-*ras*2.

The ability of the two endogenous *ras* genes to induce cellular transformation has a very important biological implication. Apparently, a mere change in the level of expression of a normal cellular gene and gene product may be sufficient to induce the transformed phenotype. This suggests that *ras* genes can influence cellular proliferation, thus suggesting a possible physiological function. In addition, the ability of these c-Ha-*ras* genes to induce cell transformation indicates that the 30S sequences are not absolutely required for this function. The relationship between the two p21 c-Ha-*ras* proteins and the v-*ras* proteins will be discussed further in the next section.

ONC PROTEIN OF *RAS*-ENCODING SARCOMA VIRUSES

As noted earlier, Ki-MuSV and Ha-MuSV share several properties with other oncogenic replication-defective retroviruses. Each virus was formed by a mechanism that led to large deletions from the genetic information of the helper-independent virus from which Ki-MuSV and Ha-MuSV derive, and each virus is a recombinant virus with cellular genetic sequences in place of the deleted information. At the time that the initial search for the *onc* protein of Ki-MuSV and Ha-MuSV was begun, RaSV had not been isolated. Because no genetic sequences of virion structural proteins remain in Ha-MuSV and Ki-MuSV, antisera to virion structural proteins could not be used to precipitate fusion proteins containing *gag* sequences and the *onc* protein, an approach used successfully for many other oncogenic retroviruses, including RaSV (65).

Translation of Ha-MuSV or Ki-MuSV viral RNA in nuclease-digested reticulocyte systems yielded a 21,000 dalton protein for each virus and an additional 50,000 dalton protein for Ki-MuSV RNA (36,51). The significance of these proteins could not be assessed until evidence had been obtained for their presence in cells transformed by Ki-MuSV or Ha-MuSV. This evidence was gained by preparing antisera to nonproducer cells transformed by Ha-MuSV and Ki-MuSV. Rats were found to be a favorable species for the successful preparation of antisera, and with such sera a 21,000 dalton protein (p21 v-*ras*) was detected in cells transformed by Ki-MuSV or Ha-MuSV (50). A two-dimensional peptide map of the methionine-containing peptides of p21 in cells transformed by Ki-MuSV or Ha-MuSV was found to be identical to the peptide map of the p21 which could be immunoprecipitated following translation of either virion RNA. These results indicated that each viral genome coded for a p21 polypeptide.

This protein was found at high levels in all cells transformed by active subgenomic fragments of Ha-MuSV or by biologically active deletion mutants of Ha-MuSV (9,10,59). In addition, the immunoprecipitability of the p21 encoded by a temperature-sensitive mutant of Ki-MuSV was found to be thermolabile (49). Thus, the p21 *ras* was identified as the *onc* protein of Ki-MuSV and Ha-MuSV, i.e., the protein required for the initiation and maintenance of transformation.

In subsequent studies, a related p29 protein (p29 *gag-ras*) was found to be encoded by RaSV (65). This protein is a *gag*-fusion protein between a part of the p15 protein of a rat type-C virus and a Ha-*ras* related (see above) p21 coding gene. No evidence exists to prove directly that the p29 is the *onc* protein of RaSV, but since the viral genome contains a p21 gene, we assume that p29 is the *onc* gene product of this virus. Recently, a mouse-derived sarcoma virus (B-MuSV) has been analyzed and also found to code for a Ha-MuSV-related p21 (v-Ha-*ras*-mouse) (2). Thus, a Ha-*ras* gene has been acquired by a mouse helper-independent virus in a mouse, a rat helper-independent virus in a rat, and mouse helper-independent viruses in rats.

In the case of the *onc* proteins of RSV (p60), Abelson virus (p120), and FeSV-Ga (p90), a protein related to the *onc* protein of each virus has been detected at low levels in certain normal cells (5,14,63). Similarly for p21, a variety of normal cells were found to express low levels of p21 (32) and one bone marrow cell line that expresses very high levels of an endogenous p21 was found (45). Until some of the genes coding for the expressed normal p21 had been cloned, we could not assess whether the endogenous p21 and various viral p21 proteins were identical. A phosphorylated form of the Ki-MuSV and Ha-MuSV p21 had been detected in cells transformed by Ki-MuSV or Ha-MuSV, and a phosphorylated form of the RaSV p29 also had been detected (50,66). However we could not detect with our sera a similarly phosphorylated form of the endogenous p21 in a variety of cells (Langbeheim, Shih, and Scolnick, *unpublished data*). In cells transformed by either of the two cloned rat genes (c-Ha-*ras*1 and c-Ha-*ras*2) homologous to the Ha-MuSV *src* gene, high levels of p21 were found (Fig. 5). Comparisons of the p21 coded for by the different p21 *ras* genes is underway and will be discussed briefly below.

The biochemical function of the p21 *ras* is not elucidated fully yet; however, certain properties have emerged. The p21 seems to have a unique affinity for guanine-containing nucleotides and a binding assay for p21 measures its ability to bind GDP or GTP (41). In addition, an autophosphorylating activity has been detected for the Ha-MuSV p21 in which the terminal phosphate of GTP is transferred to a threonine residue of p21 (47). This activity seems to be an inherent property of p21 of Ha-MuSV. A similar phospho-threonine form of Ha-MuSV has been detected in cells transformed by Ha-MuSV; in both the *in vivo* and the *in vitro* prepared forms of pp21, a single similar peptide is phosphorylated. Different forms of the p21 have been detected in pulse-chase kinetic labeling experiments, and the pp21 seems to be derived from the p21 form of the protein. Curiously, the form of p21 *ras* encoded by the c-Ha-*ras*1 gene differs from the forms encoded by the c-Ha-*ras*2 gene and the v-Ha-*ras* gene (Shih, Ellis, and Scolnick, *unpublished data*). The p21 of c-Ha-*ras*1 has guanine nucleotide binding activity; thus far, no autophosphorylating activity has been detected. Similarly, in cells transformed by this c-Ha-*ras*1 gene, no phosphorylated form of p21 has been detected, although it is possible that phosphorylation of c-Ha-*ras*1 p21 has changed its conformation in such a way that it is no longer immunoprecipitable with conventional antisera. Studies are in progress to compare the different forms of p21 encoded by the endogenous genes that might be progenitors of these viral *ras* genes. It is not known which form of p21 possesses which of the nucleotide binding or autophosphorylating activities associated with p21. However, the striking feature of the activities associated with p21 is the rigorous preference for GTP over ATP, and the fact that no phosphotyrosine-containing form of Ha-MuSV or Ki-MuSV p21 has been detected. It is clear that several other *onc* proteins of retroviruses are ATP-utilizing protein kinase enzymes that can phosphorylate tyrosine residues (5,15,16,29,33,61). Exactly how the biochemistry of p21 fits together with these other *onc* proteins in possible biochemical pathways involved in transformation is not clear yet.

At this juncture, it is clear that p21 *ras* is the transforming protein of Ha-MuSV and Ki-MuSV; p21 is found in association with the inner surface of the plasma membrane of cells transformed by Ha-MuSV or Ki-MuSV (60). A plausible hypothesis is that p21 functions as a regulatory subunit for certain enzymes important in regulating the activity of various membrane proteins. In the future, the identification of the number, functions, and target molecules for these kinases will be important tools for helping to elucidate the understanding of carcinogenesis at a molecular level. However, it is clear from studies on p21 *ras* levels in normal cells, cells transformed by Ha-MuSV or Ki-MuSV, and cells transformed by either c-Ha-*ras* gene that the mere quantitative elevation of p21, a protein normally expressed at low levels in cells, can tilt the balance of the physiology of the cell toward the malignant state.

SUMMARY

We would like to summarize some of the key observations with respect to the p21 *ras* encoding sarcoma viruses.

1. Ha-MuSV and Ki-MuSV have tripartite structures consisting of MuLV sequences (including the LTR), rat 30S sequences, and an evolutionarily conserved unique sequence cellular gene, which encodes p21 *ras*.

2. The genes in each virus encoding p21 *ras* show such extensive divergence from each other that cloned probes from these genes detect distinct sets of cellular genes in the DNA from several vertebrate species.

3. There are two rat cellular genes homologous to v-Ha-*ras*. One gene is colinear with v-Ha-*ras* whereas the other gene has three introns in its coding sequence.

4. Transfection of the ligation between the viral LTR to either c-Ha-*ras* gene results in cellular transformation and high levels of p21 *ras* expression.

5. The p21 polypeptides of v-Ha-*ras* (similar to c-Ha-*ras*2), c-Ha-*ras*1, and v-Ki-*ras* are structurally distinct.

ACKNOWLEDGMENTS

The authors gratefully acknowledge their many collaborators in the experiments described in this chapter. Among these are E. H. Chang, D. DeFeo, M. A. Gonda, T. Y. Shih, and H. A. Young. Thanks are due to L. Shaughnessy for careful preparation of this chapter.

REFERENCES

1. Aaronson, S. A., and Rowe, W. P. (1970): Nonproducer clones of murine sarcoma virus transformed BALB/3T3 cells. *Virology*, 42:9–19.
2. Andersen, P. R., Devare, S. G., Tronick, S. R., Ellis, R. W., Aaronson, S. A., and Scolnick, E. M. (1981): Generation of BALB-MuSV and Ha-MuSV by type-C virus transduction of homologous transforming genes from different species. *Cell*, 26:129–134.
3. Anderson, G. A., and Robbins, K. C. (1976): Rat sequences of the Kirsten and Harvey murine sarcoma virus genomes: Nature, origin, and expression in rat tumor RNA. *J. Virol.*, 17:335–351.
4. Andersson, P., Goldfarb, M. P., and Weinberg, R. A. (1979): A defined subgenomic fragment of in vitro synthesized Moloney sarcoma virus DNA can induce cell transformation upon transfection. *Cell*, 16:63–75.
5. Barbacid, M., Beemon, K., and Devare, S. G. (1980): Origin and functional properties of the major gene product of the Snyder-Theilen strain of feline sarcoma virus. *Proc. Natl. Acad. Sci. USA*, 77:5158–5162.
6. Barbacid, M., Lauver, A. V., and Devare, S. G. (1980): Biochemical and immunological characterization of polyproteins coded for the McDonough, Gardner-Arnstein, and Snyder-Theilen strains of feline sarcoma virus. *J. Virol.*, 33:196–207.
7. Bishop, J. M. (1978): Retroviruses. *Annu. Rev. Biochem.*, 47:35–88.
8. Brugge, J. S., and Erikson, R. L. (1977): Identification of a transformation-specific antigen induced by an avian sarcoma virus. *Nature*, 269:346–348.
9. Chang, E. H., Ellis, R. W., Scolnick, E. M., and Lowy, D. R. (1980): Transformation by cloned Harvey murine sarcoma virus DNA: Efficiency increased by long terminal repeat DNA. *Science*, 210:1249–1251.
10. Chang, E. H., Maryak, J. M., Wei, C.-M., Shih, T. Y., Shober, R., Cheung, H. L., Ellis, R. W., Hager, G. L., Scolnick, E. M., and Lowy, D. R. (1980): Functional organization of the Harvey murine sarcoma virus genome. *J. Virol.*, 35:76–92.
11. Chesterman, F. C., Harvey, J. J., Dourmashkin, R. R., and Salaman, M. H. (1966): The pathology of tumors and other lesions induced in rodents by virus derived from a rat with Moloney leukemia. *Cancer Res.*, 26:1759–1768.
12. Chien, Y. H., Lai, M., Shih, T. Y., Verma, I. M., Scolnick, E. M., Roy-Burman, P., and Davidson, N. (1979): Heteroduplex analysis of the sequence relationships between the genomes of Kirsten and Harvey sarcoma viruses, their respective parental murine leukemia viruses and the rat endogenous 30S RNA. *J. Virol.*, 31:752–760.
13. Coffin, J. M., Varmus, H. E., Bishop, J. M., Essex, M., Hardy, W. D., Martin, G. S., Rosenberg, N. E., Scolnick, E. M., Weinberg, R. A., and Vogt, P. K. (1981): A proposal for naming host cell-derived inserts in retrovirus genomes. *J. Virol.*, 40:953–957.
14. Collett, M. S., Brugge, J. A., and Erikson, R. L. (1980): Characterization of a normal avian cell protein related to the avian sarcoma virus transforming gene product. *Cell*, 15:1363–1369.
15. Collett, M. S., and Erikson, R. L. (1978): Protein kinase activity associated with the avian sarcoma virus *src* gene product. *Proc. Natl. Acad. Sci. USA*, 75:2021–2024.

16. Collett, M. S., Purchio, A. F., and Erikson, R. L. (1980): Avian sarcoma virus-transforming protein pp60^{src} shows protein kinase activity specific for tyrosine. *Nature*, 285:167–169.
17. Copeland, N. G., Zelenetz, A. D., and Cooper, G. M. (1979): Transformation of NIH/3T3 mouse cells by DNA of Rous sarcoma virus. *Cell*, 17:993–1002.
18. DeFeo, D., Gonda, M. A., Young, H. A., Chang, E. H., Lowy, D. R., Scolnick, E. M., and Ellis, R. W. (1981): Analysis of two divergent restriction endonuclease fragments homologous to the p21 coding region of Harvey murine sarcoma virus. *Proc. Natl. Acad. Sci. USA*, 78:3328–3332.
19. Dhar, R., McClements, W. L., Enquist, L. W., and Van de Woude, G. F. (1980): Nucleotide sequences of integrated Moloney sarcoma provirus long terminal repeats and their host and viral junctions. *Proc. Natl. Acad. Sci. USA*, 77:3937–3941.
20. Ellis, R. W., DeFeo, D., Maryak, J. M., Young, H. A., Shih, T. Y., Chang, E. H., Lowy, D. R., and Scolnick, E. M. (1980): Dual evolutionary origin for the rat genetic sequences of Harvey murine sarcoma virus. *J. Virol.*, 36:408–420.
21. Ellis, R. W., DeFeo, D., Shih, T. Y., Gonda, M. A., Young, H. A., Tsuchida, N., Lowy, D. R., and Scolnick, E. M. (1981): The p21 src genes of Harvey and Kirsten murine sarcoma viruses originate from divergent members of a family of normal vertebrate genes. *Nature*, 292:506–511.
22. Gilboa, E., Goff, S., Shields, A., Yoshimura, F., Mitra, S., and Baltimore, D. (1979): *In vitro* synthesis of a 9 kbp terminally redundant DNA carrying the infectivity of Moloney murine leukemia virus. *Cell*, 16:863–874.
23. Goldberg, R. J., Levin, R., Parks, W. P., and Scolnick, E. M. (1976): Quantitative analysis of the rescue of RNA sequences by mammalian type C viruses. *J. Virol.*, 17:43–50.
24. Graham, F. L., and van der Eb, A. J. (1973): A new technique for the assay of infectivity of human adenovirus 5 DNA. *Virology*, 52:456–461.
25. Hager, G. L., Chang, E. H., Chan, H. W., Garon, C. F., Israel, M. A., Martin, M. A., Scolnick, E. M., and Lowy, D. R. (1979): Molecular cloning of the Harvey sarcoma virus closed circular DNA intermediates: Initial structural and biological characterization. *J. Virol.*, 31:795–809.
26. Hanafusa, H. (1977): Cell transformation by RNA tumor viruses. In: *Comprehensive Virology, Vol. 10*, edited by H. Fraenkel-Conrat and R. R. Wagner, pp. 401–483. Plenum, New York.
27. Harvey, J. J. (1964): An unidentified virus which causes the rapid production of tumors in mice. *Nature*, 204:1104–1105.
28. Huebner, R. J., Hartley, J. W., Rowe, W. P., Lane, W. T., and Capps, W. I. (1966): Rescue of the defective genome of Moloney sarcoma virus from a non-infectious hamster tumor and the production of pseudotype sarcoma viruses with various murine leukemia viruses. *Proc. Natl. Acad. Sci. USA*, 56:1164–1172.
29. Hunter, T., and Sefton, B. M. (1980): Transforming gene product of Rous sarcoma virus phosphorylates tyrosine. *Proc. Natl. Acad. Sci. USA*, 77:1311–1315.
30. Kirsten, W. H., and Mayer, L. A. (1967): Morphologic responses to a murine erythroblastosis virus. *J. Natl. Cancer Inst.*, 39:311–335.
31. Kirsten, W. H., Mayer, L. A., Wollmann, R. L., and Pierce, M. I. (1967): Studies on a murine erythroblastosis virus. *J. Natl. Cancer Inst.*, 38:117–139.
32. Langbeheim, H., Shih, T. Y., and Scolnick, E. M. (1980): Identification of a normal vertebrate cell protein related to the p21 src of Harvey murine sarcoma virus. *Virology*, 106:292–300.
33. Levinson, A. D., Oppermann, H., Levintow, L., Varmus, H. E., and Bishop, J. M. (1978): Evidence that the transforming gene of avian sarcoma virus encodes a protein kinase associated with a phosphoprotein. *Cell*, 15:561–572.
34. Lowy, D. R., Rands, E., and Scolnick, E. M. (1978): Helper-independent transformation by unintegrated Harvey sarcoma virus DNA. *J. Virol.*, 26:291–298.
35. Oskarsson, M., McClements, W. L., Blair, D. G., and Maizel, J. V. (1980): Properties of a normal mouse cell DNA sequence *(sarc)* homologous to the src sequence of Moloney sarcoma virus. *Science*, 297:1222–1223.
36. Parks, W. P., and Scolnick, E. M. (1977): *In vitro* translation of Harvey murine sarcoma virus RNA. *J. Virol.*, 22:711–719.
37. Peters, R. L., Rabstein, L. S., Van Vleck, R., Kelloff, G. J., and Huebner, R. J. (1974): Naturally occurring sarcoma virus of the BALB/cCr mouse. *J. Natl. Cancer Inst.*, 53:1725–1729.
38. Rasheed, S., Gardner, M. B., and Huebner, R. J. (1978): *In vitro* isolation of stable rat sarcoma viruses. *Proc. Natl. Acad. Sci. USA*, 75:2972–2976.
39. Scher, C. D., Scolnick, E. M., and Siegler, R. (1975): Induction of erythroid leukemia by the Harvey and Kirsten sarcoma viruses. *Nature*, 256:225–227.

40. Scolnick, E. M., Maryak, J. M., and Parks, W. P. (1974): Levels of rat cellular RNA homologous to either Kirsten sarcoma virus or rat type C virus in cell lines derived from Osborne-Mendel rats. *J. Virol.*, 14:1435–1444.

41. Scolnick, E. M., Papageorge, A. G., and Shih, T. Y. (1979): Guanine nucleotide-binding activity as an assay for *src* protein of rat-derived murine sarcoma viruses. *Proc. Natl. Acad. Sci. USA*, 76:5355–5359.

42. Scolnick, E. M., and Parks, W. P. (1974): Harvey sarcoma virus: A second murine type-C sarcoma virus with rat genetic information. *J. Virol.*, 13:1211–1219.

43. Scolnick, E. M., Rands, E., Williams, D., and Parks, W. P. (1973): Studies on the nucleic acid sequences of Kirsten sarcoma virus: A model for formation of a mammalian RNA-containing sarcoma virus. *J. Virol.*, 12:458–463.

44. Scolnick, E. M., Vass, W. C., Howk, R. S., and Duesberg, P. H. (1979): Defective retrovirus-like 30S RNA species of rat and mouse cells are infectious if packaged by type C helper virus. *J. Virol.*, 29:964–972.

45. Scolnick, E. M., Weeks, M. O., Shih, T. Y., Ruscetti, S. K., and Dexter, T. M. (1981): Markedly elevated levels of an endogenous *sarc* protein in a hemopoietic precursor cell line. *Mol. Cell. Biol.*, 1:66–74.

46. Scolnick, E. M., Williams, D., Maryak, J., Vass, W., Goldberg, R. J., and Parks, W. P. (1976): Type C particle-positive and type C particle-negative rat cell lines: Characterization of the coding capacity of endogenous sarcoma virus-specific RNA. *J. Virol.*, 20:570–582.

47. Shih, T. Y., Papageorge, A. G., Stokes, P. E., Weeks, M. O., and Scolnick, E. M. (1980): Guanine nucleotide binding and autophosphorylating activities associated with the purified p21 *src* protein of Harvey murine sarcoma virus. *Nature*, 287:686–691.

48. Shih, T. Y., and Scolnick, E. M. (1980): Molecular biology of mammalian sarcoma viruses. In: *Viral Oncology*, edited by G. Klein, pp. 135–160. Raven Press, New York.

49. Shih, T. Y., Weeks, M. O., Young, H. A., and Scolnick, E. M. (1979): p21 of Kirsten murine sarcoma virus is thermolabile in a viral mutant temperature sensitive for the maintenance of transformation. *J. Virol.*, 31:546–556.

50. Shih, T. Y., Weeks, M. O., Young, H. A., and Scolnick, E. M. (1979): Identification of a sarcoma virus coded phosphoprotein in nonproducer cells transformed by Kirsten or Harvey murine sarcoma virus. *Virology*, 96:64–79.

51. Shih, T. Y., Williams, D. R., Weeks, M. O., Maryak, J. M., Vass, W. C., and Scolnick, E. M. (1978): Comparison of the genomic organization of Kirsten and Harvey sarcoma viruses. *J. Virol.*, 27:45–55.

52. Smotkin, D., Gianni, A. M., Rozenblatt, S., and Weinberg, R. A. (1975): Infectious viral DNA of murine leukemia virus. *Proc. Natl. Acad. Sci. USA*, 72:4910–4913.

53. Omitted in proof.

54. Tsuchida, N., Gilden, R., and Hatanaka, M. (1974): Sarcoma-virus-related RNA sequences in normal rat cells. *Proc. Natl. Acad. Sci. USA*, 71:4503–4507.

55. Tsuchida, N., and Vesagi, S. (1981): Structure and functions of the Kirsten murine sarcoma virus genome: Molecular cloning of biologically active Kirsten murine sarcoma virus DNA. *J. Virol.*, 38:720–727.

56. Van de Ven, W. J. M., Reynolds, F. H., and Stephenson, J. R. (1980): The nonstructural components of polyproteins encoded by replication-defective mammalian transforming retroviruses are phosphorylated and have associated protein kinase activity. *Virology*, 101:185–197.

57. Vogt, P. K. (1977): Genetics of RNA tumor viruses. In: *Comprehensive Virology, Vol. 9*, edited by H. Fraenkel-Conrat and R. R. Wagner, pp. 341–455. Plenum, New York.

58. Wang, L. H., Duesberg, P., Beemon, K., and Vogt, P. K. (1975): Mapping RNase T1-resistant oligonucleotides of avian tumor virus RNAs: Sarcoma specific oligonucleotides are near the poly(A) end and oligonucleotides common to sarcoma and transformation-defective viruses are at the poly(A) end. *J. Virol.*, 16:1051–1070.

59. Wei, C.-M., Lowy, D., and Scolnick, E. (1980): Mapping of transforming region of the Harvey murine sarcoma virus genome by using insertion-deletion mutants constructed *in vitro*. *Proc. Natl. Adac. Sci. USA*, 77:4674–4678.

60. Willingham, M. C., Pastan, I., Shih, T. Y., and Scolnick, E. M. (1980): Localization of the *src* gene product of the Harvey strain of MSV to plasma membrane of transformed cells by electron microscopic immunocytochemistry. *Cell*, 19:1005–1014.

61. Witte, O. H., Dasgupta, A., and Baltimore, D. (1980): Abelson murine leukaemia virus protein is phosphorylated *in vitro* to form phosphotyrosine. *Nature*, 283:826–831.

62. Witte, O. H., Goff, S., Rosenberg, N., and Baltimore, D. (1980): A transformation-defective mutant of Abelson murine leukemia virus lacks protein kinase activity. *Proc. Natl. Acad. Sci. USA*, 77:4993–4997.
63. Witte, O. N., Rosenberg, N., and Baltimore, D. (1979): A normal cell protein crossreactive to the major Abelson murine leukemia virus gene product. *Nature*, 281:396–398.
64. Young, H. A., Gonda, M. A., DeFeo, D., Ellis, R. W., Nagashima, K., and Scolnick, E. M. (1980): Heteroduplex analysis of cloned rat endogenous replication-defective (30S) retrovirus and Harvey murine sarcoma virus. *Virology*, 107:89–99.
65. Young, H. A., Rasheed, S., Sowder, R., Benton, C. V., and Henderson, L. E. (1981): Rat sarcoma virus: Further analysis of individual viral isolates and the gene product. *J. Virol.*, 38:286–293.
66. Young, H. A., Shih, T. Y., Scolnick, E. M., Rasheed, S., and Gardner, M. B. (1979): Different rat-derived transforming retroviruses code for an immunologically related intracellular phosphoprotein. *Proc. Natl. Acad. Sci. USA*, 76:3523–3527.

Advances in Viral Oncology, Volume 1,
edited by George Klein. Raven Press,
New York © 1982.

The Cellular Oncogene of the Abelson Murine Leukemia Virus Genome

*Stephen P. Goff and David Baltimore

*Center for Cancer Research and Department of Biology, Massachusetts Institute of
Technology, Cambridge, Massachusetts 02139*

BIOLOGY OF ABELSON MURINE LEUKEMIA VIRUS

Abelson murine leukemia virus (A-MuLV) is a replication-defective retrovirus capable of inducing lymphosarcomas in mice. A-MuLV was originally isolated from one of a series of mice treated with the steroid prednisolone and subsequently infected with Moloney murine leukemia virus (M-MuLV) (1,2). The usual target tissue for transformation by M-MuLV is the thymus; the resulting tumors show many of the properties of mouse T-cells. Previous treatment of animals with prednisolone, however, kills the majority of the target cells and thus prevents or delays the onset of the disease caused by M-MuLV. In one out of 159 mice in the original study, a nonthymic tumor, a lymphosarcoma, arose after a very short latent period. Filtered extracts of the tumor cells induced similar tumors in animals 3 to 6 weeks after injection. The new virus causing these tumors was termed A-MuLV. Many of the properties of the virus have previously been reviewed (16).

The tumors induced *in vivo* often could be adapted to growth *in vitro* and cloned. More importantly, primary cultures from target tissue could be prepared and then transformed *in vitro* by infection with the virus (15,17). Susceptible cells were found in fetal liver (the site of hematopoietic development in the fetal mouse) and adult bone marrow and spleen. The phenotype of the A-MuLV-induced tumor cells was found to closely resemble that of B-lymphoid cells (see later) and thus we call the process of producing these cells the *B-lymphoid transforming activity* of A-MuLV.

In addition to its B-lymphoid transforming activity, continuous fibroblastic lines such as 3T3 derived from NIH/Swiss mice can be transformed by A-MuLV (22). This latter finding is a significant experimental convenience and allows the titering of A-MuLV by focus formation on 3T3 cell monolayer cultures. We term this the

---

*Present address: Department of Biochemistry, College of Physicians and Surgeons, Columbia University, New York, New York 10032.

fibroblastic transforming activity of A-MuLV; it is not evident on all continuous cell lines and the virus will not transform primary fibroblastic cell cultures.

A-MuLV-induced tumors release both A-MuLV and M-MuLV virus into the culture medium. By infecting cells at very low multiplicity, however, transformed clones can be isolated which are free of M-MuLV; these lines, containing only A-MuLV, do not release virus (22). Thus, A-MuLV has been proven to be a replication-defective retrovirus dependent on at least one helper virus protein for its packaging and propagation. A-MuLV can be rescued from transformed nonproducers by superinfection of the cell with M-MuLV or other MuLVs; such cells release both A-MuLV and the helper virus.

A-MuLV-Transformed Cells

Immunoglobulin gene expression is the most important cell type marker of the A-MuLV-transformed lymphoid cell. Most A-MuLV tumor cells fall into one of two categories with regard to their expression of immunoglobulin: They are either "μ-only" cells, expressing cytoplasmic μ heavy chain in the absence of any detectable light chain, or they are null cells, expressing neither heavy nor light chains (11,27). Examination of the heavy and light chain genes from many of these cells has shown that generally both heavy chain alleles have undergone some DNA rearrangement preparatory to gene expression, while neither kappa nor lambda light chain genes, as a rule, are rearranged (3). Some lines derived from infection of early fetal liver cells, moreover, are unstable at the heavy chain locus and continue to rearrange their DNA in culture (3). By these criteria A-MuLV cells seem to be closely related to the pre-B-lymphocyte, an immature cell found early in the differentiation pathway leading from the stem cell to the mature immunoglobulin-producing plasma cell. A-MuLV is of interest for two reasons: as an example of a tumor virus which transforms and immortalizes a specific class of cells and as a means of isolating continuous and clonal cell lines of this important cell type (4). The tumors continue to be of great use in the study of gene rearrangement.

Proteins Encoded by A-MuLV

An A-MuLV-specific protein was first detected by immunoprecipitation of labeled proteins from A-MuLV-transformed cells using sera specific to M-MuLV proteins (13,33). All sera reactive to the *gag* gene products p12 and p15 and some sera specific to p30 were found to immunoprecipitate a protein of 120,000 daltons termed P120. This protein,or a closely related protein, was found in all A-MuLV-induced tumors, in A-MuLV-transformed lymphoid cells and in A-MuLV-transformed 3T3 cells (both producer cells and nonproducer cells which were free of M-MuLV). This result immediately suggested that the A-MuLV genome contained at least that portion of the M-MuLV genome encoding the *gag* gene products. No determinants of the *pol* or *env* genes could be found on the P120. The protein was not glycosylated, but was associated with the cell membrane. Novel antigenic determinants, however, were identified on the P120 molecule using sera from tumor-bearing animals in the process of rejecting A-MuLV-induced tumors (α-AbT sera) (31). Immunoprecipitation of the P120 by such sera was not prevented by competition with *gag* or other Moloney gene products indicating that new peptide sequences made up part of the P120 molecule.

Many A-MuLV variants have been isolated which encode proteins of sizes different than that of P120 (9,18,19). One strain, commonly considered to be the original progenitor virus, specifies a 160,000 dalton protein, A-MuLV(P160). Variants have arisen spontaneously during the passage of cell lines producing P120 which encode proteins of 100,000 daltons, A-MuLV(P100), and of 90,000 daltons, A-MuLV(P90). Finally, a strain was isolated which encodes a 92,000 dalton protein which is defective in transformation, A-MuLV(P92td). All of these proteins were immunoprecipitable with *gag*-specific sera and thus seemed to contain the same M-MuLV region. This was confirmed by analysis of the genome structure of these variants (9). The biological activity of the strains will be discussed.

Structure of the A-MuLV Genome

An understanding of the structure of these A-MuLV genomes and their relationship to the M-MuLV genome was obtained by direct analysis of viral nucleic acids. Virion RNA from stocks of A-MuLV contained both an 8.3 kb RNA contributed by the helper virus and a new 5.6 kb RNA (24). This 5.6 kb RNA was able to direct the synthesis of the P120 protein in an *in vitro* translation system (14,24) and thus could be identified as the A-MuLV genome.

Heteroduplex analysis between this RNA and full-length DNA copies of the M-MuLV genome revealed that the A-MuLV DNA contained two terminal regions of homology to M-MuLV and a large central substitution which showed no homology (24). Digestion of the hybrids with nuclease S1 released protected DNA fragments whose sizes gave the lengths of the terminal regions of homology (Fig. 1). A-MuLV thus was shown to be a hybrid virus, derived from M-MuLV by loss of part of the *gag* gene, and all of the *pol* and *env* genes and addition of new sequences specific to A-MuLV (termed V-*abl*). These V-*abl* sequences could be isolated by hydroxylapatite chromatography and used as a probe for liquid hybridization tests; homologous sequences were found in the DNA of normal BALB/c mice at an abundance corresponding to single copy genes (5).

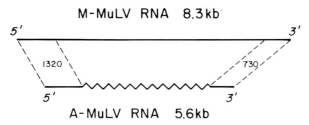

FIG. 1. Comparison of the structure of the Abelson murine leukemia virus genome and the Moloney murine leukemia virus genome.

The observed structure of the A-MuLV genome was highly satisfying because it explained so many of the unknown properties of A-MuLV. The virus, as expected, was related to M-MuLV. That the termini were conserved explained how the virus replicated; all *cis*-acting sequences needed for reverse transcription, integration, forward transcription, and viral RNA packaging are thought to be contained near the termini and thus are present in the A-MuLV genome. At least part of the *trans*-acting genes (*gag*, *pol*, and *env*) were removed by deletion, accounting for the replication defect of the virus. Finally, the 5′ terminal region of homology to M-MuLV was sufficiently large to encode the *gag*-related determinants found on P120. The novel antigenic determinants were presumably encoded by part of the 3.5 kb substitution; translation continuing in frame across the 5′ M-MuLV/V-*abl* junction would account for the properties of the P120. This general structure has been found for a wide variety of transforming retroviruses in many species (see other chapters in this book).

Molecular Cloning of the A-MuLV Genome

A more detailed analysis of the source of the new DNA sequences contained in A-MuLV required the construction of molecular clones of the viral DNA. Virus stocks were prepared from a cell line containing two different proviruses, one encoding a P90 genome and the other encoding P92t*d*; the genomes of these two A-MuLV strains were packaged and released in M-MuLV coats. This virus preparation was used to infect NIH/3T3 cells and the preintegrative viral DNA was isolated. The supercoiled DNA was purified, cleaved with Hind III and cloned in the phage vector Charon 21A (7). Because the site of cleavage by Hind III was within the V-*abl* region, each clone isolated contained a permuted copy of the A-MuLV genome; the termini of the DNA had been joined together during the formation of the circle *in vivo*. The clones were of two types: They had either one or two copies of the long terminal repeat (LTR) sequence at the site of joining of the M-MuLV encoded termini. These two types of intermediates have been identified in cells infected with most retroviruses (23,34).

In later work, cloned representations of the A-MuLV(P160) strain were produced (S. Latt and S. Goff, *unpublished observations*). Using these, a complete restriction map of the largest A-MuLV strain was produced (Fig. 2) (J. Wang and S. Goff, *unpublished observations*). Some sequence data on the clones has been obtained which has shown that when V-*abl* was inserted into M-MuLV to form A-MuLV, a precise junction was formed at either end (Fig. 3).

These data allowed subclones of the V-*abl* region to be prepared which would be free of M-MuLV sequences. A 2.3 kb segment was isolated from the A-MuLV(P90) clone after cleavage by Hind III and Bgl II and subcloned into the plasmid pBR322, to yield the plasmid pAB3sub3. This DNA could be labeled and used as a probe to detect sequences related to V-*abl*.

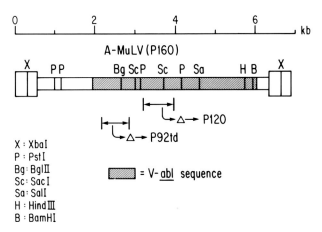

FIG. 2. Restriction enzyme sites in a DNA copy of the A-MuLV genome. These data derive from analysis of cloned representations of the A-MuLV(P160), A-MuLV(P90) and A-MuLV(P92*td*) genomes. The positions of the deletions that occurred to generate the A-MuLV(P120) and A-MuLV(P92*td*) strains are also shown.

Structure of A-MuLV Variant Genomes

Using the V-*abl* probe, the sizes of variant A-MuLV proviruses could be analyzed by hybridization to DNA fragments separated by electrophoresis and transferred to nitrocellulose. Cleavage of cellular DNA with enzymes which cut the LTR sequence (and therefore bracket the provirus) released viral fragments whose sizes were diagnostic of the genome size. In this way genomes encoding the virus-specific proteins P120, P100, and P90 were found to be indistinguishable in size and structure. Thus, the difference in the two smaller proteins from their larger parent P120 is most likely to be due to early translational terminations at point mutations or other undetectably small genetic alterations (Fig. 4; ref. 9).

The genome encoding the P92*td* protein was 700 bp shorter than the other three; this genome could be identified with smaller clones isolated in the original screen and the position of the 700 base pair (bp) deletion was determined from the structure of these clones. The site of the deletion places it well within the coding region of the V-*abl* region (Figs. 2 and 4; ref. 9). The size also correlates well with the difference in size between the P92*td* protein and its parent P120 protein. Thus, it is likely that the deletion does not alter the translational reading frame of the gene but allows read-through to the normal termination used by the P120 genome. Finally, the genome encoding the P160 protein was found to be larger than those encoding P120, P100, and P90 by approximately 800 bp (6,9). The position of the extra DNA in this genome was mapped (Figs. 2 and 4; S. Latt, J. Wang, and S. Goff, *unpublished observations*). Analysis both by heteroduplex formation between these clones and the P90 clones and by restriction enzyme mapping placed the difference near the center of V-*abl*, toward the 3' side of the deletion in the P92td strain. This DNA is also within the coding portion of V-*abl* and also roughly correlates with the larger size of the P160 protein. Thus, it is likely that in the P160 genome this

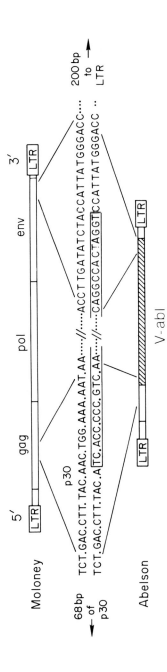

FIG. 3. Sequences at the junctions between M-MuLV and V-*abl*. The A-MuLV sequences were derived in this laboratory by R. Lee and G. Brown. The M-MuLV sequences are from the literature.

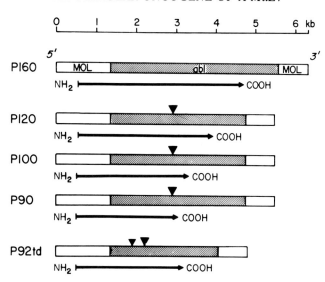

FIG. 4. The structure of variant A-MuLV genomes. The *larger arrowhead* shows the site of the deletion that produced A-MuLV(P120); the *smaller arrowhead* shows the site of the deletion that produces A-MuLV(P92*td*).

extra DNA is also translated in phase and that termination still occurs at the same site as in the P120 genome.

The isolation of these spontaneous variants points out both the remarkable genetic instability of retroviruses and the surprising plasticity of this particular gene product. Many of these variants arose during passage of the virus from cell to cell by infection. In these cases the mutations were very likely to have been introduced at one of the error prone events of the retrovirus life cycle noted previously (25): reverse transcription to synthesize viral DNA or forward transcription to synthesize viral RNA. In other cases, however, (the P90 and P100 strains) the mutations arose during the passage of cell lines, at a time when the viral DNA is merely replicated by the high fidelity cellular DNA polymerases. Thus the ease of isolating the variants makes it seem likely that some selection favors cells carrying these genomes. Indeed, the presence of the P120 genome does cause significant changes in the growth rate of fibroblast cells (G. Otto, *unpublished observations*).

It is curious that so much of the genome can be altered without serious effects on the virus. If we assume that the P160 strain was the original A-MuLV isolate, then 40,000 daltons of protein near the middle of P160 can be deleted with at most a slight change in biological activity because the resulting P120 strain is about equally as potent in transforming activity as the P160 strain. As much as 30,000 daltons at the C-terminus can be removed to yield the P90 strain without loss of transforming function in fibroblasts. There is, however, a strong reduction in biological activity in lymphoid cells and in the ability of A-MuLV(P90) to induce tumors *in vivo* from the loss of the C-terminus (18). Thus, although it is not absolutely required for transforming activity, loss of the C-terminal portion of P120 has important effects on transformation efficiency. [Recently, viruses highly trans-forming for lymphoid cells have been isolated that have proteins even smaller than P90, suggesting that the relationship between transformation and genetic structure is very complicated (N. Rosenberg, *unpublished observations*).] So much of the protein is dispensible (of the 130,000 daltons encoded by the V-*abl* region in P160 strains, only 60,000 daltons are retained in P90 strains) that it seems possible that the original protein may have several functions and that only one is required for transforming activity. Evidence to be described below suggests that the important activity of these proteins is a tyrosine-specific protein kinase activity, retained partially in the P90 molecule. The introduction of the second deletion in the P92t*d* strain, however, absolutely abolishes both transforming activity in all cell types and protein kinase activity. This result strongly points to a central role of the protein kinase activity of the P120 molecule in morphological transformation by A-MuLV.

The Normal Cell Gene Homologous to V-*abl*

The same probe used above for the analysis of proviral DNA in infected cells could also be used to search for DNA in uninfected cells homologous to the V-*abl* oncogene (6,7). Hybridization to total mouse DNA cleaved with a variety of re-striction enzymes showed a complex pattern. A single large (28 kb) Eco RI fragment was found to hybridize with the pAB3Sub3 probe; the intensity of hybridization suggested that the gene was probably unique, present once per haploid genome. Yet many fragments homologous to the probe were produced by cleavage with Bam I, Hind III, and Xba I. The sum of the size of these fragments was roughly 20 kb. Moreover, subsets of these fragments were labeled by probes specific for the 3' or 5' half of the V-*abl* region. Thus, the homology was apparently split up and spread over about 20 kb of DNA.

These results have recently been confirmed by the molecular cloning of this DNA region, termed C-*abl* (S. Goff and J. Wang, *unpublished observations*). Two over-lapping clones spanning about 30 kb were isolated; heteroduplex analysis and hybridization to electrophoretically separated DNA fragments have suggested that the homology to V-*abl* is divided into at least six blocks spread out over more than 25 kb and separated by many intervening segments (Fig. 5). C-*abl* thus seems related to V-*abl* in much the same way that a large mammalian gene is related to its mRNA: V-*abl* is probably a copy of the mRNA sequences (the exons) normally synthesized by the C-*abl* gene (containing both exons and introns). Furthermore, some of the 3' exons of C-*abl* are not present in V-*abl* (J. Wang, *unpublished observations*).

The relationship of C-*abl* to V-*abl* has implications for the mechanism by which transforming viruses are formed. It is now clear that these viruses need not always contain new DNA which was simply lifted out of the cell's genome intact. Two models for the origin of these viruses seem plausible. In one model, the recom-bination between viral and cell sequences occurs at the RNA level. Perhaps a cellular mRNA was incorporated into a virion along with the viral genome and template

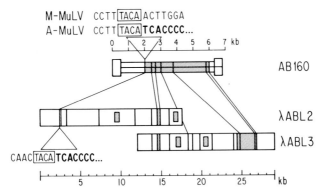

FIG. 5. The A-MuLV(P160) genome compared to clones from mouse cellular DNA. The line marked "AB160" is the viral genome and the lines marked λABL2 and λABL3 are clones from cellular DNA. Note that they are represented on different scales. The sequences at strategic places in both genomes are shown and compared to the parental Moloney MuLV. A four-base sequence *(boxed)* occurs in both the cell gene and M-MuLV at the site where V-*abl* was inserted to form A-MuLV.

switching during reverse transcription generated the recombinant. Thus, only the exons of the cellular gene (those sequences included in the mRNA) would have been incorporated into the recombinant virus. An alternative model proposes that recombination occurred at the DNA level, perhaps by integration of all or a fragment of the parental leukemia virus genome near or next to the oncogene. Then a hybrid RNA was transcribed; splicing of this RNA would remove the introns and create the new viral genome. One cycle of infection would create a DNA provirus of the new transforming virus lacking the introns of the cellular oncogene.

Recent sequencing data on V-*abl* and C-*abl* (R. Lee and J. Wang, *unpublished observations*) have shown that the 5' recombination event that generated the A-MuLV genome involved the type of 4-base homology that often occurs at sites of deletion in DNA (Fig. 5); we therefore suggest that the MuLV integrated upstream of C-*abl* and that it was joined to C-*abl* by a deletion from *gag* to a 5' exon of C-*abl*. The 3'-end of the A-MuLV genome would then have arisen by the recombinational process that rescues 5' fragments of transforming viruses (8,10).

The C-*abl* gene seems to be a unique gene in the mouse cell, present at only one copy per haploid genome. Hybridization analysis to cellular DNA, however, has often shown faint homology to restriction fragments not contained in the clones of the major C-*abl* gene. Thus, there may be one other gene with at least weak homology to the V-*abl*.

The C-*abl* gene is apparently extremely well conserved over long evolutionary times. Homology to V-*abl* is readily found in the DNA of rat, hamster, and rabbit; weaker homology can be detected in the DNA of man and chicken (6,9). Recently, using less stringent hybridization conditions, homology has even been detected in *Drosophila* DNA (26). These results suggest that C-*abl* does not encode a protein needed only in a highly specialized vertebrate tissue.

The chromosomal location of C-*abl* in the mouse genome has been determined using mouse-Chinese hamster hybrid cells; it is on chromosome 2 (S. Goff, P. D'Eustachio, F. Ruddle, and D. Baltimore, *in preparation*).

Gene Products Encoded by C-*abl*

Both the mRNA and the protein putatively encoded by the C-*abl* gene have been detected in normal cells. Total and poly(A)-containing RNA from a variety of tissues has been tested by electrophoretic separation and subsequent hybridization with the V-*abl* probe (J. Wang, *unpublished observations*). Two very large RNAs, approximately 5.3 and 6.5 kb in length, were detected in thymus and a variety of lymphoid tumors. Cell lines of the T-cell lineage, pre-B cells, and myelomas have RNAs of identical size. The RNAs are variably abundant; the intensity of hybridization suggests that there is roughly $\frac{1}{10}$ to $\frac{1}{50}$ as much RNA in these cells as there is A-MuLV RNA in an infected cell. The relationship of these two mRNAs to each other is not yet known.

Many tissues and cell lines have also been examined for the presence of protein related to the P120 protein. Labeled proteins were immunoprecipitated with the same α-AbT sera described above, sera which were specific to the V-*abl*-encoded portion of the P120 molecule (31). These sera bound to a protein of 150,000 daltons termed NCP150 found only in the thymus and spleen of normal animals (32). The protein was present at a very low level even in these tissues. In addition the protein was detected in a variety of T-cell tumor lines grown in culture. It is likely that the NCP150 protein (which was identified only by its cross-reactivity with the P120) is translated from one of the two mRNAs found in these cells.

One anomaly is that the C-*abl* mRNAs are at relatively high concentration in fibroblastic cells but NCP150 has not been detected in such cells. Whether this represents a technical problem or indicates some profound difference between the C-*abl* products in different cell types is under investigation (J. Wang and O. N. Witte, *unpublished observations*).

Antisera prepared in BALB/c mice bearing A-MuLV-induced tumors often precipitate a protein of about 50,000 molecular weight from A-MuLV-transformed cells (21). This protein is identical to the P53 protein first shown to be increased in SV40-transformed cells and now known to be increased in many tumor cells (20; see Crawford, *this volume*). It is therefore not encoded by the A-MuLV genome but its high concentration, especially in A-MuLV-transformed lymphoid cells, suggests that it may play a role in the transformation process.

Enzymatic Activities of the A-MuLV Gene Products

A complete understanding of the mechanism by which A-MuLV induces the malignant growth of pre-B-cells will ultimately require an understanding of the enzymatic activities of the P120 molecule. It has been shown that immunoprecipitated P120, even when bound to the antibody, will catalyze the transfer of phosphate from the gamma position of ATP to many tyrosine moieties on the P120 molecule itself to form a tyrosine-phosphate (29,30). We know that the A-MuLV protein itself catalyzes the reaction because even when it is expressed in *E. coli* using an expression plasmid it catalyzes its own phosphorylation on tyrosine (C. Queen and J. Wang, *unpublished observations*). Tyrosine phosphorylation reactions are carried out by the transforming gene products of other retroviruses (see other chapters). The conditions for the P120 autokinase reaction are nonphysiological; thus *in vivo* the P120 may normally kinase some other substrate and not itself. Such a hypothetical substrate has not been directly identified. Moreover, we do not know whether NCP150 is also a protein kinase.

FUTURE

Understanding A-MuLV transformation poses many intriguing, unanswered questions. The most obvious and most significant is what interactions with cellular proteins allow the transforming protein to produce its dramatic effect. It is also important to know if the transforming effect on lymphoid cells and fibroblasts is caused by the same set of events. To study these and other questions, our laboratory has tried over many years, and by many routes, to isolate temperature-sensitive mutants of A-MuLV, but without success. Why the virus has not yielded such mutants is not known, but possibly using the molecular clones of the A-MuLV genome they will prove obtainable.

Another vexing question is why the A-MuLV should have such an apparently strict target specificity. This seems not a consequence of its virion glycoprotein because that protein is supplied by the helper virus and can be varied. Under some conditions the virus does transform other blood elements (12) and has a proliferative effect on fetal erythroid cells (28), so it seems to have more potentialities than are usually realized during infection of animals or of bone marrow cells.

The target specificity in bone marrow cells, ability to transform 3T3 cells, ability to immortalize B-lymphoid cells at an immature stage of their development and tyrosine-specific protein kinase activity are all consequences of the portion of C-*abl* picked up by the A-MuLV genome. How these effects are produced and how they relate to still unknown functions of the C-*abl* product are questions for the future.

REFERENCES

1. Abelson, H. T., and Rabstein, L. S. (1970): Influence of prednisolone on Moloney leukemogenic virus in BALB/c mice. *Cancer Res.*, 30:2208–2212.
2. Abelson, H. T., and Rabstein, L. S. (1970): Lymphosarcoma: Virus-induced thymic-independent disease in mice. *Cancer Res.*, 30:2213–2222.
3. Alt, F., Rosenberg, N., Lewis, S., Thomas, E., and Baltimore, D. (1981): Organization and reorganization of immunoglobulin genes in Abelson murine leukemia virus-transformed cells: Rearrangement of heavy but not light chain genes. *Cell*, 27:391–400.
4. Baltimore, D., Rosenberg, N., and Witte, O. N. (1979): Transformation of immature lymphoid cells by Abelson murine leukemia virus. *Immunol. Rev.*, 48:3–22.
5. Baltimore, D., Shields, A., Otto, G., Goff, S., Besmer, P., Witte, O., and Rosenberg, N. (1979): Structure and expression of the Abelson murine leukemia virus genome and its relation to a normal cell gene. *Cold Spring Harbor Symp. Quant. Biol.*, 44:849–854.

6. Dale, B., and Ozanne, B. (1981): Characterization of mouse cellular deoxyribonucleic acid homologous to Abelson murine leukemia virus-specific sequences. *Mol. Cell. Biol.*, 1:731–742.

7. Goff, S. P., Gilboa, E., Witte, O. N., and Baltimore, D. (1980): Structure of the Abelson murine leukemia virus genome and the homologous cellular gene: Studies with cloned viral DNA. *Cell*, 22:777–785.

8. Goff, S. P., Tabin, C. J., Wang, J. Y-J., Weinberg, R., and Baltimore, D. (1982): Transfection of fibroblasts by cloned Abelson murine leukemia virus DNA and recovery of transmissible virus by recombination with helper virus. *J. Virol.*, 41:271–285.

9. Goff, S. P., Witte, O. N., Gilboa, E., Rosenberg, N., and Baltimore, D. (1981): Genome structure of Abelson murine leukemia virus variants: proviruses in fibroblasts and lymphoid cells. *J. Virol.*, 38:460–468.

10. Goldfarb, M., and Weinberg, R. A. (1981): Generation of novel, biologically active Harvey sarcoma viruses via apparent illegitimate recombination. *J. Virol.*, 38:136–150.

11. Pratt, D. M., Strominger, J., Parkman, R., Kaplan, D., Schwaber, J., Rosenberg, N., and Scher, C. D. (1977): Abelson virus-transformed lymphocytes: Null cells that modulate H-2. *Cell*, 12:683–690.

12. Raschke, W. C., Baird, S., Ralph, R., and Nakoinz, I. (1978): Functional macrophage cell lines transformed by Abelson leukemia virus. *Cell*, 15:261–267.

13. Reynolds, F. H., Sacks, T. L., Deobagkar, D. H., and Stephenson, J. R. (1978): Cells nonproductively transformed by Abelson murine leukemia virus express a high molecular weight polyprotein containing structural and nonstructural components. *Proc. Natl. Acad. Sci. USA*, 75:3974–3978.

14. Reynolds, R. K., van de Ven, W. J. M., and Stephenson, J. R. (1978): Translation of type C viral RNAs in *Xenopus laevis* oocytes: Evidence that the 120,000 molecular weight polyprotein expressed in Abelson leukemia virus-transformed cells is virus coded. *J. Virol.*, 28:665–670.

15. Rosenberg, N., and Baltimore, D. (1978): The effect of helper virus on Abelson virus-induced transformation of lymphoid cells. *J. Exp. Med.*, 147:1126–1141.

16. Rosenberg, N., and Baltimore, D. (1980): Abelson Virus. In: *Viral Oncology*, edited by G. Klein, pp. 187–203. Raven Press, New York.

17. Rosenberg, N., Baltimore, D., and Scher, C. D. (1975): *In vitro* transformation of lymphoid cells by Abelson murine leukemia virus. *Proc. Natl. Acad. Sci. USA*, 72:1932–1936.

18. Rosenberg, N. E., Clark, D. R., and Witte, O. N. (1980): Abelson murine leukemia virus mutants deficient in kinase activity and lymphoid cell transformation. *J. Virol.*, 36:766–774.

19. Rosenberg, N., and Witte, O. N. (1980): Abelson murine leukemia virus mutants with alterations in the virus-specific P120 molecule. *J. Virol.*, 33:340–348.

20. Rotter, V., Boss, M. A., and Baltimore, D. (1981): Increased concentration of an apparently identical cellular protein in cells transformed by either Abelson murine leukemia virus or other transforming agents. *J. Virol.*, 38:336–346.

21. Rotter, V., Witte, O. N., Coffman, R., and Baltimore, D. (1980): Abelson murine leukemia virus-induced tumors elicit antibodies against a host cell protein, P50. *J. Virol.*, 36:547–555.

22. Scher, C. D., and Siegler, R. (1975): Direct transformation of 3T3 cells by Abelson murine leukemia virus. *Nature*, 253:729–731.

23. Shank, P. R., Hughes, S. H., Kung, H-J., Majors, J. E., Quintrell, N., Guntaka, R. V., Bishop, J. M., and Varmus, H. E. (1978): Mapping unintegrated avian sarcoma virus DNA: Termini of linear DNA bear 300 nucleotides present once or twice in two species of circular DNA. *Cell*, 15:1383–1396.

24. Shields, A., Goff, S., Paskind, M., Otto, G., and Baltimore, D. (1979): Structure of the Abelson murine leukemia virus genome. *Cell*, 18:955–962.

25. Shields, A., Witte, O. N., Rothenberg, E., and Baltimore, D. (1978): High frequency of aberrant expression of Moloney murine leukemia virus in clonal infections. *Cell*, 14:601–609.

26. Shilo, B. Z., and Weinberg, R. A. (1981): DNA sequences homologous to vertebrate oncogenes are conserved in *Drosophila melanogaster*. *Proc. Natl. Acad. Sci. USA*, 78:6789–6792.

27. Siden, E. J., Baltimore, D., Clark, D., and Rosenberg, N. (1979): Immunoglobulin synthesis by lymphoid cells transformed *in vitro* by Abelson murine leukemia virus. *Cell*, 16:389–396.

28. Waneck, G. L., and Rosenberg, N. (1981): Abelson leukemia virus induces lymphoid and erythroid colonies in infected fetal cell cultures. *Cell*, 26:79–90.

29. Witte, O. N., Dasgupta, A., and Baltimore, D. (1980): The Abelson murine leukemia virus protein is phosphorylated *in vitro* to form phosphotyrosine. *Nature*, 283:826–831.

30. Witte, O. N., Ponticelli, A., Gifford, A., Baltimore, D., Rosenberg, N., and Elder, J. (1981): Phosphorylation of the Abelson murine leukemia virus transforming protein. *J. Virol.*, 39:870–878.
31. Witte, O. N., Rosenberg, N., and Baltimore, D. (1979): Preparation of syngeneic tumor regressor serum reactive with the unique determinants of the Abelson MuLV encoded P120 protein at the cell surface. *J. Virol.*, 31:776–784.
32. Witte, O. N., Rosenberg, N., and Baltimore, D. (1979): Identification of a normal cellular protein cross-reactive to the major Abelson murine leukemia virus gene product. *Nature*, 281:396–398.
33. Witte, O. N., Rosenberg, N., Paskind, M., Shields, A., and Baltimore, D. (1978): Identification of an Abelson murine leukemia virus-encoded protein present in transformed fibroblasts and lymphoid cells. *Proc. Natl. Acad. Sci. USA*, 75:2488–2492.
34. Yoshimura, F., and Weinberg, R. A. (1979): Restriction endonuclease cleavage of linear and closed circular murine leukemia viral DNAs: Discovery of a smaller circular form. *Cell*, 16:323–332.

Advances in Viral Oncology, Volume 1,
edited by George Klein. Raven Press,
New York © 1982.

The Putative *Mam* Gene of the Murine Mammary Tumor Virus

Peter Bentvelzen

Radiobiological Institute TNO, Lange Kleiweg 151, 2280 HV Rijswijk, The Netherlands

Breeding females of several mouse strains having genetically different backgrounds spontaneously develop mammary tumors at the age of 3 to 12 months (Fig. 1). This is at a young age as compared to the average life-span of two years for the majority of inbred mouse strains (29). In all strains with early mammary carcinoma, a retrovirus, the murine mammary tumor virus (MuMTV), is etiologically involved in combination with the pituitary hormone prolactin and the ovarian hormone progesterone (13,53). In most carcinogenesis studies using mice, a latency period of less than one year would be regarded as relatively short. However, in tumor virology MuMTV is regarded as a slow-acting oncogenic virus when compared with various sarcoma viruses and acute leukemia viruses, which induce fatal disease within a few weeks. Since also no *in vitro* transformation system is yet available for MuMTV, this virus is generally regarded as a somewhat poorer cousin of the retrovirus family.

The acute oncogenic viruses contain cell-derived sequences that code for a protein that causes the neoplastic transformation of the cell (11,65). Slowly acting RNA tumor viruses would lack such specific *onc* genes. In the case of avian leukosis viruses, promotor sequences in the long terminal repeat at the $3'$-end of the integrated provirus would initiate transcription of adjacent cellular sequences that are homologous to a retroviral *onc* gene (34).

Viral leukemogenesis in mice is thought to be due to the expression on the thymocyte surface of products of the leukemia virus gene, which codes for the envelope proteins. These changes in the cell surface could evoke disturbances in growth control and differentiation, eventually resulting in neoplastic transformation (40). Some viruses that are not proximate leukemogens might induce leukemia by recombining with cellular sequences resulting in an altered *env* gene product. In the same vein, Schochetman et al. (60) assumed that the products of the MuMTV gene *env*, which codes for the envelope glycoproteins gp52 and gp36, act as mitogens to mammary cells.

We have proposed that, in addition to the genes *gag*, which produces the viral core proteins, *pol*, which produces the enzyme reverse transcriptase, and *env*, MuMTV contains a transforming gene called *mam*, which causes neoplastic conversion of mammary cells (9,35). The aim of this chapter is to discuss arguments for the *mam*-gene hypothesis. It is realized that the evidence in favor of this hypothesis is not very compelling. However, we still adhere to it.

EXOGENOUS VERSUS ENDOGENOUS MuMTV

In most mouse strains with "early" mammary tumors, MuMTV is transmitted from the mother to the offspring via the milk, as was first discovered by Bittner in the A mouse strain (12). The virus can occasionally be transmitted extrachromosomally by the male (for a review, see 35). Horizontal transmission of the virus seems to occur more often (51) than we suspected (9,35), but is in our experience not involved in the appearance of tumors before one year of age.

The GR (4,8,52) and the SHN (37) mouse strains transmit a virulent MuMTV variant as a genetic factor of the host. In some sublines of high-mammary cancer strains from which the exogenous milk-borne MuMTV has been removed, mammary tumors arise at a late stage. These tumors contain typical type B particles (35). Definite proof for the oncogenic action of these virus particles has been found for the C3Hf (7,33,35,47) and the RIIIf (48) sublines. The latency period of tumors induced by these MuMTV variants on inoculation into various low-mammary tumor strains is considerably longer than of the standard milk-borne virus. These endogenous MuMTVs may be regarded as truly slow acting.

To our knowledge, every inbred strain of *Mus musculus* tested contains some proviral copies of MuMTV in its normal cellular DNA. Whether they code for virulent viruses, as we once postulated (9), remains a matter of doubt (51). The occasional detection of a virulent MuMTV in a low-mammary cancer mouse strain may be due to horizontal transmission.

In mouse strains that do not express their endogenous MuMTV spontaneously, extreme hormonal stimulation by pituitary isografts releasing prolactin induces the appearance of MuMTV RNA in mammary glands (45). These RNA molecules synthesize viral polypeptides (55). Since the viral RNA level is relatively low in the tumors induced by this endocrinological manipulation, it was assumed that virus expression was not etiologically involved in this mode of mammary carcinogenesis (45). Treatment of nonexpressor BALB/c mice with X-rays and urethane induces the production of large quantities of MuMTV RNA in mammary cells. In mammary cells of mice treated with either carcinogen alone, the MuMTV RNA quantities are low. The latency period and tumor incidences are not significantly different among the various experimental groups of mice. This would indicate that carcinogen-induced expression of endogenous MuMTV is not instrumental in the induction of mammary tumors by these agents (44).

In outbred populations derived from inbred mouse strains, several mammary tumors arose in mice that did not release virus in their milk at a young age (7); many of these tumors contained MuMTV (6). It is not clear whether this results from the switching on of endogenous MuMTV at a later age or from horizontal transmission within our colony (51). Even if the first possibility holds true, it is doubtful whether these late tumors are due to endogenous MuMTV.

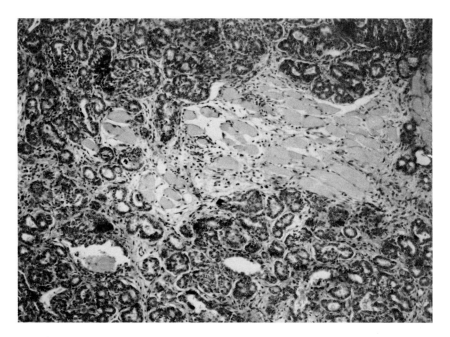

FIG. 1. Mammary adenocarcinoma type A, infiltrating in the muscle, found in a 3-month-old breeding female of the GR mouse strain.

A mammary tumor virus has been found in several colonies of wild mice (30,31, 57,58). Type-B retrovirus particles, antigenically related to MuMTV although quite distinct, have been found in the milk of several Asian species of the genus *Mus* (59,63). This suggests that the virus has been present in this genus for several million years. Proviral copies of MuMTV have been found not only in the DNA of wild *Mus musculus* (16,26,50,59) but also in that of other murine species (26,50,59), suggesting that endogenous MuMTV sequences have also occurred for a considerable length of time in this genus. However, the heterogeneity of integration sites of endogenous MuMTV in wild mice (16) suggests that the presence of germinal proviruses is of no physiological significance. The finding of some provirus-free wild mice (16,28) supports this conclusion. The absence of a provirus in these mice also implies that the putative *mam* gene of MuMTV is not homologous to a cellular mouse gene. This would be in contrast to the *onc* genes of acute oncogenic retroviruses.

BIOLOGY OF EXOGENOUS MuMTV

In susceptible mouse strains, milk-borne MuMTV can be detected in several organs at a young age (5,38). Abundant virus production is found in the salivary gland and prostate. Although we have observed thousands of mice infected with MuMTV during their whole life-span, we have not found a tumor to occur in either organ. This indicates a specific interaction of MuMTV with mammary cells with regard to neoplastic transformation.

It has been claimed that infection with MuMTV would make mammary epithelial cells more sensitive to the growth-promoting and differentiation-inducing action of mammotropic hormones (2,3,54). This is questioned by Van Nie (64). Within a few months after infection followed by hormonal stimulation, nodules of hyperplastic alveolar cells appear in mammary glands (Fig. 2). These hyperplastic cells resemble normal alveolar cells in many respects, such as hormone-dependency of proliferation and growth control by local regulatory factors (for a review, see 41). Unlike mammary tumor cells, they cannot proliferate after subcutaneous transplantation. Like normal mammary cells, they must be grafted into cleared mammary fat pads for outgrowth. These outgrowths will not expand beyond the fat pad area but, unlike normal mammary cells, they can be serially transplanted indefinitely. These immortalized hyperplasias are regarded as an intermediate stage between normal alveolar cells and adenocarcinomas. They are at considerably higher risk for tumor development than normal cells (43).

DeOme et al. (19,20) observed that inoculation of monocellular suspensions of mammary cells from infected mice into the cleared fat pad of syngeneic uninfected mice led to the rapid development of hyperplastic nodules and tumors. The infected mammary cell population of young mice contains inapparent transformed cells that

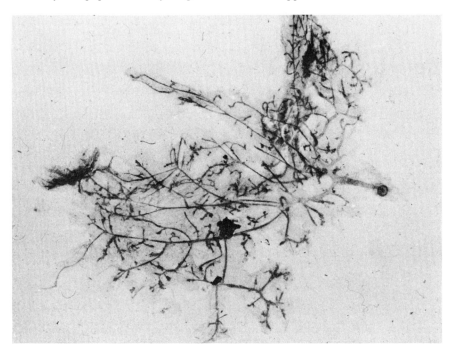

FIG. 2. Whole-mount preparation of the mammary gland from a 6-month-old virgin female of the GR mouse strain. The *black dot* is a hyperplastic alveolar nodule.

are subject to local regulatory signals but, after dissociation from normal cells, can give rise to preneoplastic and neoplastic lesions.

Hyperplastic nodules can be induced in uninfected mice by chemical carcinogens, irradiation, or strong hormonal stimulation. A nodular outgrowth line D1 of BALB/c mouse origin, showing no expression of MuMTV, produced some tumors when transplanted into BALB/c mice. When such transplantation was done in infected mice, many tumors appeared within a short time period. The virus seemed to be instrumental in the oncogenic transformation of the hyperplastic cells (42,43).

More recently, however, Ashley et al. (1) found the reverse for later passages of the D1 line. Transplantation into uninfected mice yielded a high incidence of tumors, whereas tumor incidence was considerably lower and the latency period longer in infected mice. The D1 cells proved to allow replication of MuMTV. Infection of these cells was not correlated with the appearance of tumors.

The picture emerges that viral mammary carcinogenesis is a multistep process (14) such as described for the murine sarcoma virus (49). The mammary tumor virus would induce a hyperplastic state beyond that of early passages of the D1 line but would not be necessary for the maintenance of the neoplastic state. If so, MuMTV must then be regarded as an initiating agent that causes a chain of reactions ultimately leading to the carcinomatous phenotype. The virus would not be involved in the final changes. Trisomy of chromosome 13 (24) is possibly responsible for neoplastic conversion and maintenance of the tumorous state. This would imply that to study the action of the putative *mam* gene of MuMTV, one would have to look primarily in preneoplastic mammary tissues. Furthermore, the expression of endogenous MuMTV induced by pituitary isografts in mice free of exogenous virus (45) might be instrumental in the hyperplasia induced by this endocrine manipulation (Fig. 3).

MOLECULAR BIOLOGY OF MuMTV

In mammary tumors of exogenously infected mice, new MuMTV proviral copies can be found in addition to the few endogenous proviruses. Considerable integration site heterogeneity is found among the various tumors (15,36). This suggests the clonal origin of these tumors. In tumors that developed under the influence of an endogenous MuMTV in the GR and C3Hf mouse strains, additional proviral copies are also found integrated into chromosomal DNA at varying sites (17,28). The repositioning of the germinal proviruses seems to be a prerequisite for carcinogenesis in these two strains. This is being questioned, however, by Michalides et al. (46). In the mouse strains that do not express an endogenous MuMTV spontaneously, provirus amplication is not necessary in tumors induced by nonviral agents (46). In the majority of avian lymphoid leukosis virus-induced B-cell lymphomas of chickens, long terminal repeats of the exogenous virus are inserted close to a cellular *onc*-gene (34). It must be investigated whether such a situation occurs in mammary carcinoma. The available blotting data suggest the contrary. This may be regarded as circumstantial evidence for the existence of an *onc*-gene within the MuMTV genome.

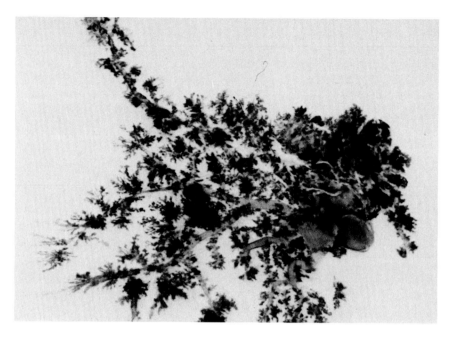

FIG. 3. Whole-mount preparation of the hyperplastic mammary gland from a 6-month-old female of the C3Hf mouse strain carrying a pituitary isograft under the kidney capsule.

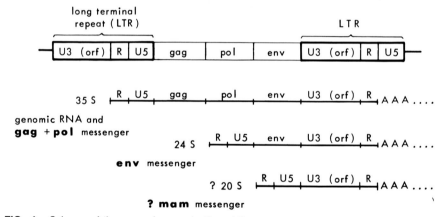

FIG. 4. Scheme of the genomic organization of the mammary tumor virus RNA, its derived provirus, and the virus-specific messenger RNAs.

If transformation of mammary cells by MuMTV was the consequence of downstream promotion of cellular genes adjacent to the acquired provirus, activation of many different cellular genes by a somatic provirus could result in oncogenic conversion, in view of the integration site heterogeneity.

MuMTV-specific messenger RNA molecules with sedimentation coefficients of 35 S and 24 S are consistently found in infected cells (27,32,56). By the use of cloned proviral DNA fragments, it could be excluded that a repeatedly reported smaller-sized viral messenger RNA (13 to 16 S) was present in addition to the 35 S and 24 S RNA molecules (27). This molecule, which has been regarded as a specific breakdown-product (32) and which we thought to be the messenger produced by the putative *mam* gene (9), is probably a cellular messenger RNA that is also present in the virions. Its presence may have physiological significance. The so-called representative cDNA probe of MuMTV-RNA would also include copies of this presumed cellular message (27) (Fig. 4).

After *in vitro* translation, the 35 S messenger yields the 73 Kd precursor polypeptide of the *gag* proteins (18,27,56,62) and occasionally readthrough products of the *gag* and *pol* genes. These products have molecular weights of 110 and 160 Kd, respectively. The 24 S messenger synthesizes *in vitro* the unglycosylated 68 Kd precursor of the envelope glycoproteins with molecular weights of 36 and 52 Kd (21,27,56,62). If this messenger contained a contiguous reading frame from its 5' toward its 3' terminus, it could have produced a polypeptide with a molecular weight higher than 100,000 daltons.

Sen et al. (61) translated *in vitro* various size classes of RNA isolated from MuMTV virions. The 35 S RNA produced, as expected, *gag*-related 75, 105, and 180 Kd polypeptides; the 24 S RNA produced nothing. The 14 S RNA yielded polypeptides of 36, 23, 21, and 20 Kd. Tryptic peptide mapping showed these four products to be related to each other but not the structural proteins of MuMTV.

Dickson and Peters (22) isolated the 35 S RNA from ^{3}H-uridine-labeled MuMTV virions and degraded this with Na_2CO_3 at 50° C. The polyadenylated fraction was fractionated on sucrose gradients. *In vitro* translation of fragments smaller than 18 S yielded polypeptides with molecular weights of 36, 24, 21, and 18 Kd, similar to the results obtained by Sen et al. (61). Peptide mapping showed these four polypeptides also to be closely related. No similarities were found between these translation products and any of the known viral structural proteins. However, their maps did not resemble those obtained by Sen et al. (61). Similarities can be noticed in the maps of the *gag*-related polyproteins as prepared by both groups. This suggests that differences in technology cannot be the principal cause of the great disparity in peptide maps of the products from the 35 S RNA-derived small fragments as compared to those from 14 S virion RNA.

Since the 14 S polyadenylated RNA molecule in the virion is probably a cellular message (27), it is not so surprising that it produces different polypeptides than the 3'- terminal fragment of the 35 S RNA as isolated by Dickson and Peters (22).

The long terminal repeat (LTR) of the MuMTV provirus is remarkably long when compared with that of other retroviruses: 1.3 to 1.4 kilobase pairs (25,39). The greatest part of this LTR (1,200 nucleotides) is constituted by sequences from the 3'- terminus of the viral genome (Fig. 3). Extensive nucleotide sequence analysis of a cloned LTR as performed by Donehower et al. (25) revealed a large open reading frame that could code for a protein of 198 amino acids.

Dickson et al. (23) have propagated the LTR cloned by Majors and Varmus (39) with the vector pAT353. The LTR was inserted at the Pst-1 cleavage site of the β-lactamase gene of this plasmid. Transcripts of that gene plus the MuMTV LTR were obtained by using *Escherichia coli* RNA polymerase and subsequently translated in the rabbit reticulocyte lysate system. The contiguous β-lactamase gene of the vector produces polypeptides, with molecular weights of 31 and 25 Kd, that can be precipitated with specific antisera. Upside down integration of the MuMTV LTR results in the synthesis of polypeptides, with molecular weights of 24 and 19 Kd, that can be precipitated with antisera to the plasmid gene product. Correct insertion of the LTR results not only in the production of 24 and 20 Kd polypeptides of plasmid origin but also in that of four unrelated ones with molecular weights of 36, 24, 21, and 18 Kd. Tryptic peptide mapping of these latter four polypeptides produced the same picture as with the four products of the 3′-terminus fragments of virion genomic RNA (22). This experiment proves convincingly that the U3 segment of the MuMTV genome contains an open reading frame, indicated as *orf*. The highest molecular weight of 36 Kd is too large for the calculated molecular weight on the basis of the reported nucleotide sequence (25). Presumably, *orf* is considerably longer than 600 nucleotides.

We have raised antisera in C3Hf mice against the mammary tumor cell line, C3HMT/cl 11, routinely used in our laboratory (66). The mice were inoculated with 10^7 lethally irradiated tumor cells at weekly intervals. All sera reacted with structural proteins of MuMTV. After repeated absorption with the virus, antibodies were retained which, at high dilutions, reacted specifically in the immunofluorescence test with mammary tumor cells. These absorbed sera no longer reacted with viral structural proteins. In immunoprecipitation tests on tumor cultures labeled for 6 hr with ^{14}C-amino acids, no known MuMTV precursor proteins were detected with the absorbed antisera. Instead, they precipitated polypeptides with molecular weights of 53, 44, 37, and 25 Kd (10). The 53 Kd protein is presumably the oncofetal antigen that is found in so many different transformed cell lines. The 44 Kd protein is assumed to be actin, which regularly contaminates immunoprecipitates. The 37 and 25 Kd proteins we thought to be the candidate *orf* products. These antisera also could precipitate the *in vitro* translation products of small-sized polyadenylated RNA fragments isolated from virion RNA. We still have to ascertain whether these precipitated polypeptides are really the products of the *orf* sequence (22,23) at the 3′ end of MuMTV RNA and not of the presumed cellular message in the virion (61).

CONCLUDING REMARKS

The existence of an open reading frame at the 3′ terminus of the MuMTV genome, which codes for nonstructural proteins, is well established. Its role in the life cycle of the virus or in the malignant or premalignant conversion of mammary alveolar cells remains unclear. It had been suggested that the products of *orf* play a role in the susceptibility of the MuMTV provirus to glucocorticoid with regard to enhanced transcription (25). The existence of a specific *onc* gene in the MuMTV genome was postulated because of the tissue specificity of MuMTV for oncogenicity but not replication. We favor the hypothesis that *orf* is synonomous to that specific *onc* gene, called *mam*.

Orf products might have been detected by us in some mammary tumor cell lines. To prove their role in oncogenesis would be a very difficult task. Comparison of the *orf* products of high-oncogenic virus strains with late-oncogenic ones present in the C3Hf or RIIIf strains might provide some clues. So far, there are no indications for enzymatic activity of the *orf* products.

Also the messenger RNA molecule producing the *orf* products must be found in infected cells. In view of a "hit and step aside" hypothesis on the multistep process of MuMTV-initiated mammary carcinogenesis, it might be worthwhile to look primarily in preneoplastic tissues for the *orf* messenger and its *in vivo* products.

If *orf* should represent the *mam* gene, we would have the unique situation that MuMTV has an *onc* gene that is not derived from cellular sequences of its natural host and that is present in the long terminal repeat of the provirus. It illustrates once more that the poorer cousin murine mammary tumor virus is nevertheless a highly interesting oncogenic retrovirus.

ACKNOWLEDGMENTS

I am grateful to many colleagues in my laboratory and the Netherlands Cancer Institute for heated discussions concerning the *mam*-gene concept. They have not yet convinced me that I was wrong. Dr. A. C. Ford is to be thanked for correcting the English text.

REFERENCES

1. Ashley, R. L., Cardiff, R. D., and Fanning, T. G. (1980): Reevaluation of the effect of mouse mammary tumor virus infection on the BALB/c mouse hyperplastic outgrowth. *J. Natl. Cancer Inst.*, 65:977–986.
2. Bardin, C., Wayne, A. G., and Liebelt, G. (1966): Mammary gland development after hypophyseal isografts in intact mice of high and low mammary cancer strains. *J. Natl. Cancer Inst.*, 36:259–275.
3. Ben-David, M., Heston, W. E., and Rodbard, D. (1969): Mammary tumor virus potentiation of endogenous prolactin effect on mammary gland differentiation. *J. Natl. Cancer Inst.*, 42:207–218.
4. Bentvelzen, P. (1968): *Genetical Control of the Vertical Transmission of the Mühlbock Mammary Tumour Virus in the GR Mouse Strain.* Hollandia, Amsterdam.
5. Bentvelzen, P., and Brinkhof, J. (1977): Organ distribution of exogenous murine mammary tumour virus as determined by bioassay. *Eur. J. Cancer*, 13:241–245.
6. Bentvelzen, P., and Brinkhof, J. (1980): Expression of mammary tumour virus in late-appearing mammary carcinomas in presumed virus-free mice. *Eur. J. Cancer*, 16:267–271.
7. Bentvelzen, P., Brinkhof, J., and Haaijman, J. J. (1978): Genetic control of murine mammary tumour viruses reinvestigated. *Eur. J. Cancer*, 14:1137–1147.
8. Bentvelzen, P., and Daams, J. H. (1969): Hereditary infections with mammary tumor viruses in mice. *J. Natl. Cancer Inst.*, 43:1025–1035.
9. Bentvelzen, P., and Hilgers, J. (1980): Murine mammary tumor virus. In: *Viral Oncology*, edited by G. Klein, pp. 311–355. Raven Press, New York.
10. Bentvelzen, P., Koornstra, W., and Dubbeld, M. A. (1982): Virus-associated tumor antigens in virally induced mouse mammary tumors which are not viral structural proteins. *(Submitted Eur. J. Cancer)*.
11. Bishop, J. M. (1981): Enemies within: The genesis of retrovirus oncogenes. *Cell*, 23:5–6.

12. Bittner, J. J. (1936): Some possible effects of nursing on the mammary tumor incidence in mice. *Science*, 84:162.

13. Boot, L. M., Kwa, H. G., and Röpcke, G. (1981): Hormonal induction of mouse mammary tumors. In: *Mammary Tumors in the Mouse*, edited by J. Hilgers and M. Sluyser, pp. 117–119. Elsevier/North-Holland, Amsterdam.

14. Cardiff, R. D., and Young, L. J. T. (1980): Mouse mammary tumor biology: A new synthesis. In: *Viruses in Naturally Occurring Cancers*, edited by M. Essex, G. Todaro, and H. zur Hausen, pp. 1105–1114. Cold Spring Harbor Laboratory, Cold Spring Harbor, New York.

15. Cohen, J. C., Shank, P. R., Morris, V. L., Cardiff, R., and Varmus, H. E. (1979): Integration of the DNA of mouse mammary tumor virus in virus-infected normal and neoplastic tissues of the mouse. *Cell*, 16:333–345.

16. Cohen, J. C., and Varmus, H. E. (1980): Endogenous mammary tumor virus varies among wild mice and segregates during inbreeding. *Nature*, 278:418–423.

17. Cohen, J. C., and Varmus, H. E. (1980): Proviruses of mouse mammary tumor virus in normal and neoplastic tissues from GR and C3Hf mouse strains. *J. Virol.*, 35:298–305.

18. Dahl, H. H. M., and Dickson, C. (1979): Cell-free synthesis of mouse mammary tumor virus pr77 from virion and intracellular mRNA. *J. Virol.*, 29:1131–1141.

19. DeOme, K. B., Miyamoto, M. J., Osborn, R. C., Guzman, R. C., and Lum, K. (1978): Detection of inapparent nodule-transformed cells in the mammary gland tissues of virgin female BALB/c fC3H mice. *Cancer Res.*, 38:2103–2111.

20. DeOme, K. B., Miyamoto, M. J., Osborn, R. C., Guzman, R. C., and Lum, K. (1978): Effect of parity on recovery of inapparent nodule-transformed mammary gland cells in vivo. *Cancer Res.*, 38:4050–4053.

21. Dickson, C., and Atterwill, M. (1980): Structure and processing of the mouse mammary tumor virus glycoprotein precursor Pr73 *Env*. *J. Virol.*, 35:349–368.

22. Dickson, C., and Peters, G. (1981): Protein-coding potential of mouse mammary tumor virus genome RNA as examined by in vitro translation. *J. Virol.*, 37:36–47.

23. Dickson, C., Smith, R., and Peters, G. (1981): *In vitro* synthesis of polypeptides encoded by the long terminal repeat region of mouse mammary tumour virus DNA. *Nature*, 291:511–513.

24. Dofuku, R., Utakoji, T., and Matsuzawa, A. (1979): Trisomy of chromosome 13 in spontaneous mammary tumors of GR, C3H and non-inbred Swiss mice. *J. Natl. Cancer Inst.*, 63:651–656.

25. Donehower, L. A., Huang, A. L., and Hager, G. L. (1981): Regulatory and coding potential of the mouse mammary tumor virus long terminal redundancy. *J. Virol.*, 37:226–238.

26. Drohan, W., and Schlom, J. (1979): Diversity of mammary tumor viral genes within the genus *Mus*, the species *Mus musculus*, and the strain C3H. *J. Virol.*, 31:53–62.

27. Dudley, J. P., and Varmus, H. E. (1981): Purification and translation of murine mammary tumor virus mRNA's. *J. Virol.*, 39:207–218.

28. Fanning, T. G., Puma, J. P., and Cardiff, R. D. (1980): Selective amplification of mouse mammary tumor virus in mammary tumors of GR mice. *J. Virol.*, 36:109–114.

29. Festings, M. F. W., and Blackmore, D. K. (1971): Life span of specified-pathogen-free (MRC category 4) mice and rats. *Lab. Anim.*, 5:179–192.

30. Fine, D. L., Arthur, L. O., and Gardner, M. B. (1978): Prevalence of murine mammary tumor virus antibody and antigens in normal and tumor-bearing fetal mice. *J. Natl. Cancer Inst.*, 61:485–491.

31. Gardner, M. B., Lund, J. K., and Cardiff, R. D. (1980): Prevalence and distribution of mammary tumor virus antigen detectable by immunocytochemistry in spontaneous breast tumors of wild mice. *J. Natl. Cancer Inst.*, 64:1251–1257.

32. Groner, B., Hynes, N. E., and Diggelman, H. (1979): Identification of mouse mammary tumor virus-specific mRNA. *J. Virol.*, 30:417–420.

33. Hageman, P., Calafat, J., and Daams, J. K. (1972): The mouse mammary tumor viruses. In: *RNA Viruses and Host Genome in Oncogenesis*, edited by P. Emmelot and P. Bentvelzen, pp. 283–300. North-Holland, Amsterdam.

34. Hayward, W. S., Neel, B. G., and Astrin, S. M. (1981): Activation of a cellular *onc* gene by promotor insertion in ALV-induced lymphoid leukosis. *Nature*, 290:475–480.

35. Hilgers, J., and Bentvelzen, P. (1978): Interaction between viral and genetic factors in murine mammary cancer. *Adv. Cancer Res.*, 26:143–195.

36. Hynes, N. E., Groner, B., Diggelman, H., Michalides, R., and Van Nie, R. (1980): Genomic location of mouse mammary tumor viral DNA in normal mouse tissue and in mammary tumors. *Cold Spring Harbor Symp. Quant. Biol.*, 44:1161–1168.

37. Imai, S., Morimoto, J., Tsubura, Y., and Hilgers, J. (1980): Mammary tumor virus antigen expression in inbred mouse strains of European origin established in Japan. *Gann.*, 71:419–424.
38. Kozma, S., Osterrieth, P. M., François, C., and Calberg-Bacq, C. B. (1980): Distribution of mouse mammary tumour virus antigens in RIII mice as detected by immunofluorescence on tissue sections and by immunoassays in sera and organ extracts. *J. Gen. Virol.*, 51:327–339.
39. Majors, J. E., and Varmus, H. E. (1981): Nucleotide sequence at host-proviral junctions for mouse mammary tumour virus. *Nature*, 289:253–258.
40. McGrath, M. S., and Weissman, I. L. (1979): AKR leukemogenesis: Identification and biological significance of thymic lymphoma receptors for AKR retroviruses. *Cell*, 17:65–75.
41. Medina, D. (1973): Preneoplastic lesions in mouse mammary tumorigenesis. *Methods Cancer Res.*, 7:3–53.
42. Medina, D., and DeOme, K. B. (1968): Influence of mammary tumor virus on the tumor-producing capabilities of nodule outgrowth free of mammary tumor virus. *J. Natl. Cancer Inst.*, 40:1303–1308.
43. Medina, D., and DeOme, K. B. (1969): Response of hyperplastic alveolar nodule outgrowth line D1 to mammary tumor virus, nodule-inducing virus, and prolonged hormonal stimulation acting simply and in combination. *J. Natl. Cancer Inst.*, 42:303–310.
44. Michalides, R., Van Deemter, L., Nusse, R., and Hageman, P. (1979): Induction of MTV-RNA in mammary tumors of BALB/c mice treated with urethane, X-irradiation and hormones. *J. Virol.*, 31:63–72.
45. Michalides, R., Van Deemter, L., Nusse, R., Röpcke, G., and Boot, L. (1978): Involvement of mouse mammary tumor virus in spontaneous and hormone-induced mammary tumors in low mammary-tumor mouse strains. *J. Virol.*, 27:351–559.
46. Michalides, R., Wagenaar, E., Groner, B., and Hynes, N. E. (1981): Mammary tumor virus proviral DNA in normal murine tissue and nonvirally induced mammary tumors. *J. Virol.*, 39:367–376.
47. Moore, D. H., Long, C. A., Vaidya, A. B., Sheffield, J. B., Dion, A. S., and Lasfargues, E. Y. (1979): Mammary tumor viruses. *Adv. Cancer Res.*, 29:347–418.
48. Moore, D. H., Merryman, C. F., Maurer, P. H., and Holben, J. A. (1978): Comparative susceptibility of hybrid mice to four mammary tumor viruses from two mouse strains. *Cancer Res.*, 38:3871–3878.
49. Morris, A. G. (1981): Neoplastic transformation of mouse fibroblasts by murine sarcoma virus: A multi-step process. *J. Gen. Virol.*, 53:39–45.
50. Morris, V. L., Medeiros, E., Ringold, G. M., Bishop, J. M., and Varmus, H. E. (1977): Comparison of mouse mammary tumor virus-specific DNA inbred, wild and Asian mice, and in tumors and normal organs from inbred mice. *J. Mol. Biol.*, 114:73–91.
51. Morris, V. L., Vlasschaert, J. E., Beard, C. L., Milazzo, M. F., and Bradburg, W. C. (1980): Mammary tumors from BALB/c mice with a reported high mammary tumor incidence have acquired new mammary tumor virus DNA sequences. *Virology*, 100:101–109.
52. Mühlbock, O., and Bentvelzen, P. (1968): The transmission of the mammary tumor viruses. *Perspect. Virol.*, 6:75–87.
53. Mühlbock, O., and Boot, L. M. (1967): The mode of action of ovarian hormones in the induction of mammary cancer in mice. *Biochem. Pharmacol.*, 16:627–630.
54. Nandi, S. (1966): Interaction among hormonal, viral and genetic factors in mouse mammary tumorigenesis. *Can. Cancer Conf.*, 6:69–81.
55. Nusse, R., Michalides, R., Röpcke, G., and Boot, L. M. (1980): Quantification of mouse mammary tumor virus structural proteins in hormone induced mammary tumors of low mammary tumor mouse strains. *Int. J. Cancer*, 25:377–383.
56. Robertson, D. L., and Varmus, H. E. (1979): Structural analysis of the intracellular RNA's of murine mammary tumor virus. *J. Virol.*, 30:576–589.
57. Rongy, R. W., Abtin, A. H., Estes, J. D., and Gardner, M. B. (1975): Mammary tumor virus particles in the submaxillary gland, seminal vesicle and nonmammary tumors of wild mice. *J. Natl. Cancer Inst.*, 54:1149–1156.
58. Rongy, R. W., Hlavackova, A., Lara, S., Estes, J., and Gardner, M. B. (1973): Type B and C RNA virus in breast tissue and milk of wild mice. *J. Natl. Cancer Inst.*, 50:1581–1589.
59. Schlom, J., Drohan, W., Teramoto, Y. A., Young, J. M., and Hand, P. H. (1980): Diversity of mammary tumor virus genes and viral gene products in rodent species. In: *Viruses in Naturally Occurring Cancers*, edited by M. Essex, G. Todaro, and H. zur Hausen, pp. 1115–1132. Cold Spring Harbor Laboratory, Cold Spring Harbor, New York.

60. Schochetman, G., Altrock, B., Lovinger, G., and Massey, R. (1980): Mouse mammary tumor virus: Role of class-specific antigenic determinants on the envelope glycoprotein in the development of autogenous immunity and binding of virus to cell receptors. In: *Viruses in Naturally Occurring Cancers*, edited by M. Essex, G. Todaro, and H. zur Hausen, pp. 1133–1148. Cold Spring Harbor Laboratory, Cold Spring Harbor, New York.

61. Sen, G. C., Racevskis, J., and Sarkar, N. H. (1981): Synthesis of murine mammary tumor viral proteins in vitro. *J. Virol.*, 37:963–975.

62. Sen, G. C., Smith, S. W., Marcus, S. L., and Sarkar, N. H. (1979): Identification of the messenger RNAs coding for the *gag* and *env* gene products of the murine mammary tumor virus. *Proc. Natl. Acad. Sci. USA*, 76:1736–1740.

63. Teramoto, Y. A., and Schlom, J. (1979): Radioimmunoassays for the 36,000 dalton glycoprotein of murine mammary tumor virus demonstrate type, group and interspecies determinants. *J. Virol.*, 31:334–340.

64. Van Nie, R. (1981): Mammary tumorigenesis in the GR mouse strain. In: *Mammary Tumors in the Mouse*, edited by J. Hilgers and M. Sluyser, pp. 201–266. Elsevier/North-Holland, Amsterdam.

65. Weinberg, R. A. (1980): Origins and roles of endogenous retroviruses. *Cell*, 22:643–644.

66. Westenbrink, F., Koornstra, W., Creemers, P., Brinkhof, J., and Bentvelzen, P. (1979): Localization of murine mammary tumor virus polypeptides on the surface of tumor cells. *Eur. J. Cancer*, 15.109–121.

Advances in Viral Oncology, Volume 1, edited by George Klein. Raven Press, New York © 1982.

The Transforming Genes of Primate and Other Retroviruses and Their Human Homologs

Flossie Wong-Staal and Robert C. Gallo

Laboratory of Tumor Cell Biology, National Cancer Institute, National Institutes of Health, Bethesda, Maryland 20205

Type-C retroviruses are associated with certain forms of naturally occurring leukemias and lymphomas of many species, including now recent evidence in humans. These viruses generally do not transform cells directly *in vitro* and apparently do not contain a specific transforming gene. In contrast, a more unusual class of retroviruses is the acutely transforming viruses (3,11). They cause diseases rapidly *in vivo*, have the capacity to transform appropriate target cells *in vitro*, and contain genomes that are usually defective for replication and include a specific transforming (v-*onc*) gene. Although there are many acutely transforming viruses isolated from avian, rodent, and feline species, the only member of this virus group isolated from primates is the woolly monkey (simian) sarcoma virus. Because of the low titer of the defective, transforming component (SSV) relative to its non-defective helper, simian sarcoma-associated virus (SSAV), the molecular biology of SSV was slow to develop. One purpose of this chapter is to follow recent developments in molecular cloning and characterization of SSV, in particular the identification of the transformation-specific gene (v-*sis*).

The *onc* genes of retroviruses, including v-*sis*, are derived from normal cellular genes of their host species of origin (3). Although the functions of these cellular gene products are not yet clearly defined, there is evidence that the viral and cellular counterparts are similar functionally, and that viral-induced transformation is sometimes correlated with enhanced level of expression of these genes. All the cellular progenitors of viral *onc* genes analyzed to date are conserved among vertebrates, suggesting an essential role of these genes in normal cellular processes. It is also reasonable to speculate that the *onc* genes may play a role in neoplasias regardless of whether viruses are involved etiologically. One of the main interests of our laboratory has been ·in the possible implication of these genes in normal and neo-plastic growth and differentiation, especially as this relates to human neoplasias. The second part of this chapter will focus on the very recent results from our laboratory on the identification, molecular cloning, and analyses of several human *onc* gene homologs, and the expression of these genes in normal and neoplastic human cells.

THE TRANSFORMING GENE OF SIMIAN SARCOMA VIRUS (V-*SIS*)

Cloning of SSV and Identification of a Transforming Gene

Two approaches have been successfully applied to cloning of the SSV genome. In one set of experiments, closed circular SSV and SSAV viral DNA intermediates were cleaved with a one-cut enzyme and ligated to phage vector arms to generate clones of complete, permuted SSV and SSAV genomes (19). Alternatively, DNA from SSV-transformed nonproducer cells was cleaved with a no-cut enzyme to yield the complete colinear SSV genome plus flanking cellular sequences. This was enriched by preparative gel electrophoresis and cloned (34). Paradoxically, the same enzyme, EcoRI, was used in both cases, suggesting that this site occurs in helper-derived sequences that are deleted in some SSV genomes without affecting their transforming capacity.

A direct comparison of the SSV and SSAV clones was made by restriction enzyme and heteroduplex mapping. The SSAV DNA genome is a 9.0 kb molecule with a long terminal repeat unit (LTR) at both ends. In the permuted SSAV genome, the two LTR units in the middle of the cloned DNA can be recognized by the tandem array of a constellation of restriction sites: Pst I, Sst I, and Kpn I (Fig. 1), and Sma I (not shown). The distance between two adjacent sites of the same enzyme (except for Sst I, which cuts twice in the LTR) is 550 bp, which marks the size of one LTR unit. Two SSV clones from viral DNA intermediates were extensively analyzed (18,19). When compared to SSAV, the two clones share three regions of

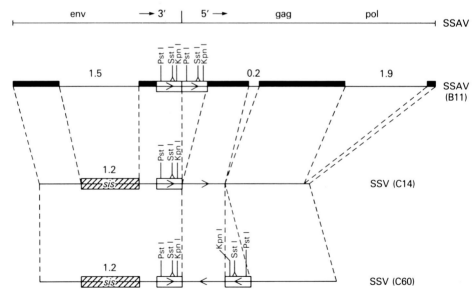

FIG. 1. Genetic structures of the SSAV and SSV clones derived from unintegrated viral DNA. *Dark bars* on the SSAV genome indicate regions conserved in SSV clones. *Dotted lines* connect corresponding regions of SSAV (BII) and the two SSV (C60 and C14) clones.

deletion and one substitution: a 0.2 kb deletion near the beginning of the *gag* gene, a 1.9 kb deletion probably comprising most of the *pol* gene, and a 1.5 kb deletion in the *env* gene where a substitution of 1.1 to 1.2 kb of SSV-specific (v-*sis*) sequences is found. In addition, one clone (C14) lacks one of the two LTRs and the other (C60) has an inversion of one LTR and 1.0 kb of adjacent sequences (Fig. 1). C14 transforms mouse fibroblasts *in vitro* (18). The SSV clone derived from the provirus of transformed rat nonproducer cells is also biologically active (34). Comparison of the restriction map of this clone with C14 and C60 revealed the same 0.2 kb *gag* and 1.5 kb *env* deletions and a slightly larger deletion of the *pol* gene, including an EcoRI site. The v-*sis* substitution of this clone has identical enzyme sites as that of C14 and C60. Labeled SSAV failed to hybridize to SSV DNA fragments within the v-*sis* substitution (18,34). This suggests that v-*sis* is SSV-specific and is the transforming gene of this virus.

Origin of v-*sis*: Recombination Between a Gibbon Ape Leukemia Virus and a Woolly Monkey Cellular Gene

The simian sarcoma virus complex (SSV/SSAV) was isolated once from the fibrosarcoma of a pet woolly monkey (41,42). The single isolate of the helper component (SSAV) is highly homologous to various Gibbon ape leukemia virus (GaLV) isolates as determined by analyses of their genomes or viral proteins such that all these viruses can be considered as one virus family (10,16). Of particular interest is the fact that the pet woolly monkey had cohabited with a gibbon ape in the same household before it developed sarcoma (43). Therefore, it is likely that SSAV was transmitted from the gibbon ape to the woolly monkey during that period. The availability of clones of the SSV genome makes it possible to determine the host species of origin of the transforming gene, v-*sis*. Using a single-stranded DNA probe derived from an M13 phage with an insert containing 250 bp of v-*sis* sequences and 900 bp of SSAV-derived sequences, Wong-Staal et al. (45) showed that under stringent liquid hybridization conditions, v-*sis* sequences are more homologous to primate DNA than to nonprimate DNA. Among the primates, the New World monkeys (woolly monkey, marmoset) contain more homologous DNA sequences to v-*sis* than the Old World apes (gibbon, humans), and near complete homology was obtained with woolly monkey DNA. These results are summarized in Table 1. In contrast, the SSAV genome has no detectable homology to primate DNA. SSAV and GaLV do have some distant homology to rodent DNA, but this can only be monitored by nonstringent hybridization conditions. We conclude that SSV arose from a recombination between a retrovirus transmitted from the gibbon to the woolly monkey and a cellular gene of the woolly monkey within the lifetime of that animal.

All Vertebrate Species Contain Genes Homologous to v-*sis*

All viral *onc* genes analyzed to date are homologous to subsets of host cellular DNA that are well conserved among vertebrates. The v-*sis* gene is no exception.

TABLE 1. *Homology between v-*sis *sequences and vertebrate DNA[a]*

	S_1 nuclease resistant (cpm)	% v-*sis* sequences hybridized
Woolly monkey	11,000	87
Marmoset	9,200	71
Gibbon	6,100	54
Human	5,500	42
Rat	1,000	8
Cat	800	6

[a]The M13 recombinant plasmid was constructed as described (45). The single-stranded phage DNA was purified, partially digested with DNase I, and labeled with [^{32}P] by polynucleotide kinase. The labeled DNA was purified by three cycles of ethanol precipitation in ammonium acetate buffer. About 400,000 cpm of the labeled probe ($\sim$12,000 cpm of v-*sis* sequence) was hybridized to 500 μg of cellular DNA to a Cot of $>10^4$. Hybridization was monitored by S_1 nuclease resistance.

When DNA from chimpanzee, humans, gibbon ape, woolly monkey, dog, and chicken were digested with Bam HI and blot hybridized to labeled pBR322-SSV plasmid, two fragments ($\sim$8.6 and 1.9 kb) were found in DNA from all four primates, one band of 4.3 kb was detected in chicken DNA and three bands of 7.3, 3.9, and 2.1 kb were detected in dog DNA (Fig. 2). These bands were obtained using moderately stringent conditions for hybrid formation (3XSSC, 50% formamide, 37° C) and detection (1XSSC, 0.5% SDS, 60° C) suggesting a strong conservation of the homologous sequences from chicken to humans (44). Therefore, although the genetic origin of v-*sis* can be traced to the woolly monkey whose tumor yielded SSV/SSAV, similar genes can be found in other vertebrate species including humans. Analysis of the human cellular *sis* (c-*sis*) gene will be presented later.

Homology of v-*sis* to Other Viral *onc* Genes

The number of acutely transforming viruses far exceed the number of cellular *onc* genes because the same cellular gene can be progenitor for different viral *onc* genes. For example, the same chicken *onc* gene (*myc*) was recovered in four independent recombination events to generate the leukemia viruses MC29, MH2, CMII, and OK10 (4). There is also one instance of a related cellular *onc* gene that has been recovered by retroviruses from different species, namely the avian sarcoma viruses (Fujinami, PRC, URI) from chickens, and feline sarcoma viruses (Snyder-Theilen and Gardner-Arnstein strains) from cats (37). Since v-*sis* is the only *onc* gene of primate origin, it would be important to define its relationship to other viral *onc* genes either to show it is a new distinct *onc* gene, or to illustrate another example of viruses of different species acquiring the same cellular gene.

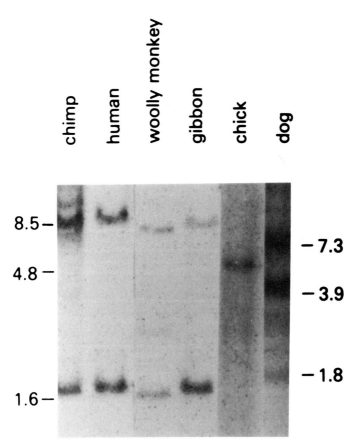

FIG. 2. Conservation of the c-*sis* gene among vertebrates. Total cellular DNA (20 μg) from chimpanzee, human, woolly monkey, gibbon, chick, and dog was digested with Bam HI, fractionated on agarose gels, transferred to nitrocellulose filters, and hybridized to [³²P]-labeled SSV DNA (43). Molecular weights are given in kilobases.

To test possible homology between v-*sis* and a number of other viral *onc* genes, we digested DNA from a recombinant phage clone of SSV with the restriction endonucleases Bgl II or a combination of Sal I and Pvu II to localize the v-*sis* sequences on a gel, and blot hybridized to ³²P-labeled plasmid clones containing *onc* sequences from different acutely transforming retroviruses (11). The filters were washed in 1XSSC, 0.5 % SDS at 60° C. As shown in the simplified map of SSV in Fig. 3, Bgl II or the combination of Sal I and Pvu II generate a 0.65 kb fragment in each case that is highly enriched in v-*sis* sequences. This fact is demonstrated by the poor detection of this fragment by the SSAV probe as compared to the homologous SSV probe (Figs. 3A and 3B). None of the other viral *onc* probes detects the 0.65 kb fragment. The HaMSV plasmid used contains the entire viral genome, and hybridization to the 2.8 kb Pvu II fragment or 3.3 kb Bgl II fragment of SSV (Fig. 3C) is most likely due to cross-reactivity of the LTR se-

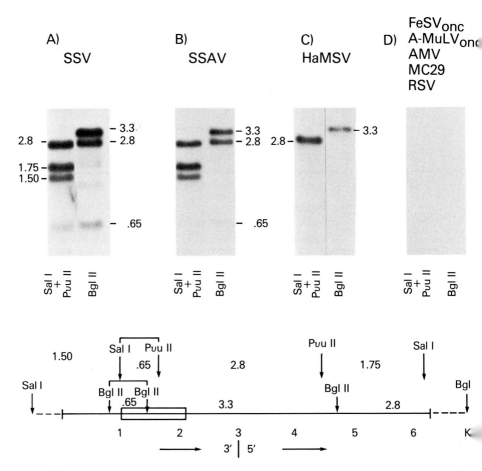

FIG. 3. Lack of homology of v-*sis* to other viral *onc* genes. DNA from a Charon 21A-SSV recombinant phage (19) was digested with Bgl II or a combination of Sal I and Pvu II. Multiple replicate filters were made and each hybridized to [³²P]-labeled cloned DNA containing *onc* sequences of a number of transforming retroviruses as indicated. The filters were washed in 1 × SSC at 60° C and autoradiography was carried out for 4 to 16 hr. A simplified map of the SSV recombinant phage with respect to the restriction sites for Bgl II, Sal I, and Pvu II is given at the bottom.

quences of the two viruses. Two other findings also suggest that v-*sis* and the *onc* gene of HaMSV (Ha-v-*ras*) are not closely related. First is the finding that v-*sis* and Ha-v-*ras* hybridized to distinct sets of sequences in human DNA (44). Second, a human gene containing all the coding sequences of v-*sis* has been cloned (9) and Ha-v-*ras* failed to hybridize to this gene using conditions of similar stringency (not shown). The other murine or feline probes do not contain helper sequences and do not hybridize detectably to any SSV DNA fragment (Fig. 3D). Although the avian viral probes do contain helper sequences, they do not show detectable homology with SSAV-derived sequences (Fig. 3D). The results of this experiment indicate that the v-*sis* gene is distinct from the *onc* genes of the transforming retroviruses tested.

HUMAN GENE HOMOLOG OF V-*SIS*

When SSV and SSAV DNA probes were blot hybridized to various human DNA samples digested with different enzymes, discrete DNA bands were detected with the SSV probe, but none with the SSAV probe. The most frequent patterns of the SSV-related fragments observed are shown in Fig. 4. Both EcoRI and Hind III gave a single high molecular weight band (>20 kbp), suggesting there is one or few copies of the v-*sis* gene in humans. Inside this region, cleavage sites for several other restriction enzymes (Bam HI, Xba I, Bgl II) are found. Survey of DNA from a large number of individuals revealed a rarer second genotype (F. Wong-Staal et al., *unpublished data*).

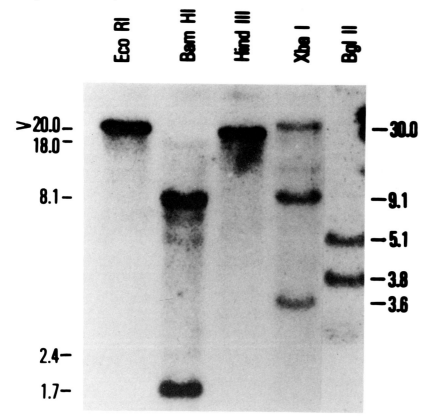

FIG. 4. Restriction enzyme digestion patterns of the human c-*sis* locus. DNA from the human cell line HL60 (7) was digested with the indicated enzymes and blot hybridized to the [32P]-labeled plasmid containing the SSV insert.

A clone of the human c-*sis* gene was isolated from a recombinant phage library (9). The DNA insert of this clone (L33) has no internal EcoRI site and contains all the coding sequences of v-*sis*. Two techniques were used to locate the regions of homology: restriction endonuclease mapping and heteroduplex formation between L33 and an SSV clone. Both analyses revealed that the 1.2 kb of v-*sis* homologous sequences in L33 span a region of 12 kb and are interrupted by four nonhomologous regions. The genetic structure of L33 and a representative heteroduplex molecule are shown in Figs. 5 and 6. The presence of intervening sequences has been shown in many eukaryotic cellular genes, and in all but one cellular *onc* gene analyzed so far (30). It is not clear whether the intervening sequences nonhomologous to v-*onc* are also noncoding for the cellular gene products. At least in the case of Rous sarcoma virus, the cellular and viral products are almost identical structurally and functionally (6), even though the cellular *src* gene has many introns (36). Therefore, it is likely that the nonhomologous sequences of c-*sis* will be processed in the corresponding mRNA, although this remains to be proven.

Another observation made with L33 was the presence in the introns of repeated sequences related to the Alu family (9). Although members of this family are abundant in the human genome (25), their presence has been found mostly at the 5' or 3' flanking regions or in the intergenic region of gene clusters, as in the case of the human β-globin gene family (12). The significance of finding these sequences in the c-*sis* introns is not known.

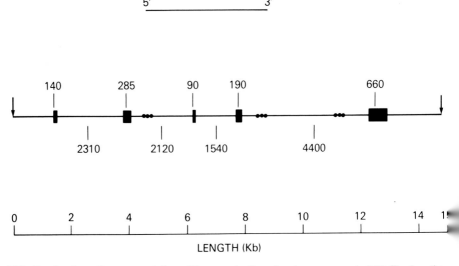

FIG. 5. A schematic representation of the organization of c-*sis* sequences in L33. The lengths of the v-*sis* homologous regions *(black boxes)* and intervening sequences *(solid lines)* are derived from both restriction enzyme mapping and heteroduplex measurements. Charon 4A DNA sequences are not shown. *Black dots* indicate the approximate position of repeated sequences of the human Alu family.

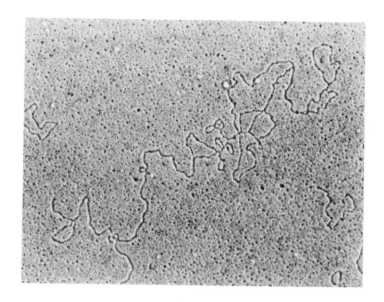

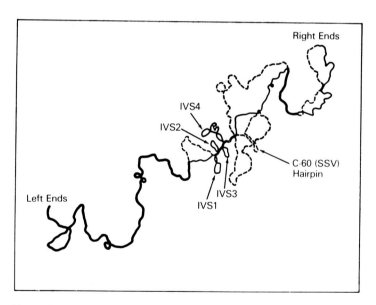

FIG. 6. Heteroduplex analysis of c-*sis* and v-*sis*. **Top:** Electron micrograph of heteroduplex structure formed by annealing λ-L33 DNA and λ C60 (SSV) DNA. **Bottom:** An interpretive drawing of the heteroduplex structure. *IV* = intervening sequences numbered in the 5′→3′ direction of c-*sis* and SSV DNA.

HUMAN GENE HOMOLOG OF THE TRANSFORMING GENE OF FELINE SARCOMA VIRUS (V-*FES*)

Feline sarcoma viruses (FeSV) were isolated from fibrosarcomas of domestic cats (17,26,38). They can induce fibrosarcomas *in vivo* and transform fibroblasts *in vitro*. Three isolates of FeSV have been characterized: the Snyder-Theilen (ST) strain, the Gardner-Arnstein (GA) strain, and the McDonough-Sarma (SM) strain. ST and GA FeSV have apparently acquired the same transforming gene (*fes*) from cats (15). Several strains of avian sarcoma virus (Fujinami, PRC II) had also acquired a homologous transforming gene from chickens (37). Restriction enzyme mapping of the cat cellular *fes* locus revealed good correspondence of restriction enzyme sites between v-*fes* and homologous sequences in c-*fes* (14). However, although v-*fes* is only 1.4 kb in size, c-*fes* spans about 4.5 kb and contains at least three intervening sequences (14).

By hybridization of recycled FeSV-specific cDNA to DNA of different species, it was previously shown that the FeSV *onc* sequences detected homologous sequences in diverse mammalian species (15). We used molecularly cloned ST-FeSV DNA as probe in Southern blot hybridization and detected a unique c-*fes* locus in DNA from chicken to humans (44). Human DNA digested with EcoRI yielded a single 14 kb band. To analyze the structure of the human c-*fes* gene further, a human DNA library was screened. Three positive clones were found to be over-lapping with each other (14a). Together they constitute >20 kb of DNA sequences inclusive of the entire 14 kb EcoRI fragment detected in total human DNA. The clones were further mapped and oriented with respect to v-*fes* using probes derived from the complete or specific regions of v-*fes*. Fig. 7 presents a map of the human c-*fes* locus. Like the cat c-*fes* locus, human c-*fes* is more complex than v-*fes* and contains three intervening sequences.

OTHER HUMAN *ONC* GENE HOMOLOGS

Accumulating evidence indicates that all viral *onc* genes are derived from phylogenetically conserved cellular genes and that human DNA is likely to contain counterparts of all the *onc* genes. In addition to SSV and FeSV, molecularly cloned genomes of Abelson-MuLV, Harvey-MSV, Balb MSV, MC29, and AMV have been reported to detect homologous genetic loci in humans (2,13,20,44). The identification of human *onc* gene homologs obviously raises the question whether they are functional genetic elements and whether they play a role in normal or neoplastic cell growth. Two major approaches are conceivable: (a) to study expression of the various *onc* genes in human normal and neoplastic cells and cells at different stages of differentiation, or (b) to study the biological effects of molecularly cloned human *onc* genes on appropriate target cells. Since molecular clones of human *onc* genes have been obtained only recently, results in the latter avenue of research are not yet available in the literature. A study on the mouse cellular gene homolog of the Moloney MSV *onc* gene demonstrated that this gene has the potential to transform mouse fibroblasts *in vitro* efficiently when ligated to viral promotor

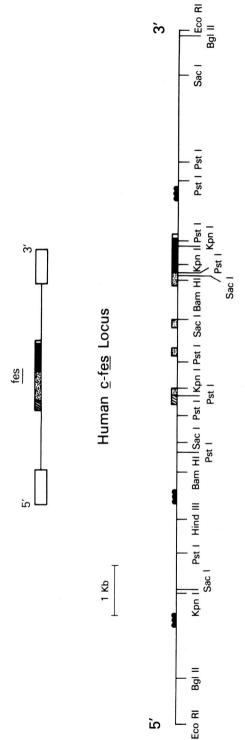

FIG. 7. Restriction enzyme map of the human c-*fes* locus. The map was derived from results analyzing three overlapping c-*fes* recombinant clones purified from a human DNA library. The *boxes* indicate the putative regions of homology to various regions of v-*fes* as designated. Placement of these regions is only approximate.

sequences (5). The next section will describe experiments carried out in our own laboratory and in collaboration with S. Aaronson and colleagues in the expression of *onc* gene homologs in human cells.

EXPRESSION OF HUMAN *ONC* GENE HOMOLOGS

Hematopoietic Cells

Considerable understanding of human hematopoietic cell differentiation has been derived from leukemic cells. Human leukemias are, in general, monoclonal diseases that have been viewed by many as specific blockages in normal hematopoiesis. Leukemic cells then are currently best viewed as equivalent to clones of normal cells "frozen" at various stages of hematopoiesis. During the past decade, a number of permanent human leukemia-lymphoma cell lines have been established and these display stable marker characteristics of the original neoplastic cells (28). Furthermore, a human promyelocytic cell line (HL60) can be induced to differentiate to granulocytes *in vitro* (7,8). The availability of these cell lines as well as fresh leukemic cells affords one with an ideal system to study gene regulation as a function of differentiation and perhaps to understand the mechanism of leukemogenesis better. We have utilized these cells or cell lines to study the expression of cellular *onc* gene homologs. The cellular genes examined correspond to the transforming genes of avian myeloblastosis virus (AMV), avian myelocytomatosis virus (MC29), Abelson murine leukemia virus (A-MuLV), Harvey murine sarcoma virus (HaMSV), and SSV. AMV causes myeloid leukemias in chickens and transforms cells of the myeloid lineage (21). MC29 induces myelocytomatosis and less frequently sarcomas and carcinomas *in vivo*, and transforms macrophage-like cells *in vitro* (21). A-MuLV causes lymphosarcomas in mice and transforms fibroblasts and cells of the B-lymphocyte series (1). HaMSV induces erythroleukemias as well as fibrosarcomas in mice (23). Finally, SSV induces sarcomas in newborn primates and seems, specifically, to transform fibroblasts (42). Genomes of these viruses have been molecularly cloned (20,22,27,39,40), and labeled probes of defined *onc*-containing segments have been shown to detect one or few genetic loci in human DNA (2,13,20,34,44). These same probes were hybridized to poly(A)-containing RNAs using RNA gel blotting techniques (41a,41b).

MC29 (myc)

The *myc* probe detected a single transcript of 2.7 kb in cells of the myeloid, lymphoid, and erythroid series at 2 to 20 copies per cell. One exception is the promyelocytic cell line HL-60 (7), which expresses >100 copies of *myc*-related sequences. Since HL60 has the unique capacity to differentiate into mature granulocytes after induction with agents such as DMSO (8) or retinoic acid, it was possible to measure modulation of *myc* expression as a function of differentiation. We found that expression of c-*myc* is drastically reduced in HL60 cells induced with either DMSO or retinoic acid. The level of reduction correlates with the fraction of cells that actually underwent differentiation. It is likely that c-*myc* is completely turned off in the terminally differentiated granulocytes.

AMV (amv)

The expression of c-*amv* is more restricted than that of c-*myc*. A single mRNA species of 4.5 kb was detected in all fresh human AML samples; lymphoid, myeloid, and erythroid precursor cells; myeloblast and promyelocyte cell lines; some pre-T-cell lines; and fresh T-cell acute lymphoblastic leukemias. However, there was little or no expression on pre-B and B cells, the more normal and leukemic mature T-cells, and, as in the case of c-*myc*, the differentiated HL60 cells.

A-MuLV (abl) and Ha-MSV (Ha-v-ras)

The human homologs of *abl* and Ha-v-*ras* are detectably expressed (1 to 5 copies per cell) in all hematopoietic cells examined, including differentiated HL60 cells. An additional contrast to c-*myc* and c-*amv* is that the *abl* and Ha-v-*ras* probes detected multiple-size species of mRNA. The positive findings in differentiated HL-60 cells with these probes also serve as a useful control for possible false negative results, e.g., with the c-*amv* probe, due to increased degradative enzymes in the more mature myeloid cells.

SSV (sis)

The *sis* gene is not detectably expressed in any hematopoietic cell with the exception of a human T-cell lymphoma cell line, HUT-102 (Clone B2, cloned by Dr. M. Maeda), which is a primary tumor cell line producing a unique human retrovirus, HTLV (31–33). HUT102 contains a 4.2 kb mRNA transcript of c-*sis*. A very closely analogous human leukemic T-cell line, but one which is virus negative, called HUT78 (31), is negative for detectable c-*sis* RNA. As will be discussed later, a 4.2 kb c-*sis* mRNA is also detected in some human solid tumors. It will be of interest to learn whether the unusual expressions of c-*sis* in HUT102 Clone B2 is a consequence of HTLV provirus integration.

In summary, the human cellular *onc* genes are functional genetic elements since they are found to be actively transcribed in human cells. Figure 8 illustrates our attempts at a preliminary correlation of *onc* gene expression and human hematopoietic cell differentiation. The *abl* and Ha-v-*ras* genes are transcribed into multiple transcripts present in all cells examined at relatively constant and low copy number. These genes probably code for proteins that have housekeeping functions for the cell. We have not come across a cell line or fresh cell sample that expresses extremely high levels of *abl* or Ha-v-*ras* genes.

The *myc* gene has been shown to be abundantly transcribed in B-cell lymphomas induced by the avian leukosis virus in a mechanism termed "downstream-promotion" (24,29). Our results showed that although this gene is expressed in human neoplastic B-cells, it is also expressed at similar levels in hematopoietic cells of other lineages.

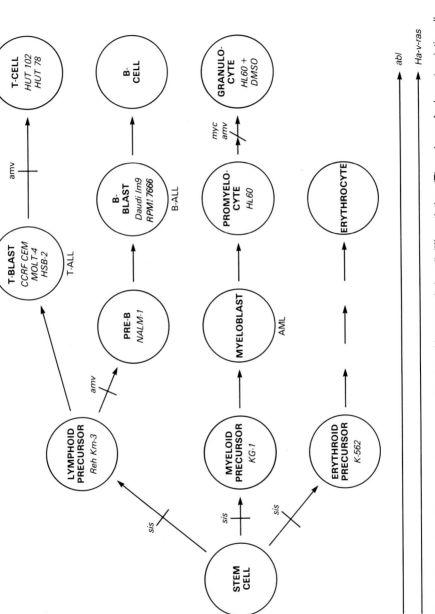

FIG. 8. Expression of human *onc* genes as a function of hematopoietic cell differentiation. (The scheme for hematopoietic cell differentiation and the assignment of cell lines in each category from Minowada et al., ref. 28.)

The highest concentration of c-*myc* transcript is found in a promyelocytic cell line (HL60). When HL60 was induced to differentiate into mature granulocytes, c-*myc* transcription is turned off.

At this point the *amv* gene appears to offer the most interest from a hemopoiesis point of view. It is expressed in the early lymphoid, myeloid, and erythroid precursor cells but there is little or no expression relatively early in B-lymphoid cells and late in T-cell or myeloid cell differentiation (see Fig. 8).

The *sis* gene is not usually transcribed in hematopoietic cell and may be a gene specifically involved in fibroblast differentiation.

Solid Tumors

A parallel study of human solid tumors and normal fibroblast cell lines was conducted by Eva et al. (13). The results are similar to those described for hematopoietic cells in that (a) the *abl* and Ha-v-*ras* genes are widely expressed (including normal fibroblast) as multiple mRNA species, and (b) the sizes of mRNA are different for different *onc* genes but are identical for a given *onc* gene among various cell types. Of interest was the finding that c-*sis* is expressed at variable levels in 5 out of 6 fibrosarcomas and 1 out of 2 glioblastomas, but not in any melanomas or carcinomas. Thus, expression of this gene shows the greatest correlation with certain specific types of neoplasias.

SUMMARY AND CONCLUSION

Acutely transforming retroviruses have been isolated from avian, rodent, feline, and primate species. The discovery that these viruses had acquired cellular sequences (c-*onc*) that conferred them their transformation potential provided a new perspective in understanding the transformation event. C-*onc* may be genes important to cell growth and the anomalous expression of these genes effected by retroviruses or even nonviral agents may lead to neoplasia. By studying these genes, basic aspects of cell growth and of leukemic transformation may be approached at the molecular level. An added boon to people interested in human leukemogenesis and hematopoietic cell differentiation is that the c-*onc* genes are phylogenetically conserved and human gene counterparts of all the viral *onc* genes irrespective of host species of origin can be detected, cloned, dissected, and studied with respect to their mode of expression in different cells and, ultimately, the nature of their gene products determined.

In this chapter, we first described the work leading to definition of the *onc* gene of the only primate-transforming virus, the simian sarcoma virus. This was accomplished by molecular cloning of the genome of the defective virus, which is usually overwhelmed in titer by the helper-associated virus. The SSV genome is approximately 5.6 kb with an *onc* gene (v-*sis*) of 1.2 kb situated near the 3' end. There are deletions in all three replicative genes (*gag*, *pol*, and *env*) derived from the helper SSAV. V-*sis* was shown to have originated from a woolly monkey that was infected by SSAV in its lifetime, almost certainly transmitted from an infected gibbon ape. Using SSV as a probe, homologous genetic loci (c-*sis*) can be detected in DNA of diverse vertebrate species including humans. A human DNA fragment comprising the entire v-*sis* homologous region was subsequently cloned. The sequences homologous to v-*sis* are found to be dispersed over a stretch of 12 kb with at least four intervening sequences.

The human c-*onc* homologous to another transforming virus, feline sarcoma virus (Snyder-Theilen), was also cloned. This gene, designated c-*fes*, is more compact than the c-*sis* gene, and spans 4.5 kb. There are at least three intervening sequences in this gene. Within a fairly short period of time, the full complement of known human *onc* genes should be available. Experiments to determine whether these genes will transform cells after appropriate manipulations, akin to the experiments with mouse c-*onc* homologous to Moloney sarcoma virus (5), may shed some light on the role of these genes in neoplastic transformation. In addition, whether high levels of expression of human c-*onc* genes are etiologically linked to the development of neoplasias can be determined. So far, the results indicate that most of the *onc* genes are transcribed in a wide variety of cells and tissues. The genes related to Harvey MSV and Abelson MuLV are transcribed at low levels as multiple RNA species in all cells examined, including human hematopoietic cells of different lineages, normal fibroblasts, and solid tumors representing a diverse spectrum of malignancies. These genes probably code for protein products that are essential for the maintenance of the cell. The gene related to MC29 is also widely transcribed, but as a single species of 2.7 kb. The size of this transcript is apparently conserved from chicken to humans, and may reflect a strong conservation in the arrangement of *onc* genes throughout evolution, or in specific processing events leading to the mature transcript.

Two *onc* genes exhibit more cell-type specificity in their expression. The gene related to SSV is not transcribed in hematopoietic cells and is only expressed in certain types of tumors (fibrosarcomas, glioblastoma). It is possible that "turning on" of this gene is etiologically linked to these neoplasias. The gene related to AMV is not transcribed in the human solid tumors and normal fibroblasts, at least not to our knowledge. Among hematopoietic cells, this gene is expressed in early precursors of lymphoid, myeloid, and erythroid lineages, but expression is blocked at different stages in different pathways. The product of this gene is probably a hematopoietic cell differentiation antigen. How this finding correlates with leukemogenesis is not known.

We are still at an early stage in understanding the mechanisms involved in human neoplastic transformation. The discovery and accessibility of cellular genes homologous to viral transforming genes may provide one means to probe at these mechanisms. Combined with recent developments, with the isolation of a replicating human retrovirus, there may be major new opportunities for viral oncology in human neoplasias.

ACKNOWLEDGMENTS

We wish to thank our colleagues for contributing to some of the experimental results described here, especially E. Westin, G. Franchini, R. Dalla Favera, E.

Gelmann, V. Manzari, and S. Arya for permission to quote their unpublished results. We are also grateful to A. Mazzuca for expert secretarial assistance.

REFERENCES

1. Abelson, H. T., and Rabstein, L. S. (1970): Lymphosarcoma: Virus-induced thymic independent disease in mice. *Cancer Res.*, 30:2208–2212.
2. Bergman, D. G., Souza, L. M., and Baluda, M. A. (1981): Vertebrate DNA contains nucleotide sequence related to the putative transforming gene of avian myeloblastosis virus. *J. Virol.*, 40:450–455.
3. Bishop, J. M.(1978): Retroviruses. *Annu. Rev. Biochem.*, 47:35–88.
4. Bister, K., Loliger, H., and Duesberg, P. H. (1979): Oligoribonucleotide map and protein of CMII: Detection of conserved and non-conserved genetic elements in avian leukemia viruses CMII, MC29 and MH2. *J. Virol.*, 32:208–219.
5. Blair, D. G., McClements, W., Oskarsson, M., Fischinger, P., and Vande Woude, G. F. (1980): The biological activity of cloned Moloney sarcoma virus DNA: Terminally redundant sequences may enhance transformation efficiency. *Proc. Natl. Acad. Sci. USA*, 77:3504–3508.
6. Collett, M. S., Brugge, J. S., and Erikson, R. L. (1978): Characterization of a normal avian cell protein related to the avian sarcoma virus transforming gene product. *Cell*, 15:1363.
7. Collins, S. J., Gallo, R. C., and Gallagher, R. E. (1977): Continuous growth and differentiation of human myeloid leukemic cells in suspension culture. *Nature*, 270:347–349.
8. Collins, S. J., Ruscetti, F. W., Gallagher, R. E., and Gallo, R. C. (1978): Terminal differentiation of human promyelocytic leukemia cells induced by dimethylsulfoxide and other polar compounds. *Proc. Natl. Acad. Sci. USA*, 75:2458–2462.
9. Dalla Favera, R., Gelmann, E. P., Gallo, R. C., and Wong-Staal, F. (1981): A human *onc* gene homologous to the transforming gene (*v-sis*) of simian sarcoma virus. *Nature*, 292:31–35.
10. Deinhardt, F. (1980): Biology of primate retroviruses. In: *Viral Oncology*, edited by G. Klein, pp. 357–398. Raven Press, New York.
11. Duesberg, P. H. (1979): Transforming genes of retroviruses. *Cold Spring Harbor Symp. Quant. Biol.*, 44:13–30.
12. Duncan, C., Biro, P. A., Chondary, P. V., Elder, J. T., Wang, R. C., Forget, B. G., Dekiel, J. K., and Weissman, S. M. (1979): RNA polymerase III transcriptional units are interspersed among human non-α-globin genes. *Proc. Natl. Acad. Sci. USA*, 76:5095–5099.
13. Eva, A., Robbins, K. C., Andersen, P. R., Srinivasan, A., Tronick, S. R., Reddy, E. P., Ellmore, N. W., Galen, A. T., Lautenberger, J. A., Papas, T. S., Westin, E. H., Wong-Staal, F., Gallo, R. C., and Aaronson, S. A. (1982): Cellular genes analogous to retroviral *onc* genes are transcribed in human tumor cells. *Nature*, 295:116–119.
14. Franchini, G., Even, J., Sherr, C. J., and Wong-Staal, F. (1981): *Onc* sequences (*v-fes*) of Snyder-Theilen feline sarcoma virus are derived from discontiguous regions of a cat cellular gene (*c-fes*). *Nature*, 290:154–157.
14a. Franchini, G., Gelmann, E. P., Dalla Favera, R., Gallo, R. C., and Wong-Staal, F. (1982): A human gene (c-*fes*) related to the *onc* sequences of Snyder-Theilen feline sarcoma virus. *J. Mol. and Cell Biol. (in press)*.
15. Frankel, A. G., Gilbert, J. H., Porzig, K. J., Scolnick, E. M., and Aaronson, S. A. (1979): Nature and distribution of feline sarcoma virus nucleotide sequences. *J. Virol.*, 30:821–827.
16. Gallo, R. C., and Wong-Staal, F. (1980): Molecular biology of primate retroviruses. In: *Viral Oncology*, edited by G. Klein, pp. 399–431. Raven Press, New York.
17. Gardner, M. B., Rongey, R. W., Arnstein, P., Estes, J. D., Sarma, P., Huebner, R. J., and Rickard, G. G. (1970): Experimental transmission of feline fibrosarcoma to cats and dogs. *Nature*, 226:807–809.
18. Gelmann, E. P., Petri, L., Cetta, A., and Wong-Staal, F. (1982): Specific regions of the genome of simian sarcoma associated virus are deleted in defective genomes and in SSV. *J. Virol.*, 41:593–604.
19. Gelmann, E. P., Wong-Staal, F., Kramer, R. A., and Gallo, R. C. (1981): Molecular cloning and comparative analyses of the genomes of simian sarcoma virus (SSV) and its helper associated virus (SSAV). *Proc. Natl. Acad. Sci. USA*, 78:3373–3377.
20. Goff, S. P., Gilboa, E., Witte, O. N., and Baltimore, D. (1980): Structure of the Abelson murine leukemia virus genome and the homologous cellular gene: Studies with cloned viral DNA. *Cell*, 22:777–785.

21. Graf, T., and Beug, H. (1978): Avian leukemia viruses: Interaction with their target cells *in vivo* and *in vitro. Biochim. Biophys. Acta*, 516:269–299.

22. Hager, G., Chang, E., Chan, H., Garon, C., Israel, M., Martin, M., Scolnick, E., and Lowy, D. (1979): Molecular cloning of the Harvey sarcoma virus closed circular DNA intermediates: Initial structural and biologic characterization. *J. Virol.*, 5:221–230.

23. Harvey, J. J. (1964): An unidentified virus which causes the rapid production of tumors in mice. *Nature*, 204:1104–1105.

24. Hayward, W. S., Neel, B. G., and Astrin, S. M. (1981): Induction of lymphoid leukosis by avian leukosis virus: Activation of a cellular "onc" gene by promotor insertion. *Nature*, 290:475–480.

25. Houck, C. M., Rinehart, F. P., and Schmid, C. W. (1979): A ubiquitous family of repeated DNA sequences in the human genome. *J. Mol. Biol.*, 132:289–306.

26. Lautenberger, J. A., Schulz, R. A., Garon, C. F., Tsichlis, P. N., and Papas, T. S. (1981): Molecular cloning of avian myelocytomatosis virus (MC29) transforming sequences. *Proc. Natl. Acad. Sci. USA*, 78:1518–1522.

27. McDonough, S. K., Larsen, S., Brodey, R. S., Stock, N. D., and Hardy, W. D., Jr. (1971): A transmissible feline fibrosarcoma of viral origin. *Cancer Res.*, 31:953–956.

28. Minowada, J., Sagawa, K., Lok, M. S., Kubonishi, I., Nakazawa, S., Tatsumi, E., Ohnuma, T., and Goldblum, N. (1980): A model of lymphoid-myeloid cell differentiation based on the study of marker profiles of 50 human leukemia-lymphoma cell lines. In: *International Symposium on New Trends in Human Immunology and Cancer Immunotherapy*, edited by B. Serrou and C. Rosenfeld, pp. 189–199. Doin Publisher, Paris.

29. Neel, B. G., Hayward, W. S., Robinson, H. L., Fang, J., and Astrin, S. M. (1981): Avian leukosis virus-induced tumors have common proviral integration sites and synthesize discrete new RNAs: Oncogenesis by promotor insertion. *Cell*, 23:323–334.

30. Oskarsson, M., McClements, W. L., Blair, D. G., Maizel, J. V., and Vande Woude, G. F. (1980): Properties of a normal mouse cell DNA sequence *(sarc)* homologous to the *src* sequence of Moloney sarcoma virus. *Science*, 207:1222–1224.

31. Poiesz, B. J., Ruscetti, F. W., Gazdar, A. F., Bunn, P. A., Minna, J. D., and Gallo, R. C. (1980): Isolation of type-C retrovirus particles from cultured and fresh lymphocytes of a patient with cutaneous T-cell lymphoma. *Proc. Natl. Acad. Sci. USA*, 77:7415–7519.

32. Poiesz, B. J., Ruscetti, F. W., Mier, J. W., Woods, A. M., and Gallo, R. C. (1980): T-cell lines established from human T-lymphocytic neoplasias by direct response to T-cell growth factor. *Proc. Natl. Acad. Sci. USA*, 77:6815–6819.

33. Reitz, M. S., Poiesz, B. J., Ruscetti, F. W., and Gallo, R. C. (1981): Characterization and distribution of nucleic acid sequences of a novel type-C retrovirus isolated from neoplastic human T-lymphocytes. *Proc. Natl. Acad. Sci. USA*, 78:1887–1891.

34. Robbins, K. C., Devare, S. G., and Aaronson, S. A. (1981): Molecular cloning of integrated simian sarcoma virus: Genome organization of infectious DNA clones. *Proc. Natl. Acad. Sci. USA*, 78:2918–2922.

35. Deleted in proof.

36. Shalloway, D., Zelenetz, A. D., and Cooper, G. M. (1981): Molecular cloning and characterization of the chicken gene homologous to the transforming gene of Rous sarcoma virus. *Cell*, 24:531–542.

37. Shibuya, M., Hanafusa, T., Hanafusa, H., and Stephenson, J. R. (1980): Homology exists among the transforming sequences of avian and feline sarcoma viruses. *Proc. Natl. Acad. Sci. USA*, 77:6536–6540.

38. Snyder, S. P., and Theilen, G. H. (1969): Transmissible feline fibrosarcoma. *Nature*, 221:1074–1075.

39. Souza, L. M., Strommer, J. N., Hillyard, R. L., Komaromy, M. C., and Baluda, M. A. (1980): Cellular sequences are present in the presumptive avian myeloblastosis virus genome. *Proc. Natl. Acad. Sci. USA*, 77:5177–5181.

40. Srinivasan, A., Reddy, E. P., and Aaronson, S. A. (1981): Abelson murine leukemia virus: Molecular cloning of infectious integrated proviral DNA. *Proc. Natl. Acad. Sci. USA*, 78:2077–2081.

41. Theilen, G. H., Gould, D., Fowler, M., and Dungworth, D. L. (1971): C-type virus in tumor tissue of a woolly monkey *(Lagothrix spp)* with fibrosarcoma. *J. Natl. Cancer Inst.*, 47:881–889.

41a. Westin, E. H., Wong-Staal, F., Gelmann, E. P., Dalla Favera, R., Papos, T. S., Lautenberger, J. A., Eva, A., Reddy, E. P., Tronick, S. R., Aaronson, S. A., and Gallo, R. C. (1982): Expression of cellular homologues of retroviral *onc* genes in human hematopoietic cells. *Proc. Natl. Acad. Sci. USA*, 79:2490–2494.

41b. Westin, E. H., Gallo, R. C., Arya, S. K., Eva, A., Sonza, L. M., Baluda, M. A., Aaronson, S. A., and Wong-Staal, F. (1982): Differential expression of the *amv* gene in human hematopoietic cells. *Proc. Natl. Acad. Sci. USA*, 79:2194–2198.

42. Wolfe, L., Deinhardt, F., Theilen, G., Kawakami, T., and Bustad, L. (1971): Induction of tumors in marmoset monkeys by simian sarcoma virus type 1 *(Lagothrix)*: A preliminary report. *J. Natl. Cancer Inst.*, 47:1115–1120.

43. Wong-Staal, F., Dalla Favera, R., Franchini, G., Gelmann, E. P., and Gallo, R. C. (1981): Three distinct genes in human DNA related to the transforming genes of mammalian sarcoma retroviruses. *Science*, 213:226–228.

44. Wong-Staal, F., Gallo, R. C., and Gillespie, D. (1975): Genetic relationship of a primate RNA tumor virus genome to genes in normal mice. *Nature*, 256:670–672.

45. Wong-Staal, F., Dalla Favera, R., Gelmann, E., Manzaei, V., Szala, S., Josephs, S., and Gallo, R. C. (1981): The transforming gene of simian sarcoma virus *(sis)*: A new *onc* gene of primate origin. *Nature*, 294:273–275.

Advances in Viral Oncology, Volume 1,
edited by George Klein. Raven Press,
New York © 1982.

Organizational Changes of Cytoskeletal Proteins During Cell Transformation

C. Bruce Boschek

Institute of Virology, Justus-Liebig-University, 6300 Giessen,
Federal Republic of Germany

Of all the characteristic differences that have been observed between normal and transformed cells, perhaps the most dramatic are the changes in cellular morphology. In addition to the altered gross shape of the cell, certain transformation-induced changes were observed in specific cellular organelles, particularly in the cytoskeletal system of actin-containing microfilaments. These structures were shown to be considerably less well organized in permanently transformed cell lines than in normal cells (52). Such structural changes were variously interpreted as possible mechanisms of altered functional characteristics, such as substrate adhesion and cellular motility.

The introduction of transformation-defective temperature-sensitive viral mutants of Rous sarcoma virus (RSV) made possible temporal studies of the various events or parameters of transformation. The breakdown of microfilament organization was shown to occur relatively late in the transformation process, roughly coinciding with the general "rounding-up" of the cell (3,20,68). Recently, by use of such viral mutants, it has been possible to show that the distribution of microfilament proteins is transiently altered much earlier after the initiation of transformation (9). In fact, a massive accumulation of these proteins within ruffle-like structures on the dorsal-cell surface is the earliest transformation-induced event yet described. Moreover, these studies have shown that the structural changes observed may be the result of a two-step mechanism or a cascade of events resulting directly or indirectly from the action of the RSV-transforming protein, pp60[src] (14,46,59).

In the next sections, a short description of the cytoskeletal organization is followed by a review of observations made on permanently transformed cell lines. The advantages and experimental strategy in using transformation-defective temperature-sensitive (td-ts) mutants to study the kinetics of transformation are then described and the results of more recent studies are presented and discussed. Finally, several hypotheses will be introduced which it is hoped will shed some light on the functional mechanisms of the changes observed as well as on the transformation process itself.

ORGANIZATION OF THE CYTOSKELETON

The following is a brief outline of a vast sum of data on the cytoskeleton. (For detailed reviews, see 16,30,41–43,54.)

The cytoskeleton is a more or less complex meshwork of fibrillar and tubular organelles distributed throughout the cytoplasm of many nonmuscle cells. As its name implies, this system has long been thought to impart and maintain the form of the cell. The presence of the major muscle proteins in the cytoskeleton, however, suggests that it may also play a role in cellular movement, i.e., translocation of organelles, changes in cell shape, and cellular locomotion. The cytoskeleton comprises three readily distinguishable systems: microfilaments, intermediate filaments, and microtubules. Since the microfilaments alone have been generally implicated in the process of cell transformation, only this system will be dealt with in detail. The organization described here principally represents that observed in cultured fibroblastic cells and differs somewhat from that in other cell types.

Microfilaments

Electron-microscopic examination of thin-sectioned fibroblasts reveals large numbers of filaments, 6 nm in diameter and of varying length (Fig. 1). They are seen to be organized in a thin-meshwork just beneath the plasma membrane (cell cortex), individually distributed throughout the medullary cytoplasm, and in large parallel sheaths or bundles within the ventral part of the cell (45). Actin (43K) is the major protein of the microfilaments (42,54), and immunofluorescence studies using antibodies against muscle actin (40) clearly show the brightly stained bundles, termed actin cables or stress fibers (Fig. 2). These tight bundles traverse the cell beneath the nucleus in a criss-cross pattern and their component microfilaments are parallel and are anchored in the substrate adhesion plaques (focal adhesions) on the ventral cell surface (1,33). Microscopic examination of living cell cultures provided evidence that the stress fibers are oriented parallel to the long axis of cell migration and appear to undergo contraction as the cell contracts. These observations were interpreted as an indication that the stress fibers may represent the major mechanism of nonmuscle cell movement (31). In contrast, however, the number of stress fibers in a given cell is inversely proportional to the motility of the cell and directly proportional to the density of the culture (35; C. B. Boschek, *unpublished observation*). The microfilaments within the "mat" in the cell cortex, on the other hand, are not parallel, but appear to be cross-linked in a complex three-dimensional network (29). In addition to the microfilaments, a portion of the cellular actin in normal fibroblasts is in the form of bound or unbound monomers (10).

Immunofluorescence and detergent-extract isolation studies have also demonstrated the presence of other mechanochemical proteins in association with the microfilaments; among them are α-actinin (110K), myosin (220K), tropomyosin (35K), vinculin (130K), and filamin (250K). This protein constellation has been considered evidence that the microfilaments are contractile elements and may play a direct role in cell motility (42,53).

The nature of the attachment of the individual microfilaments to the plasma membrane is not understood, but α-actinin (44) and vinculin (28) have both been implicated in this role as links between microfilaments and an as yet unidentified intrinsic membrane protein.

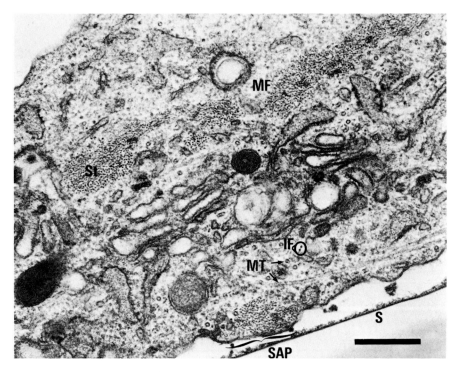

FIG. 1. Electron micrograph of a thin section through the periphery of a chick embryo cell. Numerous actin-containing microfilaments *(MF)* are seen in large bundles or cables termed stress fibers *(St)*, one of which was sectioned obliquely at the point of insertion in a substrate adhesion plaque *(SAP)*. S, substrate (surface of culture plate); *IF*, intermediate filaments; *MT*, microtubules. A long segment of a microtubule is seen running parallel to the ventral surface of the cell *(lower right)*. Cell culture was prepared according to published methods (8,58). Bar = 0.5 μm.

Intermediate Filaments

Figure 1 also shows the presence of larger diameter filaments within the cytoplasm of cultured fibroblasts. These so-called intermediate filaments, 10 nm filaments or tonofilaments, are composed primarily of the 58K protein vimentin and appear to form a cage around the nucleus (4). Although there is no direct evidence as to what their function might be, it has been speculated that they may anchor the nucleus within the cytoplasm (34) or determine the mitotic location of various organelles (4). Hynes and Destree (38) described an altered organization of intermediate filaments in herpes simplex virus-transformed NIL8 cells. (For more detailed discussions of this system of fibers, see 50.)

Microtubules

In addition to the filamentous structures described above, the cytoplasm is seen to contain microtubules, 24 nm in diameter (Fig. 1). The major structural subunit

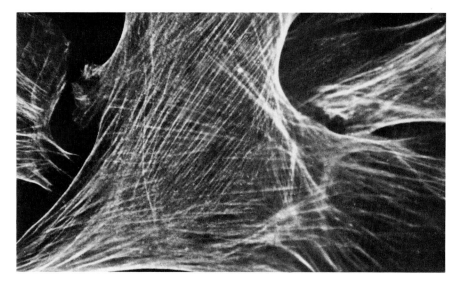

FIG. 2. Fluorescence micrograph of tsNY68-infected cell at restrictive temperature (42° C) stained with antibody to smooth-muscle actin. (For details of staining procedure, see 9.) ×750.

of microtubules is the heterodymeric protein tubulin, composed of two polypeptides, α and β, which condense into a high molecular weight polymer by self-assembly (71). Microtubules have been studied in great detail (for reviews, see 30,64) and have been implicated in a wide variety of cellular processes such as cell motility, mitosis, secretion, and molecular transport. Brinkley et al. (11–13) described the loss of microtubules in transformed cells. Osborn and Weber (51), however, demonstrated that there is no dramatic change in the number or organization of microtubules during transformation, and concluded that the differences observed are the result of altered optical properties of the cell. This latter interpretation was in turn supported by the study of numerous paired nonneoplastic and spontaneously transformed neoplastic cell lines by Tucker et al. (67).

REVIEW OF OBSERVED CYTOSKELETAL DIFFERENCES IN CELLS PERMANENTLY TRANSFORMED BY VARIOUS VIRUSES AND IN TRANSFORMED CELL LINES

In electron microscopic studies, McNutt et al. (47,48) showed differences in microfilament distribution in BALB/c 3T3 cells after SV40 transformation, whereas revertant cell lines appeared similar to uninfected, untransformed cells. Pollack et al. (52) and Weber et al. (69) verified these results by immunofluorescence techniques, showing dramatic changes in the distribution of both actin and myosin in the same cell lines. Transformed cells contained far fewer stress fibers than did their normal counterparts. Additionally, a consistent correlation between loss of stress fibers and anchorage-dependent control of cell division was demonstrated. Willingham et al. (74) in turn argued that although loss of stress fibers was related to substrate anchorage, these two parameters could be dissociated from control of cell division. These studies were extended by Tucker et al. (67) who compared various paired normal and transformed cell lines from mouse, rat, and hamster by immunofluorescence as well as by polarization microscopy of living cells. All transformed cell lines showed reduced numbers and a thinner appearance of stress fibers.

Concomitant with these morphological studies, biochemical assays of cell fractions were performed in an attempt to show changes in the cellular concentration of the various cytoskeletal proteins. A decrease in the "membrane-associated actin" of chick embryo fibroblasts was described by Wickus et al. (72), whereby the total actin content of the cell remained unchanged. Fine and Taylor (23) reported decreased synthesis of actin and tubulin in SV40-transformed 3T3 cells, as well as a change in the ratio of insoluble to soluble actin after transformation. Similar results were reported for NRK cells and their Kirsten-viral transformants by Rubin et al. (56). The absolute concentrations of the various proteins differed greatly, however, in the studies mentioned here.

TEMPERATURE-SENSITIVE MUTANTS OF ROUS SARCOMA VIRUS AS TOOLS IN THE STUDY OF TRANSFORMATION KINETICS

All of the studies described in the last section were performed on statically transformed cells. This approach has three serious drawbacks. First, it is not possible to differentiate clearly between the effects of viral infection and those of transformation. Second, due to the unknown time variables of viral adsorption, penetration, and infection, it is not feasible to perform temporal studies on the transformation event itself. Third, due to the low efficiency of these viruses to transform cells, establishment of a cell line involved strong selection. These difficulties were alleviated by use of td-ts mutants of RSV (24). Cells infected with such mutants show the transformed phenotype at the permissive temperature (35° C) but not at the restrictive temperature (42° C), whereas viral replication proceeds unaffected at both temperatures. By shifting these cultures from the restrictive down to the permissive temperature, it is possible to initiate transformation rapidly, thus making possible time-course studies of the various parameters. Appropriate control experiments ruled out the effect of temperature, so that any changes observed in such downshift experiments must be due solely to the action of the transforming gene product, pp60^{src}. Edelman and Yahara (20), Wang and Goldberg (68), and Ash et al. (3) used this td-ts system to show disruption of the stress fibers a number of hours after downshift. Furthermore, it was shown that this change did not require protein synthesis and could be reversed by shifting back to the restrictive temperature (3).

EARLY CHANGES IN THE DISTRIBUTION OF MICROFILAMENT PROTEINS

In a recent study (9), temperature downshift experiments were performed using RSV td-ts infected chick embryo cells to examine the early events in the transformation process. It could be shown that within 15 min after the initiation of transformation, actin accumulated within large whorllike structures on the dorsal cell surface (Fig. 3). By use of the scanning electron microscope (SEM) in the cathode luminescence mode (8,9), these structures were demonstrated to be identical with the plasma membrane ruffles, termed flowers, observed in earlier studies (2,68). To rule out a passive influx of monomeric actin, these experiments were repeated using a fluorescein-labeled derivative of phalloidin (FL-phalloidin). This fungal toxin is a bicyclic heptapeptide that exclusively binds to polymeric actin (73,75) when applied to prefixed cell cultures. As seen in Fig. 4, this substance brightly stains flowers, indicating that the actin within these structures is polymeric. In addition, SEM examination of tannic-acid mordanted, lead-stained cells (58,63) shows the presence of filamentous structures within flowers (Fig. 5).

In order for actin microfilaments to function as active contractile elements, they must presumably interact with certain other mechanochemical proteins (54). Indirect immunofluorescence using affinity-purified antibodies showed that flowers also contain accumulations of α-actinin, myosin, and tropomyosin (9). In addition, the 130K protein, vinculin, can be shown to be present in flowers (Fig. 6). By combined application of these antibodies, rhodamin-conjugated secondary antibody, and FL-phalloidin, these other proteins were seen to occur simultaneously with actin in every flower observed. Passive antibody trapping within these structures was ruled out by showing that they are not stained by anti-tubulin or anti-vimentin.

LATE CHANGES IN THE DISTRIBUTION OF MICROFILAMENT PROTEINS

SEM shows a release of microfilaments from the plasma membrane 4 to 6 hr after downshift (C. B. Boschek, *unpublished observation*). Between 6 and 12 hr,

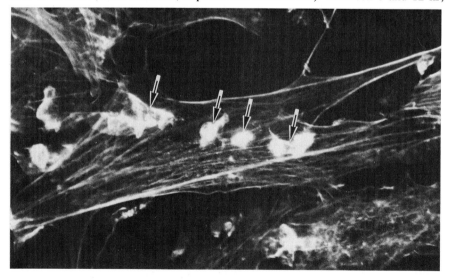

FIG. 3. Anti-actin fluorescence of tsNY68-infected cell, 15 min after downshift to permissive temperature (35° C). Note the actin-containing flowers *(arrows)* on the dorsal cell surface. × 750.

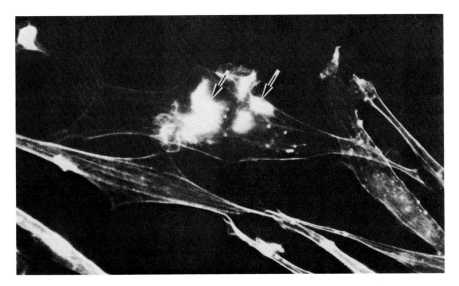

FIG. 4. Flowers *(arrows)* stain with fluorescein-conjugated derivative of phalloidin showing that actin in these structures is polymerized. See section V for details. ×1,000.

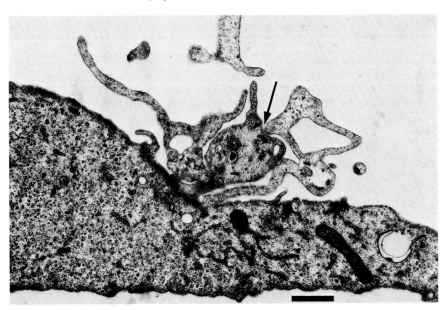

FIG. 5. Electron micrograph of a cell 30 min after downshift to permissive temperature. Dorsal surface flower is seen to contain numerous filaments *(arrow)*. Bar = 1 μm.

much of the complex system of stress fibers becomes disorganized (Fig. 7). Immunofluorescent staining of the various microfilament proteins shows a general increase in diffuse background intensity. In contrast, staining with FL-phalloidin results in a reduction of fluorescence, indicating a decrease in the degree of poly-

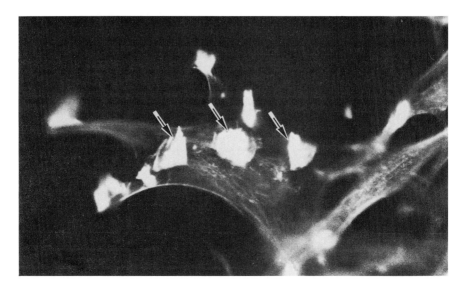

FIG. 6. Vinculin immunofluorescence of a cell 30 min after downshift to permissive temperature. Flowers are seen to contain accumulations of vinculin *(arrows).* × 850.

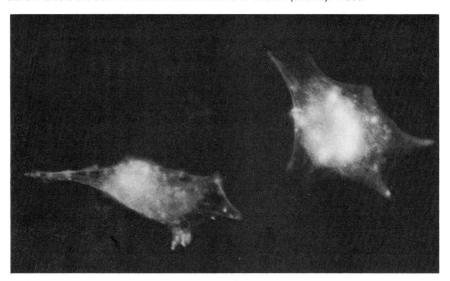

FIG. 7. Actin immunofluorescence of a culture 12 hr after downshift to permissive temperature. Note loss of stress fibers and rounded-up appearance of cells compared to Fig. 2. × 1,000.

merization of cellular actin. This observation was quantified by microfluorimetric measurements of the intensity of FL-phalloidin fluorescence (7), and showed a three- to fivefold reduction in polymerization coinciding with the time of stress fiber disorganization. These results were verified using the two-step DNase I actin inhibition assay described by Blikstad et al. (6).

All of the data described above were obtained using cells infected with the RSV viral mutant, tsNY68. Numerous other mutants have been examined as well and, although quantitative differences were measured, most mutants behaved in a qualitatively similar manner. One notable exception was the fusiform mutant, ts529 (26). Whereas most biochemical and functional transformation parameters are comparable to those observed using other mutants, this virus induces an aberrant alteration to the morphology, the cells becoming thin and elongated at the permissive temperature. Interestingly, there is no significant reduction in the number of stress fibers or in the cytoplasmic concentration of polymerized actin. By contrast, this mutant (as well as all other mutants tested) induces the formation of dorsal surface flowers, both quantitatively and qualitatively indistinguishable from the flowers seen with tsNY68.

FUNCTIONAL IMPLICATIONS

The ultimate goal of the morphological studies described here is to gain new insights into functional mechanisms of cell transformation and, in particular, the action of the RSV *src* gene product, pp60^{src} (14,46,59). This molecule was shown to be intimately associated with a protein kinase activity (18,46). More recent data provides evidence that this kinase is at least one of the intrinsic activities of pp60^{src} (21,57) and, specifically, phosphorylates tyrosine (19,22,37). Pp60^{src} has a homologous counterpart termed pp60$^{proto-src}$, which is found in extremely low concentrations in all normal vertebrate cells (17,19,49,61).

The time course of the various changes described above are summarized in Fig. 8. In td-ts mutant-infected cells at the restrictive temperature, the pp60^{src} appears to be present in a nonfunctional state (25,76) and can be reactivated by shifting to the permissive temperature. Within 15 min after downshift, the protein kinase activity reappears, accompanied by phosphorylation of the pp60^{src} itself. Since the kinase activity is likely to be one of the functions responsible for the transformation process, the correlated simultaneous reappearance of this activity and the formation of dorsal surface flowers is striking. Flower formation is the earliest observable parameter of transformation and, together with the loss of stress fibers and reactivation of kinase activity, it is among the only changes known that can take place when protein synthesis is blocked by cyclohexamide (25). Although flowers are very similar in appearance to the peripheral membrane ruffles on the lamellipodia of motile cells, the presence of myosin and tropomyosin in flowers implies that these structures are unique and specific to the transformation process (9). For these reasons, the microfilament proteins that are accumulated in flowers appear to be likely candidates as functional target molecules for pp60^{src}. To date, only vinculin, myosin heavy chain, and filamin have been found to contain measurable amounts of phosphotyrosine (37,60) and of these, only vinculin has been shown to contain elevated phosphotyrosine levels in transformed cells. For this reason there has been considerable speculation that vinculin is a potential pp60^{src}-kinase target. This speculation is supported by two additional factors known about vinculin: its presence

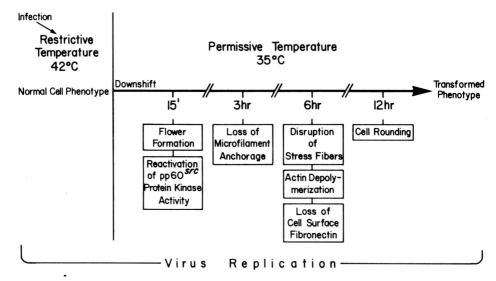

FIG. 8. Time course of various transformation-induced events. Temperature downshift experiments. Transformation-defective temperature-sensitive mutant (tsNY68) of Rous sarcoma virus-infected chick embryo cells.

within adhesion plaques (15,27) in which pp60[src] has also been reported to accumulate (55,62) and its ability to cause *in vitro* bundling of actin microfilaments (39). Vinculin has also been purported to play a role in anchoring the microfilaments into the plasma membrane. Although not an integral membrane protein itself, it has been suggested to act as a link between the microfilament and some as yet unknown protein within the membrane (27). Assuming that phosphorylation of tyrosine in vinculin results in an alteration of these properties, one can easily imagine a variety of mechanisms that would explain many of the changes in the distribution of microfilament proteins during transformation. Despite these tempting implications, the suitability of vinculin as a primary target molecule for the pp60[src] kinase is still questionable. Although the phosphotyrosine level in vinculin increases substantially during transformation (60), only a very small number of the vinculin molecules isolated from transformed cells are phosphorylated in tyrosine. If this effect is to be functionally significant, it must be assumed that either a highly specific and localized population of vinculin molecules is involved or that the turnover rate of tyrosine-phosphorylated vinculin is extremely rapid. As yet, there are no data available to support either of these assumptions directly.

Acting as a cross-linker for actin microfilaments (32,36,65) and mimicking the action of actin gelation factors (39), α-actinin appears to have a complimentary function to that of vinculin, making this also a very attractive candidate as a target molecule for pp60[src]. However, α-actinin, as well as tropomyosin, appear to be unphosphorylated in both normal and transformed cells. Whereas myosin heavy chain and filamin both contain trace amounts of phosphotyrosine, no transformation-related change in the phosphotyrosine level could be measured (60). Although actin can be readily phosphorylated *in vitro* by pp60^{src} (19), it only occurs unphosphorylated *in vivo*. In addition, the number of pp60^{src} molecules in the cell is very low, compared to the large amount of actin, so that any eventual interaction of these molecules would have to be transitory rather than stoichiometric. A microfilament-bound target of the transforming protein may, therefore, well belong to the virtually uncharacterized group of minor actin-binding proteins.

The gross alteration to cell shape (rounding up) observed in transformation mimics that observed during mitosis. It is undoubtedly the result of disruption of the stress fibers and observed reduction in the number of substrate adhesion plaques at the cell periphery (9). The occurrence of these events at a time coinciding with the loss of the cell surface protein, fibronectin (70), as well as the transmembranal relationship between actin and various surface receptors at the adhesion plaques (5), help explain the reduced substrate adhesion of the transformed cell (Fig. 8).

FL-phalloidin staining of flowers as well as the presence of filaments in electron micrographs show the polymeric state of actin in these structures, suggesting that a local polymerization may be the mechanism of flower formation. This might take place by elongation at the membrane-bound end of the microfilaments, as demonstrated by Tilney et al. (66). The rapid time course of this process suggests that microfilament elongation is a direct result of some action of pp60^{src}. Retraction of the microfilaments from the plasma membrane and the ensuing generalized depolymerization of actin in the cell occur much later (see Fig. 8), implying that these latter changes occur late in a series or cascade of transformation-induced events.

CONCLUSIONS

Although the interaction between the *src* gene product and cytoskeletal proteins remains unclear, the observations described above imply that this interaction may be a very direct one. Whereas the loss of stress fibers, the subsequent gross morphological changes, and reduced substrate adhesion may be indirect consequences of the action of pp60^{src}, the formation of surface flowers would appear to be a transformation-specific event that results directly from some action of this molecule. As more information becomes available about the additional cytoskeletal proteins and their functional properties, the exact nature of this interaction should become clear. This would provide another challenging aspect in the elucidation of the mechanisms of transformation.

ACKNOWLEDGMENTS

The author wishes to thank Ruth Back for expert technical assistance and help with preparation of the manuscript as well as Heinz Bauer, Robert Friis, Sandra Howard, and Andrew Ziemiecki for their critical reading of the manuscript and helpful suggestions. This work was supported by the Deutsche Forschungsgemeinschaft, SFB 47.

REFERENCES

1. Abercrombie, M., Heaysman, J. E. M., and Pegrum, S. M. (1971): The locomotion of fibroblasts in culture. IV. Electron microscopy of the leading lamella. *Exp. Cell Res.*, 67:359–371.

2. Ambros, V. R., Chen, L. B., and Buchanan, J. M. (1975): Surface ruffles as markers for studies of cell transformation by Rous sarcoma virus. *Proc. Natl. Acad. Sci. USA*, 72:3144–3148.

3. Ash, J. F., Vogt, P. K., and Singer, S. J. (1976): Reversion from transformed to normal phenotype by inhibition of protein synthesis in rat kidney cells infected with a temperature-sensitive mutant of Rous sarcoma virus. *Proc. Natl. Acad. Sci. USA*, 73:3603–3607.

4. Aubin, J. E., Osborn, M., Franke, W. W., and Weber, K. (1980): Intermediate filaments of the vimentin-type and the cytokeratin-type are distributed differently during mitosis. *Exp. Cell Res.*, 129:149–165.

5. Badley, R. A., Woods, A., Smith, C. G., and Rees, D. A. (1980): Actomyosin relationships with surface features in fibroblasts adhesion. *Exp. Cell Res.*, 126:263–272.

6. Blikstad, I., Markey, F., Carlsson, L., Persson, T., and Lindberg, U. (1978): Selective assay of monomeric and filamentous actin in cell extracts, using inhibition of deoxyribonuclease. *J. Cell*, 15:935–943.

7. Boschek, C. B., Friis, R. R., Grundmann, E., and Back, R. (1982): *(in preparation)*.

8. Boschek, C. B., Jockusch, B. M., Friis, R. R., Back, R., and Bauer, H. (1979): Morphological alterations to the cell surface and cytoskeleton in neoplastic transformation. *Beitr. Elektronen-mikroskop. Direktabb. Oberfl.*, 12:47–54.

9. Boschek, C. B., Jockusch, B. M., Friis, R. R., Back, R., Grundmann, E., and Bauer, H. (1981): Early changes in the distribution and organization of microfilament proteins during cell transformation. *Cell*, 24:175–184.

10. Bray, D., and Thomas, C. (1976): Unpolymerized actin in tissue cells. In: *Cell Motility*, edited by R. Goldman, T. Pollard, and J. Rosenbaum, pp. 461–473. Cold Spring Harbor Laboratory, Cold Spring Harbor, New York.

11. Brinkley, B. R., and Cartwright, J. (1975): Cold labile and cold stable microtubules in the mitotic spindle of mammalian cells. *Ann. N.Y. Acad. Sci.*, 253:428–439.

12. Brinkley, B. R., Fuller, G. M., and Highfield, D. P. (1975): Cytoplasmic microtubules in normal and transformed cells in culture: Analysis by tubulin antibody immunofluorescence. *Proc. Natl. Acad. Sci. USA*, 72:4981–4985.

13. Brinkley, B. R., Fuller, G. M., and Highfield, D. P. (1976): Tubulin antibodies as probes for microtubules in dividing and nondividing mammalian cells. In: *Cell Motility*, edited by R. Goldman, T. Pollard, and J. Rosenbaum, pp. 435–456. Cold Spring Harbor Laboratory, Cold Spring Harbor, New York.

14. Brugge, J. S., and Erikson, R. L. (1977): Identification of a transformation-specific antigen induced by an avian sarcoma virus. *Nature*, 269:346–348.

15. Burridge, K., and Feramisco, J. (1980): Microinjection and localization of a 130K protein in living fibroblasts: A relationship to actin and fibronectin. *Cell*, 19:587–595.

16. Clarke, M., and Spudich, J. A. (1977): Nonmuscle contractile proteins: The role of actin and myosin in cell motility and shape determination. *Annu. Rev. Biochem.*, 46:797–820.

17. Collett, M. S., Brugge, J. S., and Erikson, R. L. (1978): Characterization of a normal avian cell protein related to avian sarcoma virus transforming gene product. *Cell*, 15:1363–1369.

18. Collett, M. S., and Erikson, R. L. (1978): Protein kinase activity associated with the avian sarcoma virus *src* gene product. *Proc. Natl. Acad. Sci. USA*, 75:2021–2024.

19. Collett, M. S., Purchio, A. F., and Erikson, R. L. (1980): Avian sarcoma virus transformation protein pp60^{src}, shows protein kinase activity specific for tyrosine. *Nature*, 285:167–169.

20. Edelman, G. M., and Yahara, I. (1976): Temperature-sensitive changes in surface modulation assemblies of fibroblasts transformed by mutants of Rous sarcoma virus. *Proc. Natl. Acad. Sci. USA*, 73:2047–2051.

21. Erikson, R. L., Collett, M. S., Erikson, E., and Purchio, A. F. (1979): Evidence that the avian sarcoma virus transforming gene product is a cyclic AMP-independent protein kinase. *Proc. Natl. Acad. Sci. USA*, 76:6260–6264.

22. Erikson, R. L., Collett, M. S., Purchio, A. F., and Brugge, J. S. (1980): Protein phosphorylation mediated by partially purified avian sarcoma virus transforming-gene product. *Cold Spring Harbor Symp. Quant. Biol.*, 44:907–917.

23. Fine, R. E., and Taylor, L. (1976): Decreased actin and tubulin synthesis in 3T3 cells after transformation by SV40 virus. *Exp. Cell Res.*, 102:162–168.

24. Friis, R. R. (1978): Temperature-sensitive mutants of avian RNA tumor virus: A review. *Curr. Top. Microbiol. Immunol.*, 79:261–293.

25. Friis, R. R., Jockusch, B. M., Boschek, C. B., Ziemiecki, A., Rübsamen, H., and Bauer, H. (1980): Transformation defective temperature sensitive mutants of Rous sarcoma virus have a reversibly-defective *src* gene product. *Cold Spring Harbor Symp. Quant. Biol.*, 44:1007–1012.

26. Fujita, D. J., Boschek, C. B., Ziemiecki, A., and Friis, R. R. (1981): An avian sarcoma virus mutant which produces an aberrant transformation affecting cell morphology. *Virology*, 111:223–238.

27. Geiger, B. (1979): A 130K protein from chicken gizzard: Its localization at the termini of microfilament bundles in cultured chicken cells. *Cell*, 18:193–205.

28. Geiger, B., Tokuyasu, K. T., Dutton, A. H., and Singer, S. J. (1980): Vinculin, an intracellular protein localized at specialized sites where microfilament bundles terminate at cell membranes. *Proc. Natl. Acad. Sci. USA*, 77:4127–4131.

29. Goldman, R. D. (1975): The use of heavy meromyosin binding as an ultrastructural cytochemical method for localizing and determining the possible functions of actin-like microfilaments in nonmuscle cells. *J. Histochem. Cytochem.*, 23:529–535.

30. Goldman, R. D., Pollard, T., and Rosenbaum, J., eds. (1976): *Cell Motility*. Cold Spring Harbor Laboratory, Cold Spring Harbor, New York.

31. Goldman, R. D., Schloss, J. A., and Starger, J. M. (1976): Organizational changes of actin-like microfilaments during animal cell movement. In: *Cell Motility*, edited by R. Goldman, T. Pollard, and J. Rosenbaum, pp. 217–245. Cold Spring Harbor Laboratory, Cold Spring Harbor, New York.

32. Goll, D. E., Suzuki, A., Temple, J., and Holmes, G. R. (1972): Studies on purified α-actinin. I. Effect of temperature and tropomyosin on the α-actinin/F-actin interaction. *J. Mol. Biol.*, 67:469–478.

33. Heath, J. P., and Dunn, G. A. (1978): Cell to substratum contacts of chick fibroblasts and their relation to the microfilament system. A correlated interference-reflexion and high-voltage electron microscope study. *J. Cell. Sci.*, 29:197–211.

34. Henderson, D., and Weber, K. (1980): Immunoelectron microscopic studies of intermediate filaments in cultured cells. *Exp. Cell Res*, 129:441–453.

35. Herman, I. M., Crisona, N. J., and Pollard, T. D. (1981): Relation between cell activity and the distribution of cytoplasmic actin and myosin. *J. Cell Biol.*, 90:84–91.

36. Holmes, G. R., Goll, D. E., and Suzuki, A. (1971): Effect of α-actinin on actin viscosity. *Biochem. Biophys. Acta*, 253:240–253.

37. Hunter, T., and Sefton, B. M. (1980): The transforming gene product of Rous sarcoma virus phosphorylates tyrosine. *Proc. Natl. Acad. Sci. USA*, 77:1311–1315.

38. Hynes, R. O., and Destree, A. T. (1978): 10 nm filaments in normal and transformed cells. *Cell*, 13:151–163.

39. Jockusch, B. M., and Isenberg, G. (1981): Interaction of α-actinin and vinculin with actin: Opposite effects on filament network formation. *Proc. Natl. Acad. Sci. USA*, 78:3005–3009.

40. Jockusch, B. M., Kelley, K. H., Meyer, R. K., and Burger, M. M. (1978): An efficient method to produce specific anti-actin. *Histochemistry*, 55:177–184.

41. Kirschner, M. W. (1978): Microtubule assembly and nucleation. *Int. Rev. Cytol.*, 54:71–94.

42. Korn, E. D. (1978): Biochemistry of actomyosin-dependent cell motility (a review). *Proc. Natl. Acad. Sci. USA*, 75:588–599.

43. Lazarides, E. (1980): Intermediate filaments as mechanical integrators of space. *Nature*, 283:249–256.

44. Lazarides, E., and Burridge, K. (1975): α-Actinin: Immunofluorescent localization of a muscle structural protein in nonmuscle cells. *Cell*, 6:289–298.

45. Lazarides, E., and Weber, K. (1974): Actin antibody: The specific visualization of actin filaments in non-muscle cells. *Proc. Natl. Acad. Sci. USA*, 71:2268–2272.

46. Levinson, A. D., Oppermann, H., Levintow, L., Varmus, H. E., and Bishop, J. M. (1978): Evidence that the transforming gene of avian sarcoma virus encodes a protein kinase associated with a phosphoprotein. *Cell*, 15:561–572.

47. McNutt, N. S., Culp, L. A., and Black, P. H. (1971): Contact-inhibited revertant cell lines isolated from SV40-transformed cells. II. Ultrastructural study. *J. Cell Biol.*, 50:691–708.

48. McNutt, N. S., Culp, L. A., and Black, P. H. (1973): Contact-inhibited revertant cell lines isolated from SV40-transformed cells. *J. Cell Biol.*, 56:421–428.

49. Oppermann, H., Levinson, A. D., Varmus, H. E., Levintow, L., and Bishop, J. M. (1979): Uninfected vertebrate cells contain a protein that is closely related to the product of the avian sarcoma virus transforming gene *(src)*. *Proc. Natl. Acad. Sci. USA*, 76:1804–1808.

50. Osborn, M., Franke, W., and Weber, K. (1980): Direct demonstration of the presence of two immunologically distinct intermediate-sized filament systems in the same cell by double immunofluorescence microscopy. *Exp. Cell Res.*, 125:37–46.
51. Osborn, M., and Weber, K. (1977): The display of microtubules in transformed cells. *Cell*, 12:561–571.
52. Pollack, R., Osborn, M., and Weber, K. (1975): Patterns of organization of actin and myosin in normal and transformed cultured cells. *Proc. Natl. Acad. Sci. USA*, 72:994–998.
53. Pollard, T. D., Fujiwara, K., Niederman, R., and Maupin-Szamier, P. (1976): Evidence for the role of cytoplasmic actin and myosin in cellular structure and motility. In: *Cell Motility*, edited by R. Goldman, T. Pollard, and J. Rosenbaum, pp. 689–724. Cold Spring Harbor Laboratory, Cold Spring Harbor, New York.
54. Pollard, T. D., and Weihing, R. R. (1974): Actin and myosin and cell movement. *Crit. Rev. Biochem.*, 2:1–65.
55. Rohrschneider, L. R. (1979): Adhesion plaques of Rous sarcoma virus-transformed cells contain the *src* gene product. *Proc. Natl. Acad. Sci. USA*, 77:3514–3518.
56. Rubin, R. W., Warren, R. H., Lukeman, D. S., and Clements, E. (1978): Actin content and organization in normal and transformed cells in culture. *J. Cell Biol.*, 78:28–35.
57. Rübsamen, H., Friis, R. R., and Bauer, H. (1979): *Src* gene product from different strains of avian sarcoma virus: Kinetics and possible mechanism of heat inactivation of protein kinase activity from cells infected by transformation-defective temperature-sensitive mutant and wild-type virus. *Proc. Natl. Acad. Sci. USA*, 76:967–971.
58. Scholtissek, C., Rohde, W., Harms, E., Rott, R., Orlich, M., and Boschek, C. B. (1978): A possible partial heterozygote of an influenza A virus. *Virology*, 89:506–516.
59. Sefton, B. M., Beemon, K., and Hunter, T. (1978): Comparison of the expression of the *src* gene of Rous sarcoma virus in vitro and in vivo. *J. Virol.*, 28:957–971.
60. Sefton, B. M., Hunter, T., Ball, E. H., and Singer, S. J. (1981a): Vinculin: a cytoskeletal target of the transforming protein of Rous sarcoma virus. *Cell*, 24:165–174.
61. Sefton, B. M., Hunter, T., and Beemon, K. (1980): The relationship of the polypeptide products of the transforming gene of Rous sarcoma virus and the homologous gene of vertebrates. *Proc. Natl. Acad. Sci. USA*, 77:2059–2063.
62. Shriver, K., and Rohrschneider, L. (1981): Organization of pp60^{src} and selected cytoskeletal proteins within adhesion plaques and junctions of Rous sarcoma virus-transformed rat cells. *J. Cell Biol.*, 89:525–535.
63. Simionescu, N., and Simionescu, M. (1976): Galloylglucose of low molecular weight as mordant in electron microscopy. I. Procedure, and evidence for mordanting effect. *J. Cell Biol.*, 70:608–621.
64. Snyder, J., and McIntosh, J. R. (1976): Biochemistry and physiology of microtubules. *Ann. Rev. Biochem.*, 45:699–727.
65. Stromer, M. H., and Goll, D. E. (1972): Studies on purified α-actinin. II. Electron microscopic studies on the competitive binding of α-actinin and tropomyosin to Z-line extracted myofibrils. *J. Mol. Biol.*, 67:489–498.
66. Tilney, L. G., Bonder, B. M., and DeRosier, D. J. (1981): Actin filaments elongate from their membrane-associated ends. *J. Cell Biol.*, 90:485–494.
67. Tucker, R. W., Sanford, K. K., and Frankel, F. R. (1978): Tubulin and actin in paired nonneoplastic and spontaneously transformed neoplastic cell lines in vitro: Fluorescent antibody studies. *Cell*, 13:629–642.
68. Wang, E., and Goldberg, A. R. (1976): Changes in microfilament organization and surface topography upon transformation of chick embryo fibroblasts with Rous sarcoma virus. *Proc. Natl. Acad. Sci. USA*, 73:4065–4069.
69. Weber, K., Lazarides, E., Goldman, R. D., Vogel, A., and Pollack, R. (1975): Localization and distribution of actin fibers in normal, transformed and revertant cells. *Cold Spring Harbor Symp. Quant. Biol.*, 39:363–369.
70. Weber, M. J., Hale, A. H., and Losasso, L. (1977): Decreased adherence to the substrate in Rous sarcoma virus-transformed chicken embryo fibroblasts. *Cell*, 10:45–51.
71. Weisenberg, R. C. (1972): Microtubule formation in vitro in solutions containing low calcium concentrations. *Science*, 177:1104–1106.
72. Wickus, G., Gruenstein, E., Robbins, P. W., and Rich, A. (1975): Decrease in membrane-associated actin of fibroblasts after transformation by Rous sarcoma virus. *Proc. Natl. Acad. Sci. USA*, 72:746–749.

73. Wieland, T., and Faulstich, H. (1978): Amatoxins, phallotoxins, phallolysin, and antamanide: The biologically active components of poisonous *Amanita* mushrooms. *Crit. Rev. Biochem.*, 5:185–260.
74. Willingham, M. C., Yamada, K. M., Yamada, S. S., Pouyssegur, J., and Pastan, I. (1977): Microfilament bundles and cell shape are related to adhesiveness to substratum and are dissociable from growth control in cultured fibroblasts. *Cell*, 10:375–380.
75. Wulf, E., Deboben, A., Bautz, F. A., Faulstich, H., and Wieland, T. (1979): Fluorescent phallotoxin, a tool for the visualization of cellular actin. *Proc. Natl. Acad. Sci. USA*, 76:4498–4502.
76. Ziemiecki, A., and Friis, R. R. (1980): Phosphorylation of pp60^{src} and the cycloheximide insensitive activation of the pp60^{src}-associated kinase activity of transformation-defective temperature-sensitive mutants of Rous sarcoma virus. *Virology*, 106:391–394.

Advances in Viral Oncology, Volume 1,
edited by George Klein. Raven Press,
New York © 1982.

Moloney Sarcoma Virus: A Model for Transformation by Endogenous Cellular Genes

D. G. Blair and G. F. Vande Woude

Laboratory of Molecular Oncology, National Cancer Institute, National Institutes of Health, Bethesda, Maryland 20205

Acute transforming retroviruses have been isolated from a variety of avian and mammalian species. These viruses share common structural properties with competent replicating retroviruses and many have been reviewed in detail both in this volume and elsewhere (53). Acute transforming viruses induce a wide variety of tumor types *in vivo* after short latent periods and often induce morphological "transformation" in susceptible tissue culture cells. By comparison, avian and murine lymphatic leukemia viruses cause neoplastic disease *in vivo* after long latent periods and generally have no effect on cell morphology in tissue culture. The acute transforming viruses, with the sole exception of Rous avian sarcoma virus, are defective for replication and require "helper" retroviruses to provide replication functions. More significantly, the acute transforming retroviruses possess small segments of genetic information acquired from the host cell genomes. The acquired sequences are present at low or single copy levels in the genomes of the animal species from which the virus was originally isolated, and are conserved in the genomes of a wide range of other animal species as well (22,53). These acquired sequences are apparently responsible for the ability of the viruses to induce tumors in animals rapidly and to transform cells in tissue culture. Thus, sequences that cause cell transformation when introduced into cells as part of the viral genome, apparently do not normally transform when present endogenously as part of the host chromosome.

Moloney murine sarcoma virus (Mo-MSV) has been an excellent model for studying the process by which a normal cell gene with transforming potential is activated. Mo-MSV genomes isolated by recombinant DNA techniques are amenable to study by conventional DNA methodologies (37,42,49). In addition, the acquired transforming sequence *(mos)* present in the virus has been cloned from normal cellular DNA and can be tested for endogenous biological activity. (The normal cell sequence is termed c-*mos* as distinguished from v-*mos*, the viral homolog present in the Mo-MSV genome.) Like other acute transforming retroviruses, Mo-MSV apparently arose as the result of a recombination of the parental helper virus, in this case Moloney murine leukemia virus (Mo-MLV), with host cell sequences.

We have been interested in determining the molecular elements responsible for Mo-MSV transformation and in understanding the recombination events that lead to the formation of Mo-MSV. This information may ultimately allow controlled *in vitro* isolation of transforming genes. After a brief review of the biology of Mo-MSV, we will describe experimental results indicating those portions of the Mo-MSV genome essential for morphological transformation. We will also show that the combination of subgenomic cloned Mo-MuLV derived sequences and *mos* sequences can provide sufficient information to allow helper virus rescue of an acute transforming retrovirus.

Mo-MSV STRAINS

Moloney (38) reported that the inoculation of high titer Mo-MuLV into newborn Balb/c mice produced rhabdomyosarcomas at the site of injection. Cell free extracts of these tumors would also induce sarcomas when passed serially in newborn mice, and these mouse passaged stocks served as the source of most strains of Mo-MSV.

Historically, HT1-MSV was the first Mo-MSV strain to be isolated. A 6th passage Balb/c mouse tumor extract of Mo-MSV (Mo-MuLV) was used to induce tumors in newborn hamsters, and one tumor (HT1) was placed in culture after the first transplant generation. This tumor was virus negative, but rescue of infectious virus (HT1 MSV) was detected *in vitro* after the addition of infectious Mo-MuLV (29). Two additional Mo-MSV strains were derived from an uncloned, animal passaged stock propagated in 3T3 F1 cells, an outbred murine line (7). Cells were infected at low input virus multiplicity and transformed cell colonies were selected in semi-solid agar suspension (7). Two independently derived cell lines showed significant differences in reversion frequencies (20). The Mo-MSV strain with the higher reversion frequency was termed m1 MSV; the less frequently reverting strain was labeled m3 MSV (21).

The most studied Mo-MSV isolate, MSV-124, was isolated from a Balb/c mouse passaged stock of uncloned Mo-MSV (Mo-MuLV) following infection of JLS-V9 cells. A single cell clone (G8) was derived, which released high titers of infectious Mo-MSV (4), and this virus was subsequently used to infect a cell line (TB) derived from CFW/D mice (3). A single focus (clone 124) was isolated, which produced a 10- to 100-fold excess of Mo-MSV over helper Mo-MuLV. This high proportion of transforming virus has been extremely useful for biochemical studies of Mo-MSV (34), although the mechanism of excess defective virus production is still not understood. It is possible that these transformed cells were infected with multiple copies of Mo-MSV before Mo-MuLV infection established interference, and that multiply integrated Mo-MSV resulted in the production of a higher proportion of sarcoma virus. Donoghue et al. (18) have made a careful comparison of most of the known Mo-MSV strains but the above strains have been most frequently studied by recombinant techniques. Since no two Mo-MSV strains isolated to date have been identical, it is likely that the original uncloned Mo-MSV stock contained a large number of unique variants, or that some Mo-MSV configurations undergo frequent rearrangements and deletions (14).

BIOLOGICAL PROPERTIES OF Mo-MSV

All Mo-MSV isolates are defective for virus replication, and Mo-MSV transformed nonproducer cell lines established that a single Mo-MSV virus could transform cells in tissue culture. Certain nonproducer Mo-MSV transformed cells—termed $S + L -$, i.e., sarcoma positive, leukemia negative (7)—have been shown to release noninfectious particles that lack retroviral polymerase and envelope glycoprotein (6). Sequence and heteroduplex data confirm that all Mo-MSV strains studied lack most of the Mo-MuLV sequences coding for envelope *(env)* and reverse transcriptase *(pol)* functions (18,28,42,43,49,50). Moreover, some strains like HT1 MSV fail to express *gag* determinants (1,45), although they possess the genetic information coding for these peptides (18,50). The "helper" virus provides the missing functions and defective virus "rescue" really represents pseudovirion encapsidation. Infectious Mo-MSV can also be rescued by heterologous helper virus by first co-cultivating Mo-MSV transformed mouse cells with heterologous cells, and then infecting the mixed culture with a helper virus capable of growing in the heterologous cell (29). This process (transpecies rescue) probably occurs as the result of spontaneous fusion between the co-cultivated cells. Since the helper virus envelope glycoprotein determines viral host range (5,52), Mo-MSV pseudotypes can be made to infect and transform essentially all types of mammalian cells. In this way, the host range of Mo-MSV has been efficiently extended to avian cells as well (44). Since recent data indicate that retroviruses mediate their own expression through transcription recognition elements present in the ends of the viral genome (see below), the ability of Mo-MSV to transform a wide range of cells suggests that such elements are easily recognized in heterologous animal species.

BIOLOGICAL CONSEQUENCES OF Mo-MSV INFECTION

Mo-MSV induces tumors in a variety of newborn and adult animals, although tumor formation in adult animals is inefficient and rejection is usually rapid (26,32).

Mo-MSV infection of cells in tissue culture results in an altered cell phenotype. These changes include: (a) increased cell density; (b) reduced adhesion to a solid substrate; (c) ability to grow in suspension in agar or other semisolid media; (d) increases in the rate of uptake of various sugars; (e) changes in cell surface components such as the LETS (large external transformation specific) glycoprotein; (f) induction and release of plasminogen activator, sarcoma growth factor, and several high molecular weight proteins of unknown function; (g) increased agglutinibility; (h) disruption of subcellular organization, including actin fibers and microtubules; and (i) increased rates of glycolysis. Many of these phenotypic changes, however, are generally exhibited by cells transformed with a variety of both viral and chemical agents.

Mo-MSV TRANSFORMING GENE PRODUCT

Unlike many of the acute transforming retroviruses, a Mo-MSV transforming protein has not yet been identified. Despite extensive efforts by large numbers of investigators, it has been extremely difficult to produce antibodies to such a product. It is expected that new techniques, allowing more efficient eucaryotic gene expression in procaryotes or chemical synthesis of immunogenic peptides based on DNA sequences, will soon provide such reagents. Several candidates for the *mos*-specific product have been reported from *in vitro* studies (16,33,40,55) and the actual Mo-MSV nucleotide sequence (42,43,48), as well as studies with temperature-sensitive (ts) mutants (10,46), strongly argues for the existence of such a protein. *In vitro* protein synthesis, using MSV-124 virion RNA as a template, reveals several products (16,33,40). The size of the major product, 37,000 daltons, is consistent with the size of the protein predicted from the Mo-MSV *mos* sequence (49).

DESCRIPTION OF THE Mo-MSV GENOME

Figure 1a shows a schematic representation of the proviral genomes of two Mo-MSV strains that have been cloned into bacteriophage λ (50). Figure 1b shows the structures of several subgenomic clones, derived from these genomic clones, which will be discussed below. The Mo-MSV proviral genome consists of Mo-MuLV and cellular derived sequences. The Mo-MuLV sequences include the 5' and 3' 588 base pair (bp) long terminal repeats (LTR) and additional unique sequences (including the t-RNA^{pro} primer binding site and variable portions of the *gag, pol,* and *env* genes). In the m1, HT1, and MSV-124 strains, the *mos* gene is located in the Mo-MuLV *env* gene near the 5' end of the *env* region, but each of these strains possesses different portions of the 3' *env* gene sequence (18,42,50). As will be discussed, only sequences in the LTR are required for activating *mos* transformation. Many of the sequences required for infectivity, i.e., helper virus-assisted rescue and integration, are also present in the LTR (9,17,43,48). However, certain portions of the conserved unique Mo-MuLV sequences, most notably the primer binding site, are presumably also required for infectivity. It is not yet evident how much contribution the remaining *gag, pol,* and *env* sequences make to the rescue process. Studies with Harvey sarcoma virus (Ha-MSV) suggest that few of the Mo-MuLV sequences are required (23,24), but it is not clear whether rat 30S sequences in Ha-MSV provide some rescue function. Our experiments demonstrating that only the 5' LTR and *gag, pol,* and *env* sequences 5' to *mos* are necessary for rescue by Mo-MuLV will be discussed below. Some of these sequences may affect *mos* expression as well, since sub-genomic sized RNA (mRNA?) containing *mos* sequences have been identified (19).

FIG. 1. a: Genomic proviral clones of two strains of Mo-MSV have been isolated in bacteriophage λ (50). **b:** Subgenomic fragments were subsequently subcloned into the plasmid pBR322 (50,51). Recombinant clones are shown schematically with relevant restriction sites. Restriction nucleases: R-EcoR1; Bg-Bgl II; H-Hind III; B-Bam HI; S-Sal I. The origin of the DNA sequences are: ——— MSV derived; ▨ LTR; ▉ v-*mos*; ☐ c-*mos*; .... pBR322; – – – – mink cell; 0000 λ; ∿∿∿ mouse cell; ◆ target site of Mo-MSV in HT1-MSV transformed mink cells.

clone   <u>a</u>

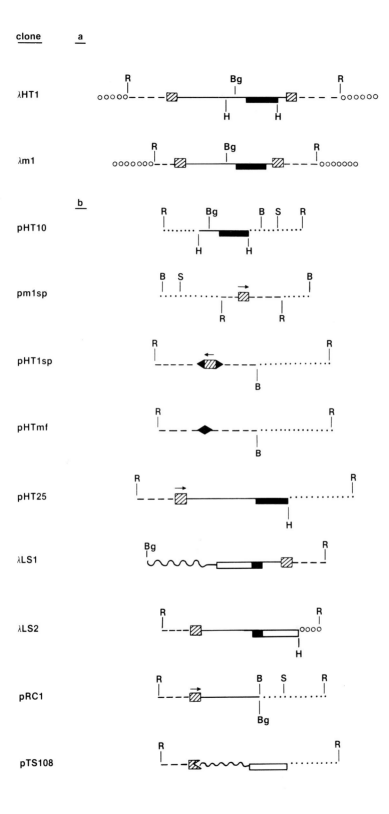

BIOLOGICAL ACTIVITY OF CLONED Mo-MSV

DNA copies and cloned proviruses of Mo-MSV have been shown to transform cultured cells morphologically in DNA transfection assays (2,11,15,52). The cloned proviruses of two Mo-MSV strains, m1 and HT1, show considerable focus forming activity ($\sim$ 40,000 ffu/p-mole) and Mo-MSV can be rescued from many of these foci following superinfection with Mo-MuLV helper virus (11). The data reviewed in Table 1 demonstrate that the *mos* and LTR sequences of Mo-MSV are responsible for morphological transformation of NIH 3T3 cells (11,12,35). Plasmid pHT10, containing v-*mos* and Mo-MuLV sequences (of *pol* and *env* origin) 5' to v-*mos*, transforms with low efficiency. Transformation efficiency is markedly stimulated in recombinants containing additional 5' or 3' portions of the provirus, as in pHT21 or pHT25. These data suggested that the LTR was responsible for enhancement, since the LTR was the only Mo-MuLV sequence common to both clones. Direct evidence for this LTR dependence was obtained from co-transfection analysis.

The plasmid recombinant pm1sp contains a single copy of the Mo-MSV LTR. The insert in this recombinant was obtained from a high frequency deletion derivative of λml that occurs during propagation of the phage recombinant in *Escherichia coli* (36). All unique Mo-MSV sequences and one LTR are deleted, whereas a single LTR and sequences flanking the integrated provirus (derived from the host) are conserved. This derivative was subcloned into pBR322 and is referred to as pm1sp. An analogous recombinant, pHT1sp was derived from λHT1 (36).

We have shown that co-transfection of plasmid recombinants containing LTR sequences with pHT10 markedly enhances v-*mos* transforming activity. The data is summarized in Table 2 (12,35) and shows that only the LTR-containing plasmids, pm1sp and pHT1sp, enhance transformation. The plasmid pHTmf (Fig. 1b), containing the unoccupied HT1-MSV integration site and lacking the Mo-MSV LTR, does not enhance the transforming activity of pHT10, whereas pHT1sp does. In addition, the data suggest that the LTR and v-*mos* co-transfected sequences must

TABLE 1. *Biological activity of intact and subgenomic Mo-MSV recombinant clones[a]*

Transfecting DNA[b]	Specific (ffu/pmole) activity[c]
Intact provirus	
m1-MSV fff 0000--------●●●●●---0000f'f'f'	46,000 ± 15,000 (17)
HT1-MSV FFFF0000----------●●●●●---0000F'F'F'F'	37,000 ± 29,000 (6)
Subgenomic fragments	
pHT10 ---●●●●●	44 ± 46 (15)
pHT25 FFFF0000----------●●●●●	7,800 ± 2,500 (2)
pm13 ---●●●●●---000f'f'f'	8,100 ± 4,100 (6)
pHT21 ---●●●●●---0000F'F'F'F'	6,900 ± 1,400 (2)

[a]Assays were performed by transfecting purified cloned DNA onto NIH 3T3 cells as previously described (11).

[b]The symbols represent: f, F = mink cell sequences; --- = Mo-MuLV derived sequences; 0000 = LTR; and ●●●●● = v-*mos*.

[c]Numbers in parenthesis indicate number of independent transfection assays. Activity is given as focus forming units per picomole of transfecting DNA.

TABLE 2. *Increased transformation following co-transfection of v-mos and LTR-containing plasmids*

Transfecting DNA[a]	Transformation efficiency[b]
pm1sp	0
pHT10	0–65
pHT10 + pm1sp (or pHT1sp)	1,700–2,200
pHT10 + pm1sp (separately precipitated)	170–450
pHT10 + pHTmf	0–43
pHT10 + pBR322	0–43

[a]200 ng plasmid per transfected dish (2.5 × 10³ NIH 3T3 cells). The plasmids were cut with either *Bam*H1 or *Sal* 1.
[b]Range of efficiencies (foci per picomole) for 4 or more separate determinations.

reassociate in the cell, since marked enhancement is only observed when both plasmids are co-precipitated with calcium. The reassociation mechanism may be analogous to that proposed for the co-transfection of nonselectable markers with the thymidine kinase gene (54).

The enhancement of pHT10 transformation by pm1sp is observed over a range from 50 to 200 ng of each plasmid transfected per plate (Fig. 2). At levels above 200 ng/plate, the number of foci/plate remains nearly constant or declines. This plateau of transforming activity appears to be due to the limitation of the system to accept high levels of specific DNA sequences. Thus, even pBR322 at high concentrations (> 200 ng/plate) will inhibit the ability of λml (at 10 to 50 ng/plate) to form foci (D. G. Blair, *unpublished observations*).

The maximum enhancement of transformation by pm1sp was determined by maintaining it at a constant level concentration while varying the concentration of pHT10 (Fig. 3). The highest efficiencies of transformation were observed when the level of pm1sp was 10 to 20 times the level of pHT10. Reduction of pm1sp relative to pHT10 results in a decrease in transformation (not shown). The low level transforming activity by pHT10 alone might be due to the acquisition of sequences with LTR-like properties during transfection from either the carrier or the host genomic DNA. If so, it is possible that such sequences could be isolated from normal cell DNA.

INFLUENCE OF VECTOR SEQUENCES ON CO-TRANSFECTION EFFICIENCY

The effect of vector sequences on the LTR enhancement of v-*mos* transformation has been analyzed by testing the effect of various restriction enzymes on co-transfection enhancement of transformation (Table 3). These analyses demonstrate that: (a) the ends of the restriction enzyme-cleaved plasmids need not be homologous (e.g., Sal I cleaved pHT10, co-transfected with BamH1 cleaved pm1sp, has the same efficiency of transformation as when both plasmids have been cut with BamH1);

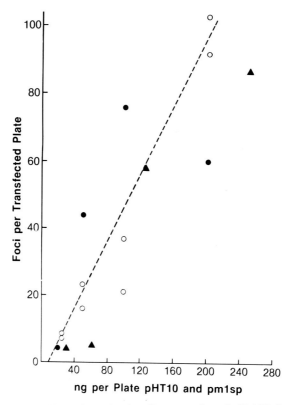

FIG. 2. The efficiency of focus formation in cells co-transfected with LTR (pm1sp) and v-*mos* (pHT10) are shown as a function of DNA added per transfected plate. All transfections were done at a molar ratio of 1. The different symbols represent independent experiments.

and (b) excision of the cloned v-*mos* sequence from the vector (as in Hind III digested pHT10) abolishes any enhancement of transforming activity whereas excision of the LTR-containing insert (pm1sp digested with *Eco*RI) reduces but does not eliminate enhancing activity. The vector sequence influence on pHT10 may be due to protection of the 3′ end open reading frame of the putative *mos* gene product. In pHT10, the Hind III site in pBR322 provides a putative translation termination signal for a *mos* product (Fig. 1b) (T. G. Wood, *unpublished observations*).

One curious feature of these analyses is that when circular DNA is transfected, enhancement is markedly reduced or virtually eliminated (Table 3). This may indicate that this DNA is either less efficiently acquired during transfection or is processed in a unique fashion compared to linearized DNA so as to exclude juxtapositioning of LTR and *mos* sequences.

The orientation of the *mos* sequence relative to the LTR in the vector has no apparent effect on the transforming activity of pHT10. Thus, pm1sp is in the opposite orientation in the vector relative to pHT1sp, but both enhance pHT10 transforming activity (Table 4) (12,35). In contrast, certain covalently linked recombinants fail

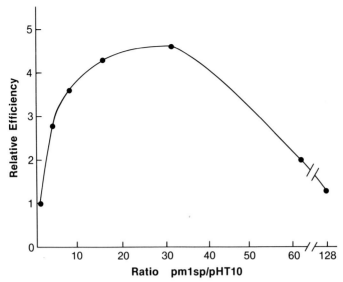

FIG. 3. The relative efficiency of focus formation in co-transfection is shown as a function of the ratio of *mos* (pHT10) to LTR (pm1sp) in the transfecting mixture. Both plasmids were cut with BamHI and were transfected in the presence of an excess (12 μg) of sheared calf thymus DNA. In all samples, the amount of pm1sp was constant (200 ng). The data shown are for a single experiment. In this experiment, 1.0 represents 2,100 ffu/pmole. Independent experiments show similar enhancements, although the absolute efficiencies vary over a two- to fourfold range.

TABLE 3. *Effect of endonuclease restriction on LTR co-transfection enhancement of v-mos transformation*

pHT10[a]	pm1sp	Transformation efficiency
Bam H1	Bam H1	1,700–2,000
Sal 1	Bam H1	1,300–1,700
Hind III	Bam H1	0
Bam H1	Eco RI	130–220
—	Bam H1	9–87
Bam H1	—	300–520
—	—	0–22

[a]200 ng of either pHT10 or pm1sp, treated with the restriction endonuclease indicated, were co-transfected onto NIH 3T3 cells. Where no enzyme is identified, uncut (circular) plasmids were used.

to transform. Thus, a hybrid recombinant containing v-*mos* with an LTR 3′ in the opposite permutation (i.e., in a position where it would effect transcription of the negative strand of the *mos* gene) is not active in the transformation assay. We expect that this arrangement occurs in co-transfected cells but does not score positively for transformation.

TABLE 4. *Effect of LTR orientation within the vector on co-transfection transformation frequencies*

mos orientation (pHT10)[a]	LTR orientation in pBR322 vector[a]	Transformation efficiency[b]
5′–3′	U3-R-U5 (pm1sp)	700–2,100
5′–3′	U5-R-U3 (pHTsp)	900–1,200

[a]200 ng plasmid per transfected dish (2.5 × 10³ NIH 3T3 cells). The plasmids were cut with either *Bam*H1 or *Sal* 1.
[b]Range of efficiencies (foci per picomole) for 4 or more separate determinations.

EFFECT OF LTR ON *MOS* EXPRESSION

We have demonstrated that an LTR placed 5′ to the normal cellular *mos* will activate its transforming potential (13,39). Hybrid recombinants with an LTR element placed in normal mouse sequences at variable distances 5′ to c-*mos* were able to transform NIH 3T3 cells at high efficiency. These results, coupled with the enhancing effect of the LTR sequences on v-*mos* transforming efficiency, suggest that the LTR functions to effect expression of adjacent sequences. The LTR can function either 5′ or 3′ to *mos*. However, in λLS1, a recombinant with the LTR 3′ to c-*mos*, the transforming efficiency is low (∼ 5 ffu/p-mole). In contrast, recombinants, where the LTR is 3′ to v-*mos*, transform efficiently (∼ 7,000 ffu/p-mole) (12,39) (Table 1). This difference in activity must reside in the differences between mouse sequences and Mo-MuLV derived sequences 5′ to *mos*. The low transformation frequency by the λLS1 recombinant may, as with pHT10 transfection, represent the low frequency acquisition of some biological function from the carrier or host DNA. With pHT10 we ascribed this to the acquisition of sequences with LTR-like transcription activation properties. However, we have not observed similar stimulation of λLS1 transforming activity when it is co-transfected with pm1sp (not shown).

At this point we can only speculate on the function of the LTR in enhancing or activating transformation by *mos*. We cannot exclude an LTR effect on stabilization and integration of *mos*, but some recombinants that lack the U⁵ and a portion of the R sequence (Fig. 4) still transform efficiently (13). It would be expected that both ends of the LTR would be necessary for it to function in integration.

The LTR activates expression of adjacent sequences (T. G. Wood, *unpublished observations*) and it is likely that this function is responsible for its co-transforming activity with *mos*. Putative transcription control sequences are present in the LTR (17,43), but these signals apparently serve only to align or start RNA transcription. A signal that appears to be associated with activation of transcription is the 72 base pair (bp) duplication (Fig. 4) (17). A 72 bp duplication exists in SV40 (8,25) with no sequence homology to the Mo-MSV LTR duplication but both are located the same distance upstream from sequences encoding the 5′ end of the mRNA (21). When this duplication is removed from SV40, the virus is prevented from replicating

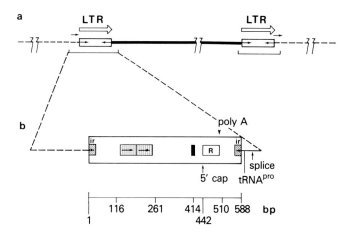

FIG. 4. The size and important structural features of the Mo-MSV proviral LTR are shown. ■ Hogness box; 72 bp direct repeats. The figure is drawn from data of Dhar et al. (17).

(25). Levinson et al. (31) have replaced the SV40 72 bp duplication with the Mo-MSV 72 bp duplication and demonstrated restoration of SV40 transcription and replication.

The evidence that we have presented previously (11,12,35) and reviewed here (Table 1) show that v-*mos* recombinants with the LTR 3′ to *mos* transform as efficiently as when the LTR is 5′ to *mos* (e.g., pHT21 versus pHT25) (Table 1). The RNA transcribed in cells transformed with recombinants such as pHT21 and pHT25 has been examined, and the sequence complexity of the transcript is consistent with the structure of the transfected DNA (T. G. Wood, *unpublished observations*). Thus, the LTR apparently activates transcription just as well 3′ to *mos* as it does 5′ to *mos*. It is not clear how such sequences activate expression. One of the pTS series has been modified to contain only the 72 bp repeats (pTS 108, Fig. 1b) of the Mo-MSV LTR, and preliminary experiments indicate that this recombinant transforms with low efficiency even though the entire 5′ RNA coding sequences have been removed.

RESCUE OF TRANSFORMING VIRUS

The above experiments demonstrated that only the LTR and *mos* elements are required for transformation. An understanding of how sequences like *mos* are transduced by retroviruses may provide a means for duplicating this scheme *in vitro*. As mentioned earlier, Goldfarb and Weinberg (24) have demonstrated that transforming virus can be rescued from cells transformed with 5′ subgenomic portions of Ha-MSV. They showed that the rescued Ha-MSV virus had acquired 3′ retroviral sequences, presumably from recombination with the helper Mo-MuLV 3′ sequences. Our experience with rescue of transforming virus from cells transformed with 5′ subgenomic fragments of Mo-MSV or with analogous recombinants containing c-*mos* instead of v-*mos* are summarized in Table 5. Plasmid pHT25 and the c-*mos* recombinant λLS$_2$ (Fig. 1b) both transform at high efficiency.

Mo-MuLV infection of either pHT25 or λLS$_2$ transformed cell clones results in the rescue of a low titer transforming virus from many of the independent clones. Secondary virus transformants yield normal titers and ratios of focus forming to helper virus units. As mentioned earlier, the RNA expressed in the parental pHT25 and λLS$_2$ transformants does not contain 3' retroviral sequences (T. G. Wood, *unpublished observations*). It is expected that the viral RNA in secondary foci have regenerated 3' viral sequences in a manner analogous to the rescue of subgenomic Ha-MSV fragments (24).

The enhancement of pHT10 transformation by co-transfection with LTR elements is presumably due to the juxtaposition of plasmids in the transformed cells. To test this, we asked whether plasmid pRC1 (containing the LTR and *gag* sequences derived from the 5' end of Mo-MuLV) would enhance transformation as well as provide sufficient Mo-MuLV information for transforming viruses to be rescued. The experiments have been performed in two ways: the recombinant plasmids pRC1 and pHT10 were digested with Bgl II and then were either ligated prior to transfection (before the addition of carrier DNA) or were mixed with carrier DNA and co-transfected. The results (Table 5) show that the enhancement by pRC1 is significant, relative to the transforming activity of pHT10 alone, in both the ligated and co-transfected samples. The enhancement of the co-transfected sample might be expected to be considerably lower because of dilution by carrier DNA, but this was not observed. The co-transfected DNA must reassociate in the transfected cell since many of the individual foci were rescuable. Surprisingly, we find only a twofold difference in the number of rescuable transformants whether the samples were ligated or co-transfected, and the fraction of rescuable foci is similar to those observed with pHT25 or λLS$_2$ transformants. These experiments suggest that it may be possible to "rescue" a variety of selectable phenotypes from genomic DNA.

CONCLUSIONS

Rescue-Transduction of c-*onc*

The models presented in Fig. 5 were developed from our experiments and the results of Hayward et al. (27) and Payne et al. (41). They suggest both how

TABLE 5. *Recovery of infectious Mo-MSV from cells transformed by subgenomic fragments*

	pHT25	λLS2	pRC1 + pHT10	
			Ligated	Unligated
DNA infectivity (ffu/pmole)	7,800	2,700	670	400
Rescuable foci	9/33	4/6	6/9	7/24
Titer of MSV released by 1° foci[a]	2–30	800	4–50	10–20
Ratio Mo-MSV/Mo-MLV in 1° foci	3–5 × 10^{-4}	NT	<10^{-4}	<10^{-4}
Titer of Mo-MSV released by 2° foci	10^3–10^5	3 × 10^4	>10^3	>10^3

[a]Titer is given as focus forming units per ml.

Integration

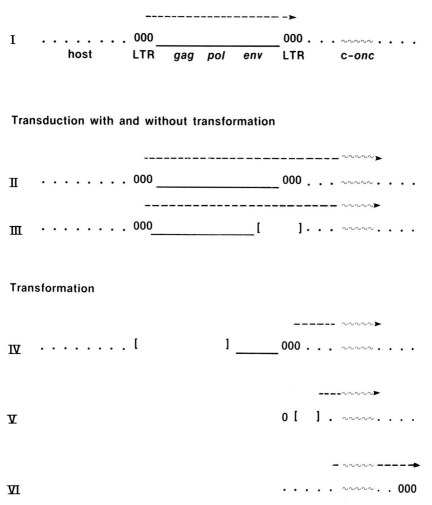

FIG. 5. Models for mechanisms of viral-induced transformation and translation of cellular oncogenes. The sequence c-*onc* represents any cellular sequence with transforming potential. The *broken line* (––– >) indicates the extent and polarity of RNA synthesis off the indicated DNA sequence.

nontransforming retroviruses can activate cell genes with transforming potential and how they might transduce these genes into viruses. Retroviruses integrate at multiple sites in the host chromosome (30,47). These models show retrovirus integration adjacent to a cellular gene with transforming potential (c-*onc*; line I, Fig. 5). The most abundant expression occurs between the LTR elements, yielding viral transcripts (line I, Fig. 5). Although the possibility exists for the expression of adjacent sequences—downstream promotion (27)—sufficient expression of c-*onc* to produce cellular transformation may not always occur. Nevertheless, a c-*onc* containing RNA transcript could be encapsidated into virions. Subsequent deletion (loss of 3′ LTR or U3-sequences) and recombination (acquisition of helper-derived U3 sequences 3′ to c-*onc*) could occur during infection and integration to yield a transforming retrovirus. This virus could infect other target cells (perhaps of a different cell type from the one in which the transcript was produced) and result in neoplastic transformation as a result of elevated c-*onc* expression (line III, Fig. 5). This sequence could only be rescued as a virus if the cell was expressing a second competent helper virus. Since an *env* gene product would prevent reinfection with a helper virus either the cell would have to be dually infected at the time of integration or expression of the *env* gene product by the provirus would also have to be abolished to allow superinfection and rescue by a competent helper virus. The line III model is consistent with the Ha-MSV rescue (23) and Mo-MSV rescue in experiments with pHT25, λLS$_2$, and pRC1-v-*mos* (Table 5).

Transformation

A deletion of the 5′ LTR (line IV, Fig. 5) could result in elevated expression of c-*onc*. This arrangement was observed most frequently in the bursal lymphoma tumors by Hayward et al. We have stated that preliminary data suggests the 72 bp duplication in the LTR (pTS108) may be sufficient to activate c-*mos*. This is shown in line V (Fig. 5). Another arrangement of LTR and c-*onc* has been observed, which may be analogous in some ways to the model shown in line V. Payne et al. (41) have found a bursal tumor in which the LTR of RAV-2 is inserted in the opposite permutation (direction) from that shown in line III or IV. It is possible that the transcription activation sequence in the RAV-2 LTR, equated with the 72 bp repeat, enhances c-*myc* expression. We have also discussed activation by LTRs located 3′ to v-*mos* and c-*mos*. This is depicted in line VI (Fig. 5) and is analogous to one arrangement of the RAV-2 LTR and c-*myc* reported by Payne et al. (41) in bursal lymphomas. There may be other arrangements that result in neoplastic transformation or retrovirus transduction of cellular genes. Further analysis of spontaneous and virus-induced tumors coupled with model studies utilizing retroviral transforming and transcription control elements such as we have described should produce an understanding of the neoplastic transformation process. The study of transformation by the activation of cellular sequences may already show many similarities between oncogenesis by both viral and nonviral agents.

ACKNOWLEDGMENTS

We thank T. Wood, P. Gruss, B. Levinson, G. Khoury, G. Payne, J. M. Bishop, and H. Varmus for communicating their results to us prior to publication. We also thank C. Cooper and M. Tainsky for reviewing the manuscript, and K. Cannon and K. Barry for preparing the manuscript.

REFERENCES

1. Aaronson, S. A., Bassin, R. H., and Weaver, C. (1972): Comparison of murine sarcoma viruses in nonproducer and S⁺L⁻ transformed cells. *J. Virol.*, 9:701–704.
2. Andersson, P., Goldfarb, M. P., and Weinberg, R. A. (1979): A defined subgenomic fragment of an *in vitro* synthesized Moloney sarcoma virus DNA can induce cell transformation upon transfection. *Cell*, 16:63–75.
3. Ball, J. K., Hub, T. Y., and McCarter, J. A. (1964): On the statistical distribution of epidermal papillomata in mice. *Brit. J. Cancer*, 18:120–123.
4. Ball, J. K., McCarter, J. A., and Sunderland, S. M. (1973): Evidence for helper independent murine sarcoma virus. I. Segregation of replication-defective and transformation-defective viruses. *Virology*, 56:268–284.
5. Baltimore, D. (1974): Tumor viruses. *Cold Spring Harbor Symp. Quant. Biol.*, 39:1187–1200.
6. Bassin, R. H., Phillips, L. A., Kramer, M. J., Haapala, D. K., Peebles, P. T., Nomura, S., and Fischinger, P. J. (1971): Transformation of mouse 3T3 cells by murine sarcoma virus: Release of virus-like particles in the absence of replicating murine leukemia helper virus. *Proc. Natl. Acad. Sci. USA*, 68:1520–1524.
7. Bassin, R. H., Tuttle, N., and Fischinger, P. J. (1970): Isolation of murine sarcoma virus-transformed mouse cells which are negative for leukemia virus from agar suspension cultures. *Int. J. Cancer*, 6:95–107.
8. Benoit, C., and Chambon, P. (1981): In vivo sequence requirements of the SV40 early promoter region. *Nature*, 239:304–310.
9. Benz, E. W., Jr., Wydro, R. M., Nadal-Genard, B., and Dina, D. (1980): Moloney murine sarcoma proviral DNA is a transcriptional unit. *Nature*, 288:665–669.
10. Blair, D. G., Hull, M. A., and Finch, E. A. (1979): The isolation and preliminary characterization of temperature-sensitive transformation mutants of Moloney sarcoma virus. *Virology*, 95:303–316.
11. Blair, D. G., McClements, W. L., Oskarsson, M. K., Fischinger, P. J., and Vande Woude, G. F. (1980): Biological activity of cloned Moloney sarcoma virus DNA: Terminally redundant sequences may enhance transformation efficiency. *Proc. Natl. Acad. Sci. USA*, 77:3504–3508.
12. Blair, D. G., Oskarsson, M., McClements, W. L., and Van de Woude, G. F. (1981): The long terminal repeat of Moloney sarcoma provirus enhances transformation. In: *Haematology and Blood Transfusion, Modern Trends in Human Leukemia IV* edited by R. Neth, R. C. Gallo, T. Graff, K. Mannweiler, and K. Winkler, Vol. 26, pp. 460–466. Springer-Verlag, Berlin, Heidelberg.
13. Blair, D. G., Oskarsson, M., Wood, T. G., McClements, W. L., Fischinger, P. J., and Vande Woude, G. F. (1981): Activation of the transforming potential of a normal cell sequence: A molecular model for oncogenesis. *Science*, 212:941–943.
14. Canaani, E., and Aaronson, S. A. (1980): Isolation and characterization of naturally occurring deletion mutants of Moloney murine sarcoma virus. *Virology*, 105:456–466.
15. Canaani, E., Robbins, K. C., and Aaronson, S. A. (1979): The transforming gene of Moloney murine sarcoma virus. *Nature*, 282:378–383.
16. Cramer, K., Reddy, E. P., and Aaronson, S. A. (1981): Translational products of Moloney murine sarcoma virus RNA: Identification of proteins encoded by the murine sarcoma virus *src* gene. *J. Virol.*, 38:704–711.
17. Dhar, R., McClements, W., Enquist, L., and Vande Woude, G. F. (1980): Nucleotide sequences of integrated Moloney sarcoma virus long terminal repeats and their viral and host junctions. *Proc. Natl. Acad. Sci. USA*, 77:3937–3941.
18. Donoghue, D. J., Sharp, P. A., and Weinberg, R. A. (1979): Comparative study of different isolates of murine sarcoma virus. *J. Virol.*, 32:1015–1027.
19. Donoghue, D. J., Sharp, P. A., and Weinberg, R. A. (1979): An MSV-specific subgenomic fragment of an *in vitro* synthesized Moloney sarcoma virus DNA can induce cell transformation upon transfection. *Cell*, 16:63–75.
20. Fischinger, P. J., Nomura, S., Peebles, P. T., Haapala, D. K., and Bassin, R. H. (1972): Reversion of murine sarcoma virus-transformed cells: Variants without a rescuable sarcoma virus. *Science*, 176:1033–1035.
21. Fischinger, P. J., Nomura, S., Tuttle-Fuller, N., and Dunn, K. J. (1974): Revertants of mouse cells transformed by murine sarcoma virus. III. Metastable expression of virus functions in revertants retransformed by murine sarcoma virus. *Virology*, 59:217–229.

22. Frankel, A. E., and Fischinger, P. J. (1977): Rate of divergence of cellular sequences homologous to segments of Moloney sarcoma virus. *J. Virol.*, 21:153–160.

23. Goldfarb, M. P., and Weinberg, R. A. (1981): Structure of the provirus within NIH 3T3 cells transfected with Harvey sarcoma virus DNA. *J. Virol.*, 38:125–135.

24. Goldfarb, M. P., and Weinberg, R. A. (1981): Generation of novel, biologically active Harvey sarcoma viruses via apparent illegitimate recombination. *J. Virol.*, 38:136–150.

25. Gruss, P., Dhar, R., and Khoury, G. (1981): Simian virus 40 tandem repeated sequences as an element of the early promoter. *Proc. Natl. Acad. Sci. USA*, 78:943–947.

26. Harvey, J. J., and East, J. (1971): The murine sarcoma virus. *Int. Rev. Exp. Pathol.*, 10:265–360.

27. Hayward, W., Neel, B., and Astrin, S. (1981): Activation of a cellular *onc* gene by promoter insertion in ALV-induced lymphoid leukosis. *Nature*, 290:475–480.

28. Hu, S., Davidson, N., and Verma, I. (1977): A heteroduplex study of the sequence relationships between the RNAs of M-MSV and M-MLV. *Cell*, 10:469–477.

29. Huebner, R. J., Hartley, J. W., Rowe, W. P., Lane, W. T., and Capps, W. I. (1966): Rescue of the defective genome of Moloney sarcoma virus from a noninfectious hamster tumor and the production of pseudotype sarcoma viruses with various leukemia viruses. *Proc. Natl. Acad. Sci. USA*, 56:1164–1169.

30. Hughes, S., Shank, P., Spector, D., Kung, H. J., Bishop, J., Varmus, H., Vogt, P., and Breitman, M. (1978): Proviruses of avian sarcoma virus are terminally redundant, co-extensive with unintegrated linear DNA and integrated at many sites. *Cell*, 15:1397–1410.

31. Levinson, B., Khoury, G., Vande Woude, G., and Gruss, P. (1981): Activation of the SV40 genome by the 72 base pair tandem repeat of Moloney sarcoma virus. *Nature (in press)*.

32. Levy, J. P., and Leclerc, J. C. (1977): The murine sarcoma virus-induced tumor: Exception or general model in tumor immunology? *Adv. Cancer Res.*, 24:1–66.

33. Lyons, D. D., Murphy, E. C., Mong, S. M., and Arlinghaus, R. B. (1980): The translation products of Moloney murine sarcoma virus-124 RNA. *Virology*, 105:60–70.

34. Maisel, J., Dina, D., and Duesberg, P. H. (1977): Murine sarcoma viruses: The helper independence reported for a Moloney variant is unconfirmed. Distinct strains differ in the size of their RNAs. *Virology*, 76:295–312.

35. McClements, W. L., Dhar, R., Blair, D. G., Enquist, L., Oskarsson, M., and Vande Woude, G. F. (1981): The long terminal repeat of Moloney sarcoma provirus. *Cold Spring Harbor Symp. Quant. Biol.*, 45:699–705.

36. McClements, W. L., Enquist, L. W., Oskarsson, M., Sullivan, M., and Vande Woude, G. F. (1980): Frequent site-specific deletion of coliphage λ murine sarcoma virus recombinants and its use in the identification of a retrovirus integration site. *J. Virol.*, 35:488–497.

37. McClements, W. L., and Vande Woude, G. F. (1981): Cloning retroviruses: Retrovirus cloning? In: *Genetic Engineering*, edited by J. K. Setlow and A. Hollaender, pp. 89–107. Plenum Press, New York.

38. Moloney, J. B. (1966): Biological studies on a lymphoid leukemia virus extracted from sarcoma S37. I. Origin and introductory investigations. *Natl. Cancer Inst. Monogr.*, 22:139–142.

39. Oskarsson, M., McClements, W. L., Blair, D. G., Maizel, J. V., and Vande Woude, G. F. (1980): Properties of a normal mouse cell DNA sequence *(sarc)* homologous to the *src* sequence of Moloney sarcoma virus. *Science*, 207:1222–1224.

40. Papkoff, J., Hunter, T., and Beemon, K. (1980): In vitro translation of virion RNA from Moloney murine sarcoma virus. *Virology*, 101:91–103.

41. Payne, G. S., Bishop, J. M., and Varmus, H. E. (1981): Multiple arrangements of viral DNA and an activated host oncogene (c-*myc*) in bursal lymphomas. *Cell (in press)*.

42. Reddy, E. P., Smith, M. J., and Aaronson, S. A. (1981): Complete nucleotide sequence and organization of the Moloney murine sarcoma virus genome. *Science*, 214:445–450.

43. Reddy, E. P., Smith, M. J., Canaani, E., Robbins, K. C., Tronick, S. R., Zain, S., and Aaronson, S. A. (1980): Nucleotide sequence analysis of the transforming region and large terminal redundancies of Moloney murine sarcoma virus. *Proc. Natl. Acad. Sci. USA*, 77:5234–5238.

44. Robey, W. G., Kuenzel, W. J., Vande Woude, G. F., and Fischinger, P. J. (1982): Growth of murine sarcoma and murine xenotropic leukemia viruses in Japanese quail. I. Induction of tumors and development of continuous tumor lines. *Cancer Res. (in press)*.

45. Robey, W. G., Oskarsson, M. K., Vande Woude, G. F., Naso, R. B., Arlinghaus, R. B., Haapala, D. K., and Fischinger, P. J. (1977): Cells transformed by certain strains of Moloney sarcoma virus contain murine p60. *Cell*, 10:79–89.

46. Somers, K., and Kit, S. (1973): Temperature-dependent expression of transformation by a cold-sensitive mutant of murine sarcoma virus. *Proc. Natl. Acad. Sci. USA*, 70:2206–2210.
47. Steffen, D., and Weinberg, R. (1978): The integrated genome of murine leukemia virus. *Cell*, 15:1003–1010.
48. Sutcliffe, J. G., Shinnick, T. M., Verma, I. M., and Lerner, R. A. (1980): Nucleotide sequence of Moloney leukemia virus: 3' end reveals details of replication, analogy to bacterial transposons and an unexpected gene. *Proc. Natl. Acad. Sci. USA*, 77:3302–3306.
49. Van Beveren, C., Goddard, J. G., Jonas, V., Berns, A. J. M., Doolittle, R. F., Donoghue, D. J., and Verma, I. (1981): The nucleotide sequence and formation of the transforming gene of a mouse sarcoma virus. *Nature*, 289:258–262.
50. Vande Woude, G. F., Oskarsson, M., Enquist, L. W., Nomura, S., Sullivan, M., and Fischinger, P. J. (1979): Cloning of integrated Moloney sarcoma proviral DNA sequences in bacteriophage λ. *Proc. Natl. Acad. Sci. USA*, 76:4464–4468.
51. Vande Woude, G. F., Oskarsson, M., McClements, W., Enquist, L., Blair, D., Fischinger, P., Maizel, J., and Sullivan, M. (1980): Characterization of integrated Moloney sarcoma provirus and flanking sequences cloned in bacteriophage lambda. *Cold Spring Harbor Symp. Quant. Biol.*, 44:735–746.
52. Verma, I. M., Lai, M-H. T., Bosselman, R. A., McKennet, M. A., Fan, H., and Berns, A. (1980): Molecular cloning of unintegrated Moloney mouse sarcoma virus DNA in bacteriophage λ. *Proc. Natl. Acad. Sci. USA*, 77:1773–1777.
53. Weiss, R. A., Teich, N. M., Varmus, H., and Coffin, J. M. (eds.) (1982): *RNA Tumor Viruses, Monograph 10C, Part 3, Molecular Biology of Tumor Viruses*. Cold Spring Harbor Laboratory, New York.
54. Wigler, M., Sweet, R., Sim, G. K., Wold, B., Pellicer, A., Lacy, E., Moniatis, T., Silverstein, S., and Axel, R. (1979): Transformation of mammalian cells with genes of prokaryotes and eukaryotes. *Cell*, 16:777–785.
55. Wood, T. G., Peltier-Horn, J., Robey, W. G., Blair, D. G., and Arlinghaus, R. B. (1980): Characterization of virus-specified proteins present in NRK cells infected with a temperature-sensitive transformation mutant of Moloney murine sarcoma virus. *Cold Spring Harbor Symp. Quant. Biol.*, 44:747–754.

Note added in proof

Papkoff et al. (*Cell*, 27:109–119, 1981; *Cell*, 1982, *in press*) have recently identified a 37,000 dalton protein made *in vitro* off MSV-124 viral RNA and present in MSV-124 transformed cells. This protein was detected using an antisera made against a synthetic polypeptide whose sequence represents the C-terminal 12 amino acids deduced from the MSV-*mos* DNA sequence. It appears to represent the product of the *mos* gene.

Advances in Viral Oncology, Volume 1,
edited by George Klein. Raven Press,
New York © 1982.

Avian Leukosis Viruses: Activation of Cellular "Oncogenes"

*William S. Hayward, **Benjamin G. Neel, and †Susan M. Astrin

*Sloan-Kettering Institute for Cancer Research, New York, New York 10021; **The Rockefeller University, New York, New York 10021; and †The Institute for Cancer Research, Fox Chase Cancer Center, Philadelphia, Pennsylvania 19111

The avian leukosis viruses (ALVs) belong to a class of RNA tumor viruses of both avian and mammalian origin that lack oncogenes. Although often classified as "nontransforming" viruses because of their inability to induce morphologic transformation at a detectable frequency in tissue culture cells, these viruses induce neoplastic disease at high frequency in experimentally infected animals and in nature. Neoplasms appear, however, only after a long latent period of several months or more. Thus, these viruses can be more accurately classified as "slowly transforming" retroviruses. In contrast, the "rapidly transforming" retroviruses, such as Rous sarcoma virus and the acute leukemia viruses, induce neoplastic disease within weeks after infection, and cause rapid transformation of target cells in tissue culture. Viruses of this type contain oncogenes (or "onc" genes), which encode transforming proteins.

The absence of onc genes in ALV and other slowly transforming retroviruses has stimulated considerable interest in this class of viruses. Recent studies with ALV suggest that these viruses exert their oncogenic potential by activating specific cellular genes—cellular counterparts of the known oncogenes of rapidly transforming retroviruses. In this chapter we will discuss some of the biological and genetic properties of the avian leukosis viruses. The major focus, however, will be on the mechanism by which these viruses induce neoplastic disease.

IDENTIFICATION OF GENETIC SEQUENCES INVOLVED IN VIRAL ONCOGENESIS

All of the rapidly transforming retroviruses contain genetic information that is not present in the slowly transforming viruses. In most cases, these sequences have been shown, by a combination of genetic and biochemical experiments, to encode proteins that are directly responsible for transformation (see chapters by Goff and Baltimore; Ellis, Lowy, and Scolnick; Moscovici and Gazzolo; Wong-Staal and Gallo). More than a dozen such genes, which are called collectively viral "onc" (v-onc) genes, have been identified in different virus isolates from avian or mammalian sources (25). The prototype is the transforming gene of Rous sarcoma virus, v-*src*, which encodes a 60K protein (17,88) that possesses a protein kinase activity (28,69) with specificity for tyrosine residues (29,61). As first demonstrated in the Rous sarcoma virus (RSV) system (114), there is a cellular gene (c-*onc*) corresponding to each of the v-*onc* genes (7,21,22,42,80,94,100,102,103,104,108,112; for reviews, see refs. 11,41,51). The v-*onc* genes of rapidly transforming viruses have apparently been derived from the cellular genes through some as yet unknown recombination mechanism (48,64,125).

The normal functions of the c-*onc* genes are unknown, but these genes are highly conserved in all vertebrates (7,94,100,104,112), and even in some invertebrates (R. Weinberg, *personal communication*), suggesting that they play an essential role in the host cell. The c-*onc* genes are expressed at low levels in most normal cells (7,21,52,102,104,111,126; for a review, see ref. 11). However, Chen (21) has reported an elevated expression of one such gene (c-*myb*) in certain early hematopoietic cells, and other groups have recently found tissue-specific expression of several c-*onc* genes (cf. ref. 104; C.-K. Shih et al., *unpublished*; T. Gonda, *personal communication*; D. Stehelin, *personal communication*). It is possible that the c-*onc* genes play a role in the differentiation or growth regulation of specific cell lineages.

With the exception of RSV (and the closely related B-77 virus), all of the rapidly transforming viruses are defective. In the defective transforming viruses, internal viral sequences that encode proteins required for replication have been replaced by the cellular sequences. The location, size, and genetic content of the insert varies (see Fig. 1), but all of these viruses have retained at least some viral sequences at the 5' and 3' ends of their genomes—sequences that encode important recognition sites involved in replication, transcription, packaging, and integration.

The slowly transforming viruses, which include the avian and mammalian lymphoid leukosis viruses [e.g., ALV, murine leukemia virus (MuLV), feline leukemia virus (FeLV)] as well as the murine mammary tumor virus (MMTV), do not appear to contain transforming genes. The prototypes for this class of viruses are the avian leukosis viruses (ALVs), first described by Ellerman and Bang in 1908 (40). Since many ALV strains were originally isolated as helper viruses associated with the defective Bryan strain of Rous sarcoma virus, ALV isolates have often been called Rous associated viruses (RAV). Similar helper viruses have been found associated with acute leukemia viruses—for example, MCAV (MC29-associated virus), EAV (avian erythroblastosis virus-associated virus), and MAV (myeloblastosis virus-associated virus). More obscure nomenclature has also been used, including RPL (regional poultry laboratory) and YAV ("yet another virus"). Deletion mutants of RSV ("transformation defective" or "td" viruses), which have lost the *src* gene and the ability to induce rapidly developing sarcomas, are still able to induce slowly developing neoplasms (10,85).

Although most exogenous ALVs induce neoplastic disease, the endogenous ALV, RAV-0, appears to be essentially nononcogenic in chickens (36,72). A comparison of the genomes of exogenous ALVs and RAV-0 revealed differences primarily near the 3' end of the genome (within the *env* and "c" regions) (24,52,57,76; S. Hughes,

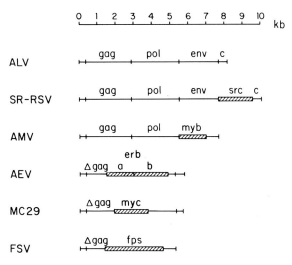

FIG. 1. Genomic RNAs of the slowly transforming retrovirus, ALV, and of representative rapidly transforming avian retroviruses. Rapidly transforming retroviruses include Schmidt-Ruppin strain of Rous sarcoma virus (SR-RSV), avian myeloblastosis virus (AMV), avian erythroblastosis virus (AEV), myelocytomatosis virus-29 (MC29), and Fujinami sarcoma virus (FSV). Viral genes encode the structural proteins (*gag* gene), reverse transcriptase (*pol*), and the envelope glycoprotein *(env)*. The "c" region, which apparently does not encode a protein, includes sequences (U3 + R) that form part of the long terminal repeat (LTR) of proviral DNA (see Fig. 2), plus other sequences of unknown function. Oncogenes of the rapidly transforming viruses, shown in *cross-hatched* boxes, are labeled according to recently adopted nomenclature (25). These sequences are of cellular origin, apparently acquired by recombination. (Adapted from ref. 54.)

personal communication). Since all known endogenous ALVs have envelope glycoprotein with the same host range specificity (subgroup E) (91), it seemed possible that this specificity had some role in oncogenesis.

The possible role of the ALV *env* gene in oncogenesis was tested by examining the oncogenicity and genetic composition of RAV-60 type virus isolates (35,92,121). These viruses, originally isolated from chicken cells infected with various exogenous viruses (50), are recombinants (53,107) which have acquired most of their genetic information from the exogenous virus, but have acquired the *env* gene, with subgroup E host range, from endogenous proviruses. All RAV-60 isolates tested, unlike RAV-0, caused lymphomas in susceptible chickens (35,92). Thus, the oncogenic potential was not related to the subgroup E envelope specificity.

Comparison of RAV-60 genomes with those of the exogenous and endogenous parents demonstrated that all of these recombinants had "c" region information from the exogenous parent (35,92,121). This region does not appear to encode a protein (37; S. Hughes, *personal communication*). The "c" region, as originally defined (124), includes sequences encoding portions of the long terminal repeat (LTR) (U3 + R) plus some additional sequences (located upstream from U3) of unknown function. Although it is tempting to speculate that the low oncogenicity of RAV-0 reflects an inability of the endogenous virus promoter (located within the U3 region) to activate a c-*onc* gene (92,121) (see later), this explanation may not be satisfactory. Weiss and Frisby (127) have recently shown that RAV-0 induces lymphomas with high frequency (approximately 50%) in Sonnerat Junglefowl. RAV-0, which replicates poorly in most hosts (49), replicates to high titers in the Junglefowl. The rather variable replication ability of RAV-0 in different hosts, which appears to be influenced by the "c" region (35,121), certainly plays some role in its oncogenicity. But other viral and host-related factors may also be important (J. Coffin and H. Robinson, personal communication).

PATHOGENICITY OF ALV

Avian leukosis viruses induce a variety of neoplastic and nonneoplastic diseases. The most common neoplasm is B-cell lymphoma, but other neoplasms such as fibrosarcomas, nephroblastomas, and erythroblastosis are also induced in some ALV-infected birds (85,86).

The incidence and spectrum of diseases can vary widely, depending on such factors as virus titer, site of injection, age of the bird at the time of infection, and genetic makeup of the virus and host. In general, the incidence of neoplasia is highest (often as high as 80–90%) in birds that are infected either in the embryo, or during the first few weeks after hatching. This presumably reflects a greater susceptibility to virus infection at early stages, when the immune system is not yet fully developed. Burmester et al. (19) have reported both age-dependent and virus titer-dependent differences in the incidence of specific neoplasms. Using RPL-12 virus (a field isolate, containing a mixture of ALVs), they observed a high incidence of erythroleukemia in birds infected with high virus titers, or at early times (within one week after hatching). Lower virus titers, or later times of infection, favored development of lymphomas. Bacon et al. (5) observed a high incidence (up to 25%) of erythroleukemia in line 15I chickens infected with RAV-1, a virus that induces primarily B-cell lymphomas in most birds. These studies indicated that the incidence of erythroleukemia was strongly influenced by the B-haplotype of the chicken. As mentioned above, the endogenous virus RAV-0 induces neoplastic disease with low efficiency in chickens (36,72), but induces lymphomas at high frequency in Sonnerat Junglefowl (127).

Development of B-cell lymphomas in ALV-infected birds appears to be a multistage process (32,77). The first morphologic change observed is the appearance of "transformed follicles" in the bursa at about 2 months of age in birds infected shortly after hatching. As many as 10 to 100 such follicles per bursa have been reported (77). At later times, most of these follicles regress, possibly as a result of the normal physiologic regression of the bursa at 4 to 6 months of age. Transformed nodules (one or a few per bird) are observed at about 3 months, followed by clearly defined tumors and metastasis to other organs such as liver, kidney, and spleen. Death usually occurs only after extensive metastasis. Tumor cells contain surface IgM (33), suggesting that the target cell is an immature B-cell; apparently, transformation causes a differentiation block prior to the switch from IgM to IgG or IgA.

B-cell lymphomas are not induced in bursectomized animals, though other neoplasms occur (18,83,84,87). Bursectomy as late as 12 weeks after infection prevents development of metastatic tumors (32), and bursectomy as late as 5 months greatly reduces the incidence of metastasis in most birds (84). Thymectomy has no apparent influence on lymphoma development (83).

Little is known about the early stages in development of other ALV-induced neoplasms, such as nephroblastomas, fibrosarcomas, and leukemias.

Osteopetrosis, a proliferative disease affecting the bones, is often found at later times in ALV-infected birds (86). Smith and Ivanyi (109), however, have isolated a "helper" virus, MAV-2(0), from AMV stocks, which induces a high incidence of osteopetrosis, with very short latency (2–6 weeks). Recent studies (R. E. Smith, *personal communication*) indicate that the agent responsible for this disease is a minor component of the MAV-2(0) population. It is interesting to note that the high incidence and rapid appearance of osteopetrosis occurs only when virus is injected into early embryos.

Tsichlis and Coffin (121) have isolated a recombinant virus, NTRE-7, which induces few early lymphomas, but causes a low incidence of a variety of neoplasms at late times (> 12 months) (J. M. Coffin and H. Robinson, *personal communication*). Neither of the parent viruses (RAV-0 and a tdPR-B isolate) induces lymphomas at early times (< 12 months), but tdPR-B causes a high incidence of osteopetrosis and induces a low incidence of a variety of neoplasms at late times.

Other diseases associated with ALV infection include anemia, cachexia, and a "nonneoplastic syndrome" (NNS) that appears early (6–12 weeks) after infection. NNS appears to be an autoimmune disease, characterized by a variety of lesions, including ascites, shrunken heart and liver, hepatitis, atrophy of the bursa, and death (34). Interestingly, the disease is found only in birds that are not expressing endogenous proviral information. Up to 50% of such birds die within 12 weeks. The disease may be caused by a hyperimmune response directed against viral antigens. Birds expressing endogenous viral genes may have a degree of tolerance and, therefore, do not develop a strong immune response against the viral antigens.

Birds that lack endogenous proviruses (*ev*-negative; ref. 2) are particularly susceptible to NNS. However, a normal incidence of lymphoma (30–40%) was observed among ALV-infected *ev*-negative birds that survived longer than 12 weeks (*unpublished data*).

ACTIVATION OF A CELLULAR *ONC* GENE BY ALV

Certain characteristics of the virus life cycle have suggested a mechanism by which ALV and other slowly transforming viruses might activate a potentially oncogenic cellular gene. As an essential part of their life cycle, retroviruses synthesize a double-stranded DNA copy of the RNA genome (6,120). The DNA then becomes integrated into the host cell chromosome, where it is stably associated with the cellular DNA. Integration occurs at many sites within the host cell chromosome—possibly at random (4,26,59,70,89,90,105,113,119).

An important characteristic of the integrated viral DNA (provirus) is the presence of LTR sequences flanking the coding sequences of the virus (58,59,96,98). Located within the LTRs are recognition signals involved in, among other things, initiation of transcription and poly(A) addition (9,37,39,63,70,105,106,115,116,122,129; for review, see ref. 54). Synthesis of viral mRNA (and genomic RNA) initiates within the left LTR, and poly(A) addition occurs within the right LTR. The LTR contains a sequence similar to the TATA box, which is thought to be involved, in some way, in the proper positioning of RNA polymerase II (for reviews, see refs. 54,130). Other sequences upstream from the TATA box are probably involved in polymerase binding and in regulation of transcriptional activity.

Since the left and right LTRs are identical, it might be expected that initiation would also occur within the right LTR. Transcription from the right LTR, and reading into adjacent cellular sequences, could cause enhanced expression of the cellular gene. Thus, if the provirus integrated adjacent to a cellular gene with oncogenic potential (a c-*onc* gene), transcriptional activation of this gene might induce neoplastic transformation. This model, which we have called the "promoter insertion" model for oncogenesis (55,56,73), is illustrated schematically in Fig. 2.

Initial experiments designed to test this hypothesis were based on the following predictions of the model:

1. Tumors should be clonal. Since the provirus integrates at many sites, possibly at random, integration at a site capable of activating a c-*onc* gene would be a rare event, probably occurring only once or a few times in a single animal. Spread of neoplastic disease would occur primarily by proliferation of the initial target cell, rather than by spread of virus (as occurs with Rous sarcoma virus and other viruses that carry their own oncogene).

2. Independently derived ALV-induced tumors should contain proviruses integrated at common sites. The number of cellular genes that possess the potential to

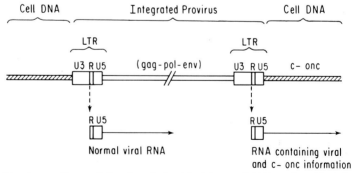

FIG. 2. Structure and transcriptional products of the integrated ALV provirus. The LTRs, shown greatly enlarged to emphasize structural details, are approximately 350 base pairs (bp) in length, and are composed of sequences derived from the 5′ (U5) and 3′ (U3) ends of genomic RNA, and a short sequence (R) present at both ends of genomic RNA. Synthesis of viral genomic and messenger RNAs initiates within the *left* LTR. Initiation within the *right* LTR could result in elevated transcription of adjacent cellular sequences. If, as a rare event, the provirus integrated adjacent to a potentially oncogenic cellular gene ("c-*onc*"), transcriptional activation of this gene could lead to neoplastic transformation.

cause cell transformation, if expressed constitutively, should be small. Thus, examination of the proviral integration sites in a large number of independently derived tumors should reveal integration sites common to more than one tumor.

3. The tumors should contain new RNA transcripts consisting of viral R + U5 sequences (approximately 100 nucleotides; see Fig. 2) covalently linked to nonviral sequences. Again, assuming a limited number of potential cellular genes, transcripts from independent tumors should be similar.

ANALYSIS OF LYMPHOMA DNA

The cellular DNA adjacent to the integrated proviruses in ALV-induced lymphomas was characterized by restriction endonuclease analysis, using the Southern transfer technique (110). Restriction fragments containing viral R + U5 sequences (see Fig. 2) were detected with a probe (cDNA$_{5'}$) specific for this region. The restriction endonuclease Eco RI makes several cuts in the ALV provirus, including a single cut in the U3 region (see Fig. 2) of the LTR (16,58,59,98). A complete integrated provirus will thus yield two Eco RI fragments detectable with cDNA$_{5'}$: an internal fragment containing part of the left LTR and the *gag* gene, and a "junction" fragment containing a portion of the right LTR plus adjacent cellular sequences.

Distinct junction fragments were detected in all tumor DNAs tested (43,73,78,82). This suggests that the tumors are clonal (i.e., derived from a single initially infected cell), since junction fragments would appear as distinct bands only if all, or a majority, of the cells in the tumor contain proviruses integrated at the same chromosomal site. In many tumors, more than one junction fragment was detected. The pattern observed in primary (bursal) tumors was also found in metastatic tumors (spleen, kidney, and liver) from the same animal. Thus, the metastatic tumors are apparently derived from the same clonal population. Such clonality has also been observed in tumors induced by MuLV (62,113,123) and MMTV (26).

Of even greater significance was the observation that many independent tumors, from different ALV-infected birds, contained proviruses integrated at common sites (73,82). Neel et al. (73) were able to place most tumors into four classes, based on the size of the RI junction fragment. Further restriction analyses of tumor DNAs from one of these classes (six independent tumors), using Eco RI in conjunction with other restriction enzymes, showed that the adjacent cellular sequences from each of these tumors possessed identical restriction maps. Payne et al. (82) analyzed three tumor DNAs with restriction endonucleases and concluded that two of these contained proviruses at similar chromosomal sites. A third appeared to contain a provirus integrated at approximately the same site, but in a different orientation relative to the cellular sequences (see later). Since there is no known specificity in the integration process, these observations suggest that neoplastic transformation results only after integration at one of a limited number of cellular sites. Subsequent studies (discussed later) showed that the different classes of junction fragments reflected integrations at slightly different locations adjacent to the same cellular gene.

A surprisingly high proportion of the tumors contained only defective proviruses. Approximately half of the tumors analyzed by Neel et al. (73) and Fung et al. (43) lacked the diagnostic internal fragment of proviral DNA, and in most cases where this fragment was detectable, it was present at substantially less than one copy per cell, suggesting that it represented proviruses introduced in a minority of cells at later stages in tumor development. All three of the integrated proviruses analyzed by Payne et al. (82) contained at least one deletion. Subsequent experiments (discussed later) suggest that perhaps all of the proviruses directly involved in gene activation are defective.

LYMPHOMA RNAs

Poly(A) RNA from tumor cells was analyzed by the "Northern" (1) transfer technique, using cDNA probes corresponding to the total viral genome ($cDNA_{rep}$) or to the R + U5 sequences ($cDNA_{5'}$). Normal viral mRNAs (35S and 21S) (52,128), or any defective viral RNAs that contained significant amounts of viral coding information, would be detected by both probes. RNAs transcribed from the viral promoter in the right LTR, and reading into adjacent cellular sequences, would be detected only with $cDNA_{5'}$.

More than 50% of lymphomas tested did not contain detectable amounts of the normal viral mRNAs, suggesting that expression of viral genes is not necessary for maintenance of transformation (73,82). These tumors contained defective proviruses.

Nearly all tumors contained at least one new tumor-specific RNA transcript detectable with $cDNA_{5'}$ (73,82). Most of these tumor-specific RNAs were in the range of 2.5 to 2.9 kb, although larger RNAs were detected in some tumors. The tumor-specific RNAs did not hybridize to $cDNA_{rep}$, and thus did not contain significant amounts of viral coding information. These RNAs were fairly abundant (100 to 200 copies/cell) in ALV-induced lymphomas, compared to the levels of c-*onc* RNAs in most normal tissues (1–5 copies/cell) (56,73).

IDENTIFICATION OF A CELLULAR GENE ACTIVATED BY ALV

The strategy employed to identify the cellular gene (or genes) activated by proviral insertion was based on the possibility that this gene might be the cellular counterpart of one of the known v-*onc* genes. The v-*onc* genes of rapidly transforming viruses are known to induce cell transformation. Furthermore, Hanafusa and his colleagues (48,64,125) demonstrated that c-*src* sequences, acquired by recombination between partial td viruses and cellular sequences, were capable of inducing transformation; some v-*src* sequences, however, may have been contributed by the parental td viruses. More direct evidence for the oncogenic potential of a c-*onc* gene was provided by Vande Woude and his colleagues (15,80) who demonstrated transformation of NIH/3T3 cells transfected with cloned c-*mos* DNA that was linked to a viral LTR.

Screening for possible c-*onc* participation in lymphomagenesis was performed by analyzing c-*onc*-specific mRNA levels in normal tissues and in tumors (55,56). Five different *onc* probes, corresponding to the cell-derived sequences of Rous sarcoma virus (the *src* gene), Fujinami sarcoma virus *(fps)*, avian erythroblastosis virus *(erb)*, avian myeloblastosis virus *(myb)*, and myelocytomatosis virus MC29 *(myc)* (see Fig. 1), were prepared by differential hybridization techniques.

The c-*onc* genes were expressed at low levels (1–5 copies of mRNA per cell) in normal tissues. Four of these genes (c-*src*, c-*fps*, c-*erb*, and c-*myb*) were expressed at similarly low levels in ALV-induced lymphomas. However, c-*myc* was expressed at elevated levels in nearly all (approximately 85%) of the lymphomas examined (56). The levels of c-*myc* RNA (approximately 100 –300 copies/cell) were at least 30-fold higher than in normal tissues (see Table 1). In a cell line derived from an ALV-induced tumor, approximately 1,000 copies/cell of *myc* RNA were found. This cell line also exhibited a somewhat elevated level of c-*myb* expression (40 copies/cell), but the significance of this is unknown.

The *myc*-specific RNAs from the lymphomas co-migrated in Northern gels with the 2.5 or 2.9 kb tumor-specific RNAs previously detected with cDNA$_{5'}$, suggesting that the c-*myc* and viral 5' sequences were present on the same RNA transcripts. Since these RNAs were not detected with cDNA$_{rep}$ (73), or with probes corresponding to individual viral genes *(gag, pol, env,* or "c") (56; B. Neel, *unpublished*), they apparently contained only the approximately 100 nucleotides of viral information encoded within the R + U5 sequences of the LTR. Five abundant *myc*-specific RNAs were detected in the lymphoma cell line—all corresponding to RNAs detected with cDNA$_{5'}$. The smallest, and most abundant, of these was a 2.9 kb transcript.

In normal cell DNA the c-*myc* coding sequences are present on a single Eco RI restriction fragment of approximately 14 kb (56,102). In lymphoma DNA,

TABLE 1. *c*-onc-*specific mRNAs in normal tissues and in ALV-induced lymphomas*[a]*

Sample no.	Tissue	RNA (copies/cell)				
		src	fps	erb	myb	myc[b]
12B	Normal bursa	3	1	2	3	3
31L	Normal liver	2	1	4	1	2
7K	Lymphoma (kidney)	4	1	6	5	110
11B	Lymphoma (bursa)	3	2	2	4	180
23L	Lymphoma (liver)	5	1	2	3	330
9B	Lymphoma (bursa)	5	1	4	2	230
22L	Lymphoma (liver)	4	2	ND[c]	5	90
RP9	Lymphoma cell line	3	1	3	40	1,000

[a]Data from ref. 56. Tissues were from 3–6 month old birds.
[b]In a larger screening, 13 of 15 ALV-induced lymphomas showed elevated expression of c-*myc* (56).
[c]ND = not determined.

however, *myc* information was found on smaller RI restriction fragments, (usually in the range of 2.7 to 3.5 kb) (56). This would be predicted from the model in Fig. 2, since integration of the provirus would introduce new Eco RI restriction sites adjacent to this gene. Each of the new *myc*-specific fragments corresponded to a restriction fragment detected with cDNA$_{5'}$, suggesting strongly that the viral and c-*myc* sequences are covalently linked in the tumor DNA. Direct evidence for this was obtained for two tumors by cloning Eco RI junction fragments (74). The cloned junction fragments contained both c-*myc* and viral 5' information (see later). Of 36 tumors analyzed, 30 were found to contain rearrangements involving proviral integrations in the vicinity of the c-*myc* gene (3). The finding that proviral information is integrated adjacent to the c-*myc* gene in ALV-induced lymphomas has been confirmed in several laboratories (31,43,81).

Among the six tumors that lacked apparent integrations near c-*myc*, two had been analyzed for *myc* expression. Both contained only low levels of *myc*-specific RNA (56). All six of these tumors contained integrated proviral information. It is possible that the proviruses in these tumors are integrated next to other c-*onc* genes. Alternatively, these tumors may have originally contained proviruses next to c-*myc*, but have lost these during tumor development. The second explanation might be possible if *myc* expression is required only as an early "initiating" event, but not for maintenance of transformation.

The finding that the c-*myc* gene was involved in most ALV-induced lymphomas was somewhat surprising, since the rapidly transforming viruses that carry the v-*myc* gene have not been reported to induce lymphomas (44). Recent experiments (C. Moscovici, C.-K. Shih, and W. Hayward, *unpublished*), however, have demonstrated a fairly high incidence ($\sim$ 20%) of lymphoma in MC29-infected chickens. The lymphomas developed more slowly (1–3 months) than the leukemias (which often caused death within 3–6 weeks). The possibility that the lymphomas were induced by the helper virus, MCAV, was excluded in two ways: (a) No lymphomas were observed during the first four months in birds infected only with MCAV; and (b) the lymphomas expressed high levels of 5.5 kb MC29 RNA, which was readily distinguishable by Northern analysis from the 2.5 to 2.9 kb *myc*-specific RNA in ALV-induced tumors.

IS A SECOND CELLULAR GENE INVOLVED?

Cooper and Neiman (30) used an entirely different approach toward identifying possible cellular genes involved in ALV-induced lymphomagenesis. Tumor DNA was analyzed by transfection to test for its ability to induce morphologic transformation of NIH/3T3 cells (see chapter by Cooper et al.). DNA from ALV-induced tumors caused transformation of recipient cells with a frequency substantially higher than that found with normal cell DNA. However, viral LTR or coding sequences were not detected in the DNA of the recipient transformed cells. This led the authors to propose that proviral DNA sequences were not directly involved in the transformation process (30).

Following the observation that the c-*myc* gene is activated in ALV-induced lymphomas (56), Cooper and Neiman (31) analyzed the transformants to test for the possible transfer of this gene in the transfection experiments. Tests of the DNA and RNA from donor lymphoma cells confirmed the presence of proviral integrations adjacent to c-*myc*, and the presence of RNA transcripts containing both viral 5' and c-*myc* information. However, no new c-*myc* sequences were detected in the DNA of the transformed recipient cells transfected with the lymphoma DNA.

To reconcile these apparently conflicting observations, the authors proposed that two cellular genes are involved in lymphomagenesis: the c-*myc* gene, activated by proviral integration (56), and a second, unlinked gene, activated by some unknown mechanism that does not involve direct proviral integration (31). One possibility is that the activated c-*myc* gene causes, either directly or indirectly, further rearrangements of cellular genes at sites distal to the provirus, and that one such rearrangement results in activation of the cellular gene that is detected in the transfection assay. This is consistent with biological evidence that lymphoma development in ALV-infected birds is a multistage process (32,77). It is possible, however, that the activity detected in the transfection assay reflects a secondary consequence of c-*myc* expression that is not directly involved in lymphomagenesis.

DEFECTIVENESS OF THE INTEGRATED PROVIRUS

Most, and perhaps all, of the proviruses integrated in the vicinity of c-*myc* are defective. As mentioned previously, a high proportion of tumors lack an internal restriction fragment representing the left one-third of the provirus, and more than half of the tumors do not contain detectable amounts of normal viral mRNAs (73,82). In every case where only a single integrated provirus was detected, the provirus was found to be defective either by the criteria mentioned above or on the basis of more complete restriction analysis (3,43,73,81,82). Many tumors with multiple integrations also lacked the internal Eco RI fragment of the provirus, and in a large proportion of those that contained this fragment, it was present at substantially less than one copy per cell (as estimated from band intensity). The internal fragments in these tumors probably represented proviruses introduced by secondary infections of a minor portion of the cells at some later stage in tumor development. In many tumors only one of the two proviral LTRs was detected.

Several tumors contained multiple proviruses integrated at different sites, and in roughly equimolar amounts. Since none of the integration sites, other than those adjacent to c-*myc*, appeared to be common to more than one tumor, it seemed likely that only those proviruses integrated near c-*myc* were relevant to neoplastic transformation. The structure of these proviruses could be examined by analyzing proviral sequences covalently linked to the c-*myc* gene (i.e., by identifying restriction fragments that contained both *myc*-specific and viral sequences). All of the proviruses identified in this way contained substantial deletions, which ranged in length from 0.5 kb to more than 7 kb (3). The minimum amount of viral information found in any of the lymphomas was about 0.35 kb—approximately the size of the LTR—suggesting that only LTR sequences are required for c-*myc* activation (3,43).

The unusually high frequency of deletions within these proviruses suggests that defectiveness may play an essential role in ALV-induced lymphomagenesis. One possible explanation is that cells lacking a complete provirus (and thus not expressing viral antigens) might be more likely to escape detection by the host immune system. This possible advantage, however, would not apply to the tumors that contain complete proviruses at other sites and synthesize apparently normal viral mRNA, although it is possible that these viral mRNAs are synthesized by proviruses that were introduced into the cells at more advanced stages in tumor development, or that the mRNAs are defective in ways not discernible by the hybridization techniques used. A second explanation is that the viral promoter within the right LTR cannot be used efficiently if normal transcription (from the left LTR) is taking place. During normal viral RNA synthesis, chain elongation proceeds into the right LTR, beyond the site where polymerase would bind (54), and thus might block the binding of polymerase or other proteins required for transcription from the right LTR.

It is not known if the observed defectiveness is generated before or after integration of the provirus. Thus far no common features have been found among the different defective proviruses that might suggest a specific mechanism for generating these deletions. It is clear, however, that if defectiveness is an essential step in ALV-induced transformation, the probability that infection would lead to tumor formation would be substantially reduced. This would then be another factor contributing to the long latency of this disease. If the deletions occur after integration, this might also contribute to the apparent multistage nature of lymphoma induction.

ORIENTATION OF THE INTEGRATED PROVIRUS

In the majority of ALV-induced lymphomas analyzed thus far, the provirus is integrated in an orientation that would permit transcription from the viral promoter into the c-myc gene (as shown in Fig. 2). Payne et al. (81), however, have identified several tumors in which the provirus is integrated in other orientations. Of 13 tumors in which orientation could be determined, four were found to contain proviruses integrated upstream from c-myc but in the opposite transcriptional orientation. An additional tumor contained a provirus integrated in the same transcriptional orientation, but downstream from the c-myc gene. Several of these tumors were shown to contain elevated levels of myc-specific RNA that was not linked to viral 5' sequences, suggesting that transcription of c-myc did not initiate on the viral promoter.

It appears, therefore, that sequences within the provirus can exert a regulatory influence over c-myc without providing the initiation site. In the tumor in which integration had occurred downstream from c-myc, this regulatory influence is apparently exerted at a distance of several kilobases from the initiation site (presumably a cellular promoter). It should be noted, however, that the viral LTR encodes signals that function at both the 5' end (regulation, polymerase binding, initiation) and 3' end [poly(A) addition and, possibly, chain termination] of the viral transcriptional unit. In the tumor in which the provirus is downstream from c-myc, the c-myc transcript appears to terminate within the LTR of the virus. Thus it is possible that c-*myc* activation in this tumor results from a different mechanism, related to poly(A) addition or termination signals in the LTR.

The above observations are reminiscent of several studies in which "promoter" sequences have been linked in different arrangements with coding sequences of viral or cellular genes. Vande Woude and his collaborators (14,15,80) have cloned the transforming gene (v-*mos*) of Moloney murine sarcoma virus (MoMSV), and its cellular counterpart, c-*mos*. These cloned DNAs do not induce transformation at significant frequency when transfected into NIH/3T3 cells. However, when either c-*mos* or v-*mos* DNAs are linked to the LTR of MoMSV, transformation occurs at high frequency. With v-*mos*, enhancement of transforming activity was observed when the LTR was linked either upstream or downstream from the coding sequences (14). With c-*mos*, however, high frequency transformation was achieved only when the LTR was located upstream from the coding sequences (15,80).

Grosschedl and Birnstiel (45) have reported that sequences located upstream from the initiation site of the H2A histone gene exert a positive influence on the expression of this gene. Similarly, several groups (8,46,71) have identified a 72 base pair repeat, located about 115 bases upstream from the initiation site of the SV40 early region, that appears to be required for active expression of these genes *in vivo*. The 72 base pair repeat appears to function in a bidirectional manner (71). If the sequence is removed and reinserted at the same location but in the opposite orientation, active expression is observed. This effect, however, is sensitive to location. When the repeat sequence was positioned at more distal sites (as much as 4 kb from the initiation site), some enhancement occurred, but at a much lower level. Little is known about the mechanism by which these sequences exert their influence on gene expression.

The promoter region of the retroviruses has been less well characterized than that of SV40. Both the initiation site and "enhancer" or "regulator" sequences appear to be located within the LTR, since the LTR alone is sufficient to activate a cellular gene in genetically engineered plasmids (14,15,38; P. Luciw, *personal communication*). Similarly, in ALV-induced lymphomas, activation of the c-*myc* gene appears to require only LTR sequences, since some tumors contain little or no viral information other than the LTR (3,43). A majority [60% (81) to greater than 90% (3, H. J. Kung, *personal communication*)] of the proviruses integrated adjacent to c-*myc* are located upstream from this gene and in the same transcriptional orientation. It thus appears that this configuration provides the most efficient means for activating the c-*myc* gene. It is possible that "productive" integrations can occur at a larger number of potential sites when the viral initiation site is provided in the proper orientation, since transcription would not be dependent on the cellular promoter (i.e., integration could occur downstream from the cellular promoter). Alternatively, this orientation may induce a higher level of c-*myc* expression, because the initiation site and "enhancer" sequences of the viral LTR are provided as a unit, in their normal juxtaposition.

STRUCTURE OF THE C-*MYC* GENE IN NORMAL AND IN ALV-TRANSFORMED CELLS

The c-*myc* gene from normal cells has been cloned in several laboratories (74; D. Sheiness et al.; T. Robins, et al., *personal communications*). As previously mentioned, most or all of the c-*myc* gene is contained within a single Eco RI fragment of about 14 kb. The restriction map of a portion of this restriction fragment (a 10 kb fragment extending from an Alu I or Hae III site at the left to the Eco RI site at the right) is shown in Fig. 3 (74). All of the coding information detectable with a v-*myc* probe (from MC29 virus) is located within the terminal 2.5 kb at the right end of the c-*myc* clone (74). The coding information within this region appears to be localized in two exons, 0.7 to 0.8 kb in length, separated by an intron of approximately 1 kb. The cellular promoter for the c-*myc* gene has not been precisely localized, though preliminary studies indicate that it is located approximately 4 kb from the right end of the clone (B. G. Neel, C.-K. Shih, and W. S. Hayward *unpublished*).

With one exception, discussed previously, all of the proviruses integrated in the vicinity of c-*myc* have been found to be located upstream from the major coding portion of this gene. Most integrations were within an 0.8 kb region (approximately 2.6–3.4 kb to the left of the RI site, between the putative c-*myc* promoter and the first exon) (73), but in several tumors the proviruses were integrated further upstream, as much as 2 kb from this region (3,43).

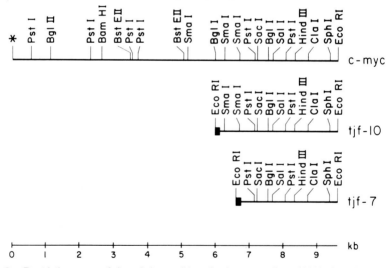

FIG. 3. Restriction maps of cloned virus-cell junction fragments from ALV-induced lymphomas, and a c-*myc* fragment from normal cells. Sequences homologous to v-*myc* are encoded in two exons, within a 2.5 kb region at the extreme right of the c-*myc* clone (74). Tumor junction fragments (tjf-7 and tjf-10) were cloned from two independent tumors (tumors 7 and 10) (see refs. 56,73), and selected by screening with a probe specific for viral LTR sequences (R + U5) (74). LTR sequences in the tumor junction fragments are represented by *solid boxes*. The left end of the c-*myc* clone is defined by a Hae III or Alu I site *(asterisk)*.

Within the 0.8 kb region, integrations appear to be clustered into several distinct groups (73). Whether or not these clusters represent integration events at the same nucleotide is not known. It seems more likely that the clusters represent locations that are favorable for efficient activation of the c-*myc* gene. One possibility is that integration must occur within exons, so that the cellular sequences can provide splice donor sites for generating appropriately processed mRNAs (see later). It should be noted that the LTR does not contain such sites.

Eco RI restriction fragments, containing sequences at the virus/cell junction, were cloned from two ALV-induced lymphomas (74). The cloned tumor junction fragments ("tjf"; see Fig. 3) were selected by screening with viral cDNA$_5'$ probe, but also hybridized to cDNA$_{myc}$, confirming the covalent linkage of viral and c-*myc* sequences in the tumor DNAs. The restriction maps of the two tumor junction fragments are identical to that of the coding portion (right end) of the c-*myc* clone from normal cells, except for the addition of an Eco RI site at the left, located within the LTR of the integrated provirus (see Fig. 3). Thus, there were no apparent rearrangements or deletions within the coding portion of the c-*myc* gene in these tumors. In both clones the LTR was oriented such that transcription from the viral promoter would read into c-*myc*.

Payne et al. (81) have cloned DNA from a tumor in which the provirus was located upstream from c-*myc*, but in the opposite transcriptional orientation. Unlike the tumor DNAs described above, the DNA from this tumor appears to have sustained a deletion within the cellular sequences, between the integrated provirus and the coding region of the c-*myc* gene.

The sequence arrangements at the virus-cell junctions of the two tumor DNAs depicted in Fig. 3 were analyzed by sequencing the extreme left end of the tumor junction fragments (74). The first 156 nucleotides of both clones matched exactly with the known sequence to the right of the Eco RI site in the viral LTR, as expected, and were followed immediately by cellular sequences (which differed in the two clones, since the proviruses were integrated at different sites, roughly 0.5 kb apart). The last two bases of the LTR were absent. Deletion of the terminal two nucleotides of the LTR has been observed in earlier analyses of integrated proviruses (39,63,105,122), and probably reflects a normal feature of the integration process. In both tumors the LTR was located just upstream from cellular sequences similar to the "consensus" splice donor sequence of eukaryotes (68,93). These sequences may serve as splice sites for processing the primary transcript of the c-*myc* gene in normal cells. If so, this suggests the presence of at least two small exons upstream from the major coding region—possibly encoding the leader sequence of the c-*myc* mRNA.

The absence of the two terminal bases of the LTR, and of further viral information downstream from the LTR, provides strong evidence that the c-*myc* sequences are linked to the right LTR of the provirus. Since both of the tumors from which these clones were isolated contained only a single LTR, it is reasonable to assume that the tumor-specific RNA transcripts in these lymphomas initiated within these LTR sequences, and would thus contain no viral information other than the approximately

100 bases (R + U5) that form part of the leader sequence of viral mRNA. This is consistent with analyses of the RNA from these tumors (tumors 7 and 10; see refs. 56,73). The tumor-specific RNAs hybridized to cDNA$_{5'}$ and cDNA$_{myc}$, but not to probes specific for other regions of the viral genome *(gag, pol, env,* or "c"*)*. Thus, the predicted translation product of the c-*myc* gene in these tumors would not contain any virus-encoded peptides, unlike the *myc* protein of MC29 virus, which is a *gag-myc* fusion protein (12,51).

It is interesting that, although the integrated proviruses in different tumors are located at widely separated sites upstream from the c-*myc* gene, the major *myc*-specific mRNAs in most of these tumors are similar in size (2.5–2.9 kb), and contain viral 5′ sequences. This suggests that most of the cellular sequences located between the LTR and the coding region of the c-*myc* gene are spliced out to generate the active mRNA. Intervening sequences between the two c-*myc* exons would presumably also be spliced out. In Northern analyses of tumor RNAs, several minor RNAs detectable with both cDNA$_{5'}$ and cDNA$_{myc}$ could be seen after long auto-radiographic exposures (74). These RNAs, which were larger than the more abundant 2.5–2.9 kb RNAs, may be precursors or processing intermediates of the spliced mRNAs.

MYC GENE EXPRESSION IN ALV- AND MC29 VIRUS-INDUCED TUMORS

Figure 4 compares the structures and patterns of expression of the ALV/c-*myc* complex, and of the rapidly transforming virus, MC29, which contains the v-*myc*

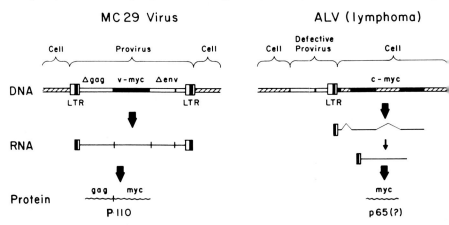

FIG. 4. Strategies of *myc* gene expression in ALV- and MC29 virus-induced tumors. The site of integration does not play a major role in transformation by MC29, since the oncogene (v-*myc*) is carried by the viral genome. Transformation by ALV, on the other hand, occurs only when the provirus is inserted adjacent to a c-*onc* gene. A defective ALV provirus is shown integrated in an orientation such that transcription of c-*myc* can initiate on the viral promoter, as found in most ALV-induced lymphomas. The putative product of the c-*myc* gene (p65) has not been isolated. Its size is estimated from the apparent coding capacity of the gene.

gene. The ALV provirus is depicted as found in the majority of tumors (i.e., upstream from c-*myc* and in the same transcriptional orientation).

Several important features distinguish these two viral systems:

1. The site of integration does not play a major role in transformation by MC29. Since the *myc* gene is present in the viral genome, essentially all cells infected with MC29 become transformed. Transformation by ALV, on the other hand, would occur only in those rare cases when the provirus integrates in the vicinity of the c-*myc* gene (or other c-*onc* gene).

2. The mRNA for the v-*myc* gene of MC29 is a molecule of genome length—apparently unspliced (51,101). The mRNA for the ALV-activated c-*myc* gene is apparently a spliced message, derived from a larger precursor.

3. Whereas the RNA of MC29 can serve as a viral genome, which is packaged in virus particles and reverse-transcribed in the presence of an appropriate helper virus, the *myc*-specific mRNA in the ALV-induced tumor cannot. The latter RNA lacks the essential viral sequence at its 3' end (U3 + R) required for reverse transcription, for transcription, and (presumably) for integration; it also lacks the tRNA primer binding site, located near the 5' end of the genome, just downstream from U5 (117,118), and sequences in the same region that are thought to be required for packaging (99). It should also be noted that the structure of the c-*myc* gene in ALV-induced tumors could not be derived by reverse transcription of the MC29 RNA, or of the processed mRNA of the ALV-activated c-*myc* gene, since there would be no mechanism for regenerating the intervening sequences.

4. The v-*myc* gene product of MC29 virus is a fusion protein containing both viral *(gag)* and *myc* encoded portions (12,51,66). The c-*myc* protein from ALV-induced tumors has not yet been isolated. However, analyses (described previously) of the DNA and RNA of these tumors indicate that, at least in most tumors, no viral information other than the R + U5 sequences is present in the mRNA. The predicted protein would thus lack viral peptides and would be essentially identical to the c-*myc* protein in the uninfected cell. The possibility that some portion of the amino-terminus of the c-*myc* protein is deleted because of the proviral integration cannot be excluded. However, it is unlikely that this is true in all tumors, since integrations within a 2 to 3 kb region upstream from c-*myc* are capable of inducing transformation.

Thus, the *gag* portion of the MC29 transforming protein (P110$^{gag-myc}$) is apparently not essential for cell transformation, at least in lymphocytes. Consistent with this conclusion is the observation that the *myc* gene is inserted at different locations in the genomes of four independently isolated acute leukemia viruses (MC29, MH2, CMII, and OK10) (23,51,66). In OK10, *myc* is located near the 3' end of the genome, and is almost certainly not expressed as a *gag-myc* fusion protein (23). The possibility that the *myc* protein of OK10 contains other virus-encoded sequences (e.g., *env*) has not been excluded. The viral portions of these v-*myc* proteins could play some role in the transport or intracellular localization of the proteins, but there is no evidence for this at present.

HOW WIDESPREAD IS THE GENE ACTIVATION MECHANISM?

The finding that c-*myc* is activated in ALV-induced lymphomas has prompted surveys of other ALV-induced neoplasms. While the data are not extensive at this time, several observations are worth noting.

Fung, Crittenden, and Kung *(personal communication)* have analyzed erythroblasts from leukemic line 15I chickens infected with ALV. As mentioned previously, ALV induces a high incidence of erythroblastosis in this chicken line. Proviruses were found to be integrated in the vicinity of the c-*erb* gene in erythroblasts from approximately 50% of the leukemic chickens. Levels of *erb*-specific RNA were elevated in these cells, though a complete analysis of the transcripts has not yet been performed. It is interesting that erythroleukemias are the major neoplasms induced by the rapidly transforming virus AEV, which carries the v-*erb* gene. The observation that c-*erb* rather than c-*myc* is involved in ALV-induced erythroleukemias is important, since it indicates that c-*onc* gene activation by ALV is not restricted to the c-*myc* gene. Rather, the particular gene involved appears to be related more to the target tissue.

One ALV-induced fibrosarcoma was analyzed in our laboratory. This tumor contained elevated levels of *fps*-specific RNA (55), but it became clear from subsequent studies that a different mechanism was involved (75). A defective acute virus (termed 16L virus) was recovered from the tumor and shown to be capable of inducing foci in tissue culture fibroblasts and of inducing rapidly developing sarcomas in infected chickens. Oligonucleotide fingerprint analysis showed that the *fps*-related insert in 16L virus is similar (but not identical) to those in Fujinami virus and UR1. The virus-derived sequences, however, were clearly acquired from the particular ALV strain used for infection of the chickens. It seems likely, therefore, that 16L virus was generated by recombination between the infecting virus (ALV) and the cellular gene (c-*fps*). Such a recombination event between viral and cellular sequences, to generate a rapidly transforming retrovirus, would be a second (more indirect) mechanism by which slowly transforming retroviruses could induce neoplastic disease.

To date, evidence supporting a gene activation mechanism has been demonstrated with only one other virus, the reticuloendotheliosis virus (REV). REV (helper virus) induces a long latency B-cell lymphoma in birds, similar to that induced by ALV. Noori-Daloii et al. (79) have recently found that REV-induced lymphomas, like ALV-induced lymphomas, contain proviruses integrated in the vicinity of the c-*myc* gene. Although expression of the c-*myc* gene was not analyzed, it seems likely that c-*myc* is activated by REV in the same way as by ALV. It is also of interest that several REV-induced tumors appeared to have increased numbers of c-*myc* gene copies, suggesting some type of gene amplification. Although REV has a structure similar to that of ALV, it is unrelated by nucleic acid homology. This virus, in fact, appears to be more closely related to certain mammalian viruses (27,60).

As yet, no strong evidence is available demonstrating a gene activation mechanism in any of the mammalian retroviruses. It would be surprising, though, if this mechanism did not operate in slowly transforming retroviruses of mammals since they are similar to ALV in their basic structure and their lack of a transforming gene. Several studies with mammalian retroviruses demonstrate parallels with the ALV system. Kettman et al. (65), for example, have found that tumors induced by bovine leukemia virus contain apparently defective proviruses, and do not express viral mRNA. As with ALV, the tumors are clonal with respect to viral integration sites, but integration at specific sites, or activation of cellular genes has not been demonstrated. H. Varmus and his colleagues *(personal communication)* have found that a high percentage of MMTV-induced tumors contain proviruses integrated within a single 20 kb domain. Expression of cellular sequences within this region, however, has not been demonstrated.

The experiments of Oskarsson et al. described previously have demonstrated that c-*mos*, the cellular counterpart of the transforming gene of Moloney MSV, can induce cell transformation when linked to a viral LTR (80). No other viral sequences are required (15). This structure, constructed *in vitro*, is analogous to that found *in vivo* in the ALV-induced lymphomas. Similarly, De Feo et al. (38) demonstrated transformation in cells transfected with cloned DNA containing the c-*ras* gene (the cellular counterpart of the Harvey MSV transforming gene) linked to LTR sequences.

Gene activation by a "promoter insertion" type mechanism is not restricted to c-*onc* genes. Quintrell et al. (89) found RNA transcripts containing both viral 5' and nonviral sequences in some biologically cloned mammalian cells transformed by RSV. Since transformation in these cells was induced by the viral oncogene (v-*src*), and the proviruses in different cloned populations were integrated at different sites, the cellular sequences in these RNAs presumably represented cellular genes that did not play any role in the transformation process. A heterogeneous population of such virus/cell mRNAs was found in cells randomly infected with RAV-2 (W. S. Hayward, *unpublished*). The heterogeneity of the cellular portion of these RNAs presumably reflected the fact that proviruses were integrated at many different sites. It seems likely that, with an appropriate selection procedure, activation of specific (nontransforming) cellular genes could be demonstrated. In the case of the ALV-induced lymphoma, selection occurs naturally within the host animal, since activation of the c-*myc* gene confers a strong selective advantage to the cell, by inducing malignant transformation.

CONCLUSIONS AND FURTHER SPECULATIONS

Activation of the c-*myc* gene by provirus integration has been observed in nearly all ALV-induced lymphomas tested. Although there is as yet no formal proof, the conclusion that c-*myc* activation is directly responsible for lymphomagenesis seems inescapable. Integration of the ALV provirus is known to occur at many chromosomal sites. Thus, proviruses might be expected to integrate near any one of the hundred thousand or so genes in the cell. Yet, nearly all ALV-induced lymphomas contain proviruses integrated adjacent to a single gene, c-*myc*, which is then expressed at elevated levels in these cells. The fact that the activated cellular gene is homologous to a viral gene (v-*myc*) of known oncogenic potential cannot be attributed to coincidence. This conclusion is strengthened by recent data demonstrating involvement of c-*myc* in REV-induced lymphomas, and of c-*erb* in ALV-induced erythroleukemias. It seems likely that other slowly transforming retroviruses will prove to induce neoplastic disease by a similar mechanism.

The precise nature of the viral promoter region, and the mechanism by which these sequences induce enhanced transcriptional activity, are not known. Likewise, little is known about the mechanism by which the *myc* protein (either c-*myc* or v-*myc*) initiates the chain of events leading to cell transformation. Many cellular changes are associated with transformation (for reviews, see refs. 44,47). Yet, at least in the case of many rapidly transforming viruses, it is clear that a single gene product can induce (directly or indirectly) the many alterations in cellular structure and metabolism. The functions of the c-*onc* genes in normal cells are unknown. It seems clear that they must play an essential role—possibly in cell growth regulation or differentiation—since they have been highly conserved throughout evolution in all vertebrates and apparently also in some invertebrates.

Although many v-*onc* proteins appear to act as protein kinases, there is as yet no evidence for kinase activity in the *myc* protein (13,97). Recent evidence, in fact, indicates that the *myc* protein of MC29 virus is located in the nucleus (R. Eisenman; K. Moelling, *personal communications*), rather than on the cell membrane (as is the *src* protein), and may function by an entirely different mechanism that involves interaction with cellular DNA. This is interesting in light of the suggestion of Cooper and Neiman that ALV-induced lymphomagenesis might involve additional genetic alterations at a second site, unlinked to the c-*myc* gene. It is conceivable, in fact, that the c-*myc* protein is directly responsible for the postulated additional chromosomal alteration. In normal birds the c-*myc* gene appears to be expressed at somewhat higher levels in cells and tissues that are undergoing genetic rearrangements within the immunoglobulin gene (T and B cells; early hematopoietic tissues) (T. Gonda et al., *personal communication*; C.-K. Shih and W. Hayward, *unpublished*).

The long latency of tumor induction by ALV and other slowly transforming viruses is only partly explained by the low probability of integration events that could lead to activation of a potentially oncogenic cellular gene. Host factors, such as the immune response to viral antigens, may also be involved. Several other factors that may influence latency include the following: (a) If, as appears to be true, proviral defectiveness is essential for c-*onc* gene activation, this would decrease the probability of obtaining a "productive" integration, and hence increase the latent period. (b) If further chromosomal arrangements are required after c-*myc* activation, as suggested by Cooper and Neiman (30,31), the long latency could reflect, in part, this two-step process. (c) It is possible that target cells are susceptible to neoplastic transformation by c-*onc* gene activation only at specific stages in their development. For example, if integration occurs preferentially within transcriptionally active regions, integration in the vicinity of a particular c-*onc* gene would occur only during those stages when this gene is normally expressed. This "window" would then influence not only the timing of the neoplastic event, but also the "selection" of the particular target cell, and of the c-*onc* gene involved. Alternatively, the "target" molecule for a specific c-*onc* protein might be present only in certain cells, or at specific stages of development.

The data accumulated thus far suggest that the important factor in transformation by an activated c-*onc* gene (or a v-*onc* gene in a rapidly transforming virus) is the "inappropriate" expression of a normal cellular gene. By this we mean either an abnormally high level of expression, or expression at a time when this gene would normally be inactive (or both). Presumably the c-*onc* genes are under tight regulatory control in the normal cell, and are turned on and off at specific stages in normal development. Integration of the ALV provirus, however, results in constitutive expression of the gene, since the gene is placed under the control of viral regulatory sequences, which do not respond to the normal cellular signals that modulate expression of the gene.

Of particular interest is the possibility that other, nonviral carcinogens could induce the same types of regulatory alterations. Since the critical factor appears to be a change in gene expression rather than in protein structure, it seems likely that physical or chemical agents could cause alterations (point mutations, deletions, transpositions, or translocations) within the regulatory sequences of c-*onc* genes that would result in their constitutive expression. Specific chromosomal rearrangements are correlated with many neoplastic diseases in both humans and experimental animals (for reviews, see refs. 20,67,95). Any such rearrangement that joined an active regulatory element to the coding sequences of a c-*onc* gene could cause activation of the gene. Screening for involvement of these genes in nonviral cancers is currently in progress in many laboratories. Two approaches are currently being used: (a) screening for elevated expression and genetic rearrangements of known c-*onc* genes, as described in this chapter; and (b) identification of potentially oncogenic cellular genes by transfection assays (see chapters by Weinberg and Cooper et al.). These two approaches are complementary and may in many cases identify different sets of cellular genes involved in neoplastic transformation.

It seems likely that the common denominator in all cancers, both virus-induced and chemically-induced, is the involvement of specific cellular genes, the so-called c-*onc* genes. The study of this class of cellular genes—their role in normal cells and in both viral and nonviral cancers, the factors that alter their expression, and the enzymatic activities of their gene products—will be a major focus for research in the near future.

ACKNOWLEDGMENTS

We would like to thank our many colleagues, cited in the text, for permission to quote unpublished data. Work in our laboratories was supported by NIH grants CA-16668 and CA-18213, and the Flora E. Griffin Fund (W. S. H.), and by NSF grant CA-06927 and ACS grant PCM 76-09721 (S. M. A.). B. G. N. is a biomedical fellow in the Medical Scientist Training Program of the National Institutes of Health.

REFERENCES

1. Alwine, J. C., Kemp, D. J., and Stark, G. R. (1977): Method for detection of specific RNAs in agarose gels by transfer to diazobenzyloxymethyl-paper and hybridization with DNA probes. *Proc. Natl. Acad. Sci. USA*, 74:5350–5354.

2. Astrin, S. M., Buss, E. G., and Hayward, W. S. (1979): Endogenous viral genes are nonessential in the chicken. *Nature*, 82:339–341.

3. Astrin, S. M., Neel, B. G., Rogler, C., Rovigatti, U., Skalka, A. M., and Hayward, W. S. (1982): Characterization of integrated proviruses in ALV-induced lymphomas. *(Submitted.)*

4. Bacheler, L. T., and Fan, H. (1979): Multiple integration sites for Moloney leukemia virus in productively infected mouse fibroblasts. *J. Virol.*, 30:657–667.

5. Bacon, L. D., Witter, R. L., Crittenden, L. B., Fadly, A. M., and Motta, J. (1981): B-haplotype influence on Marek's disease, Rous sarcoma, and lymphoid virus-induced tumors in chickens. *Poul. Sci.*, 60:1132–1139.

6. Baltimore, D. (1970): RNA-dependent DNA polymerase in virions of RNA tumor viruses. *Nature*, 226:1209–1211.

7. Baltimore, D., Shields, A., Otto, G., Goff, S., Besmer, P., Witte, O., and Rosenberg, N. (1980): Structure and expression of the Abelson murine leukemia virus genome and its relationship to a normal cell gene. *Cold Spring Harbor Symp. Quant. Biol.*, 44:849–854.

8. Benoist, C., and Chambon, P. (1981): *In vivo* sequence requirements of the SV40 early promoter region. *Nature*, 290:304–310.

9. Benz, E. W., Wydro, R. M., Nadal-Ginard, B., and Dina, D. (1980): Moloney murine sarcoma proviral DNA is a transcriptional unit. *Nature*, 288:665–668.

10. Biggs, P. M., Milne, B. S., Graf, T., and Bauer, H. (1973): Oncogenicity of non-transforming mutants of avian sarcoma viruses. *J. Gen. Virol.*, 18:399–403.

11. Bishop, J. M. (1981): Enemies within: The genesis of retrovirus oncogenes. *Cell*, 23:5–6.

12. Bister, K., Hayman, M., and Vogt, P. K. (1977): Defectiveness of avian myelocytomatosis virus MC29: Isolation of long term non-producer cultures and analysis of virus-specific polypeptide synthesis. *Virology*, 82:431–448.

13. Bister, K., Lee, W. -H., and Duesberg, P. H. (1980): Phosphorylation of the nonstructural proteins encoded by avian acute leukemia viruses and by avian Fujinami sarcoma virus. *J. Virol.*, 36:617–621.

14. Blair, D. G., McClements, W. L., Oskarsson, M. K., Fischinger, P. J., and Vande Woude, G. F. (1980): Biological activity of cloned Moloney sarcoma virus DNA: terminally redundant sequences may enhance transformation efficiency. *Proc. Natl. Acad. Sci. USA*, 77:3504–3508.

15. Blair, D. G., Oskarsson, M., Wood, T. G., McClements, W. L., Fischinger, P. J., and Vande Woude, G. F. (1981): Activation of the transforming potential of a normal cell sequence: A molecular model for oncogenesis. *Science*, 212:941–943.

16. Boone, L. R., and Skalka, A. M. (1981): Proviral DNA synthesized *in vitro* by avian retrovirus particles permeabilized with mellitin. II. Evidence for a strand displacement mechanism in (+) strand synthesis. *J. Virol.*, 37:117–126.

17. Brugge, J. S., and Erikson, R. L. (1977): Identification of a transformation-specific antigen induced by an avian sarcoma virus. *Nature*, 45:346–348.

18. Burmester, B. R. (1969): The prevention of lymphoid leukosis with androgens. *Poult. Sci.*, 48:401–408.

19. Burmester, B. R., Gross, M. A., Walter, W. G., and Fontes, A. K. (1959): Pathogenicity of a viral strain (RPL 12) causing avian visceral lymphomatosis and related neoplasms. II. Host-virus interrelations affecting responses. *J. Natl. Cancer Inst.*, 22:103–127.

20. Cairns, J. (1981): The origin of human cancers. *Nature*, 289:353–357.

21. Chen, J. -H. (1980): Expression of endogenous avian myeloblastosis virus information in different chicken cells. *J. Virol.*, 36:162–170.

22. Chien, Y. -H., Lai, M., Shih, T. Y., Verma, I. M., Scolnick, E. M., Roy-Burman, P., and Davidson, N. (1979): Heteroduplex analysis of the sequence relationships between the genomes of Kirsten and Harvey sarcoma viruses, their respective parental murine leukemia viruses, and the rat endogenous 30S RNA. *J. Virol.*, 31:752–760.

23. Chiswell, D. J., Ramsay, G., and Hayman, M. J. (1981): Two virus-specific RNA species are present in cells transformed by defective leukemia virus OK10. *J. Virol.*, 40:301–304.

24. Coffin, J. M., Champion, M., and Chabot, F. (1978): Nucleotide sequence relationships between the genomes of an endogenous and an exogenous avian tumor virus. *J. Virol.*, 28:972–991.

25. Coffin, J. M., Varmus, H. E., Bishop, J. M., Essex, M., Hardy, W. D., Martin, G. S., Rosenberg, N. E., Scolnick, E. M., Weinberg, R. A., and Vogt, P. K. (1981): A proposal for naming host cell-derived inserts in retrovirus genomes. *J. Virol.*, 49:953–957.

26. Cohen, J. C., Shank, P. R., Morris, W. L., Cardiff, R., and Varmus, H. E. (1979): Integration of the DNA of mouse mammary tumor virus in virus-infected normal and neoplastic tissue of the mouse. *Cell*, 16:333–345.

27. Cohen, R. S., Wong, T. C., and Lai, M. M. C. (1981): Characterization of transformation- and replication-specific sequences of reticuloendotheliosis virus. *Virology*, 113:672–685.

28. Collett, M. S., and Erikson, R. L. (1978): Protein kinase activity associated with the avian sarcoma virus *src* gene product. *Proc. Natl. Acad. Sci. USA*, 75:2021–2024.

29. Collett, M. S., Purchio, A. F., and Erikson, R. L. (1980): Avian sarcoma virus transforming protein pp60^{src} shows protein kinase activity for tyrosine. *Nature*, 285:656–659.

30. Cooper, G. M., and Neiman, P. E. (1980): Transforming genes of the neoplasms induced by avian lymphoid leukosis viruses. *Nature*, 287:656–659.

31. Cooper, G. M., and Neiman, P. E. (1981): Two distinct candidate transforming genes of lymphoid leukosis virus induced neoplasms. *Nature*, 292:857–858.

32. Cooper, M. D., Payne, L. N., Dent, P. B., Burmester, B. R., and Good, R. A. (1968): Pathogenesis of avian lymphoid leukosis. I. Histogenesis. *J. Natl. Cancer Inst.*, 41:373–389.

33. Cooper, M. D., Purchase, H. G., Brockman, D. E., and Gathings, W. E. (1974): Studies on the nature of the abnormality of B cell differentiation in avian lymphoid leukosis: Production of heterogeneous IgM by tumor cells. *J. Immunol.*, 113:1210–1222.

34. Crittenden, L. B., Fadly, A. M., and Smith, E. J. (1981): Effect of endogenous leukosis virus genes on response to infection with avian leukosis and reticuloendotheliosis viruses. *Avian Dis.* *(in press)*.

35. Crittenden, L. B., Hayward, W. S., Hanafusa, H., and Fadly, A. M. (1980): Induction of neoplasms by subgroup E recombinants of exogenous and endogenous avian retroviruses (Rous-associated virus Type 60). *J. Virol.*, 33:915–919.

36. Crittenden, L. B., Witter, R. L., and Fadley, A. M. (1979): Low incidence of lymphoid tumors in chickens continuously producing endogenous virus. *Avian Dis.*, 23:646–653.

37. Czernilofsky, A. P., DeLorbe, R., Swanstrom, R., Varmus, H. E., Bishop, J. M., Tischer, E., and Goodman, H. M. (1980): The nucleotide sequence of an untranslated but conserved domain at the 3' end of the avian sarcoma virus genome. *Nucleic Acids Res.*, 8:2967–2984.

38. DeFeo, D., Gonda, M. A., Young, H. A., Chang, E. H., Lowy, D. R., Scolnick, E. M., and Ellis, R. W. (1981): Analysis of two divergent rat genomic clones homologous to the transforming gene of Harvey murine sarcoma virus. *Proc. Natl. Acad. Sci. USA*, 78:3328–3332.

39. Dhar, R., McClements, W. L., Enquist, L. W., and Vande Woude, G. F. (1980): Nucleotide sequences of integrated Moloney sarcoma provirus long terminal repeats and their host and viral junctions. *Proc. Natl. Acad. Sci. USA*, 77:3937–3941.

40. Ellermann, V., and Bang, O. (1908): Experimentelle Leukämie bei Huhnern, *Zentralbl. Bacteriol.*, 46:595–609.

41. Erikson, R. L. (1981): The transforming protein of avian sarcoma viruses and its homologue in normal cells. *Curr. Top. Microbiol. Immunol.*, 91:25–40.

42. Frankel, A. E., and Fischinger, P. J. (1976): Nucleotide sequences in mouse DNA and RNA specific for Moloney sarcoma virus. *Proc. Natl. Acad. Sci. USA*, 73:3705–3709.

43. Fung, Y.-K., Fadly, A. M., Crittenden, L. B., and Kung, H.-J. (1981): On the mechanism of retrovirus-induced avian lymphoid leukosis: Deletion and integration of the proviruses. *Proc. Natl. Acad. Sci. USA*, 78:3418–3422.

44. Graf, T., and Beug, H. (1978): Avian leukemia viruses. Interaction with their target cells *in vivo* and *in vitro*. *Biochem. Biophys. Acta Rev. Cancer*, 516:269–299.

45. Grosschedl, R., and Birnstiel, M. L. (1980): Identification of regulatory sequences in the prelude sequences of an H2A histone gene by the study of specific deletion mutants *in vivo*. *Proc. Natl. Acad. Sci. USA*, 77:1432–1436.

46. Gruss, P., Dhar, R., and Khoury, G. (1981): Simian virus 40 tandem repeated sequences as an element of the early promoter. *Proc. Natl. Acad. Sci. USA*, 78:943–947.

47. Hanafusa, H. (1977): Cell transformation by RNA tumor viruses. In: *Comprehensive Virology*, Vol. X, edited by H. Fraenkel-Conrat and R. R. Wagner, pp. 401–483. Plenum Press, New York.

48. Hanafusa, H., Halpern, C. C., Buchhagen, D. L., and Kawai, S. (1977): Recovery of avian sarcoma virus from tumors induced by transformation-defective mutants. *J. Exp. Med.*, 146:1735–1747.

49. Hanafusa, H., Hayward, W. S., Chen, J. -H., and Hanafusa, T. (1975): Control of expression of tumor virus genes in uninfected chicken cells. *Cold Spring Harbor Symp. Quant. Biol.*, 39:1139–1144.

50. Hanafusa, T., Hanafusa, H., and Miyamoto, T. (1970): Recovery of a new virus from apparently normal chick cells by infection with avian tumor viruses. *Proc. Natl. Acad. Sci. USA*, 67:1797–1803.

51. Hayman, M. J. (1981): Transforming proteins of avian retroviruses. *J. Gen. Virol.*, 52:1–14.

52. Hayward, W. S. (1977): Size and genetic content of viral RNAs in avian oncovirus-infected cells. *J. Virol.*, 24:47–63.

53. Hayward, W. S., and Hanafusa, H. (1975): Recombination between endogenous and exogenous RNA tumor virus genes as analyzed by nucleic acid hybridization. *J. Virol.*, 15:1367–1377.

54. Hayward, W. S., and Neel, B. G. (1981): Retroviral gene expression. *Curr. Top. Microbiol. Immunol.*, 91:217–276.

55. Hayward, W. S., Neel, B. G., Fang, J., Robinson, H. L., and Astrin, S. M. (1981): Avian lymphoid leukosis is correlated with the appearance of discrete new RNAs containing viral and cellular genetic information. In: *Modern Trends in Human Leukemia*, Vol. IV, edited by R. Neth and R. Gallo, pp. 439–444. Bergmann-Verlag, Munich.

56. Hayward, W. S., Neel, B. G., and Astrin, S. M. (1981): Activation of a cellular *onc* gene by promoter insertion in ALV induced lymphoid leukosis. *Nature*, 290:475–480.

57. Hishinuma, F., DeBona, P. J., Astrin, S., and Skalka, A. M. (1981): Nucleotide sequence of the acceptor site and termini of integrated avian endogenous provirus evl: Integration creates a 6 bp repeat of host DNA. *Cell*, 23:155–164.

58. Hsu, T. W., Sabran, J. L., Mark, G. E., Guntaka, R. V., and Taylor, J. M. (1978): Analysis of unintegrated avian RNA tumor virus double-stranded DNA intermediates. *J. Virol.*, 28:810–818.

59. Hughes, S. H., Shank, P. R., Spector, D. H., Kung, H. -J., Bishop, J. M., Varmus, H. E., Vogt, P. K., and Breitman, M. L. (1978): Proviruses of avian sarcoma virus are terminally redundant, co-extensive with unintegrated linear DNA, and integrate at many sites. *Cell*, 18:347–359.

60. Hunter, E., Bhown, A. S., and Bennett, J. C. (1978): Amino terminal amino acid sequence of the major structural polypeptides of avian retroviruses: Sequence homology between reticuloendotheliosis virus p30 and p30s of mammalian retroviruses. *Proc. Natl. Acad. Sci. USA*, 75:2708–2712.

61. Hunter, T., and Sefton, B. M. (1980): Transforming gene product of Rous sarcoma virus phosphorylates tyrosine. *Proc. Natl. Acad Sci. USA*, 77:1311–1315.

62. Jahner, D., Stuhlmann, H., and Jaenisch, R. (1980): Conformation of free and of integrated Moloney leukemia virus proviral DNA in preleukemic and leukemic BALB/Mo mice. *Virology*, 101:111–123.

63. Ju, G., and Skalka, A. M. (1980): Nucleotide sequence analysis of the long terminal repeat (LTR) of avian retroviruses: Structural similarities with transposable elements. *Cell*, 22:379–386.

64. Karess, R. E., Hayward, W. S., and Hanafusa, H. (1979): Cellular information in the genome of recovered avian sarcoma virus directs the synthesis of transforming protein. *Proc. Natl. Acad. Sci. USA*, 76:3154–3158.

65. Kettmann, R., Marbaix, G., Clueter, Y., Portetelle, D., Mammerickx, M., and Burny, A. (1981): Genomic integration of Bovine Leukemia provirus and lack of viral RNA expression in the target cells of cattle with different responses to BLV infection. *Leuk. Res.*, 4:509–519.

66. Kitchener, G., and Hayman, M. J. (1980): Comparative tryptic peptide mapping studies suggest a role in cell transformation for the *gag*-related protein of avian erythroblastosis virus and avian myelocytomatosis virus strains CM II and MC29. *Proc. Natl. Acad. Sci. USA*, 77:1637–1641.

67. Klein, G. (1981): Changes in gene dosage and gene expression: A common denominator in the tumorigenic action of viral oncogenes and non-random chromosomal changes. *Nature*, 294:313–318.

68. Lerner, M. R., Boyle, J. A., Mount, S. M., and Steitz, J. A. (1980): Are snRNPs involved in splicing? *Nature*, 283:220–224.

69. Levinson, A. D., Oppermann, H., Levintow, L., Varmus, H. E., and Bishop, J. M. (1978): Evidence that the transforming gene of avian sarcoma virus encodes a protein kinase associated with a phosphoprotein. *Cell*, 15:561–572.

70. Majors, J. E., and Varmus, H. E. (1981): Nucleotide sequence at host-proviral junctions for mouse mammary tumor virus. *Nature*, 289:253–257.

71. Moreau, P., Hen, R., Wasylyk, B., Everett, R., Gaub, M. P., and Chambon, P. (1981): The SV40 72 base pair repeat has a striking effect on gene expression both in SV40 and other chimeric recombinants. *Nucleic Acids Res.*, 9:6047–6068.

72. Motta, J. V., Crittenden, L. B., Purchase, H. G., Stone, H. A., Okazaki, W., and Witter, R. L. (1975): Low oncogenic potential of avian endogenous RNA tumor virus infection or expression. *J. Natl. Cancer Inst.*, 55:685–689.
73. Neel, B. G., Hayward, W. S., Robinson, H. L., Fang, J., and Astrin, S. M. (1981): Avian leukosis virus-induced tumors have common proviral integration sites and synthesize discrete new RNAs: Oncogenesis by promoter insertion. *Cell*, 23:323–334.
74. Neel, B. G., Rogler, C. E., Gasic, G. P., Skalka, A. M., Papas, T., Astrin, S. M., and Hayward, W. S. (1981): Molecular cloning of virus-cell junctions from ALV-induced lymphomas: Comparison with the normal c-*myc* gene. *J. Virol. (in press)*.
75. Neel, B. G., Wang, L. -H., Hanafusa, T., Mathey-Prevot, B., Hanafusa, H., and Hayward, W. S. (1981): Isolation of a new acute transforming virus from an ALV-induced fibrosarcoma. *Proc. Natl. Acad. Sci. USA (in press)*.
76. Neiman, P. E., Das, S., Macdonnell, D., and McMillen-Helsel, C. (1977): Organization of shared and unshared sequences in the genomes of chicken endogenous and sarcoma viruses. *Cell*, 11:321–329.
77. Neiman, P. E., Jordan, L., Weiss, R., and Payne, L. N. (1980): Malignant lymphoma of the bursa of Fabricius and analysis of early transformation. *Cold Spring Harbor Conf. Cell Prolif.*, 7:519–528.
78. Neiman, P. E., Payne, L. N., and Weiss, R. A. (1980): Viral DNA in bursal lymphomas induced by avian leukosis virus. *J. Virol.*, 34:178–186.
79. Noori-Daloii, M. R., Swift, R. A., Kung, H. -J., Crittenden, L. B., and Witter, R. L. (1981): Specific integration of REV proviruses in avian bursal lymphomas. *Nature*, 294:574–575.
80. Oskarsson, M., McClements, W. L., Blair, D. G., Maizel, J. V., and Vande Woude, G. F. (1980): Properties of a normal mouse cell DNA sequence *(sarc)* homologous to the *src* sequence of Moloney sarcoma virus. *Science*, 207:1222–1224.
81. Payne, G. S., Bishop, J. M., and Varmus, H. E. (1982): Multiple arrangements of viral DNA and an activated host oncogene (c-myc) in bursal lymphomas. *Nature*, 295:209–213.
82. Payne, G. S., Courtneidge, S. A., Crittenden, L. B., Fadly, A. M., Bishop, J. M., and Varmus, H. E. (1981): Analyses of avian leukosis virus DNA and RNA in bursal tumors: Viral gene expression is not required for maintenance of the tumor state. *Cell*, 23:311–322.
83. Peterson, R. D., Burmester, B. R., Fredrickson, T. N., Purchase, H. G., and Good, R. A. (1964): Effect of bursectomy and thymectomy on the development of visceral lymphomatosis in the chicken. *J. Natl. Cancer Inst.*, 32:1343–1354.
84. Peterson, R. D., Purchase, H. G., Burmester, B. R., Cooper, M. D., and Good, R. A. (1966): Relationships among visceral lymphomatosis, bursa of Fabricius, and bursa-dependent lymphoid tissue of the chicken. *J. Natl. Cancer Inst.*, 36:585–595.
85. Purchase, H. G., Okazaki, W., Vogt, P. K., Hanafusa, H., Burmester, B. R., and Crittenden, L. B. (1977): Oncogenicity of avian leukosis viruses of different subgroups and of mutants of sarcoma viruses. *Infect. Immun.*, 15:423–428.
86. Purchase, H. G., and Burmester, B. R. (1978): Neoplastic diseases: Leukosis/sarcoma group. In: *Diseases of Poultry*, 7th edition, edited by M. S. Hofstad, B. W. Calnek, C. F. Helmboldt, W. M. Reid, and H. W. Yoder, Jr., pp. 418–468. Iowa State University Press, Ames, Iowa.
87. Purchase, H. G., and Gilmore, D. G. (1975): Lymphoid leukosis in chickens chemically bursectomized and subsequently inoculated with bursa cells. *J. Natl. Cancer Inst.*, 55:851–855.
88. Purchio, A. F., Erikson, E., Brugge, J. S., and Erikson, R. L. (1978): Identification of a polypeptide encoded by the avian sarcoma virus *src* gene. *Proc. Natl. Acad. Sci. USA*, 75:1567–1571.
89. Quintrell, N., Hughes, S. H., Varmus, H. E., and Bishop, J. M. (1980): Structure of viral DNA and RNA in mammalian cells infected with avian sarcoma virus. *J. Mol. Biol.*, 143:363–393.
90. Ringold, G. M., Shank, P. R., Varmus, H. E., Ring, J., and Yamamoto, K. R. (1979): Integration and transcription of mouse mammary tumor virus DNA in rat hepatoma cells. *Proc. Natl. Acad. Sci. USA*, 76:665–669.
91. Robinson, H. L. (1978): Inheritance and expression of chicken genes that are related to avian leukosis sarcoma virus genes. *Curr. Top. Microbiol. Immunol.*, 83:1–36.
92. Robinson, H. L., Pearson, M. N., DeSimone, D. W., Tsichlis, P. N., and Coffin, J. M. (1980): Subgroup-E avian-leukosis virus-associated disease in chickens. *Cold Spring Harbor Symp. Quant. Biol.*, 44:1133–1142.
93. Rogers, J., and Wall, R. (1980): A mechanism for RNA splicing. *Proc. Natl. Acad. Sci. USA*, 77:1877–1879.

94. Roussel, M., Saule, S., Lagrou, C., Rommens, C., Beug, H., Graf, T., and Stehelin, D. (1979): Three new types of viral oncogene of cellular origin specific for haematopoietic cell transformation. *Nature*, 281:452–455.

95. Rowley, J. D. (1980): Chromosome abnormalities in human leukemia. *Annu. Rev. Genet.*, 14:17–39.

96. Sabran, J. L., Hsu, T. W., Yeater, C., Kaji, A., Mason, W. S., and Taylor, J. M. (1979): Analysis of integrated avian RNA tumor virus DNA in transformed chick, duck, and quail fibroblasts. *J. Virol.*, 29:170–178.

97. Sefton, B. M., Hunter, T., Beemon, K., and Eckhart, W. (1980): Evidence that phosphorylation of tyrosine is essential for cellular transformation by Rous sarcoma virus. *Cell*, 20:807–816.

98. Shank, P. R., Hughes, S. H., Kung, H. -J., Majors, J. E., Quintrell, N., Guntaka, R. V., Bishop, J. M., and Varmus, H. E. (1978): Mapping unintegrated avian sarcoma virus DNA: Termini of linear DNA bear 300 nucleotides present once or twice in two species of circular DNA. *Cell*, 15:1383–1395.

99. Shank, P. R., and Linial, M. (1980): An avian oncovirus mutant (SE21Q1B) deficient in genomic RNA: Characterization of a deletion in the provirus. *J. Virol.*, 36:450–456.

100. Sheiness, D., and Bishop, J. M. (1979): DNA and RNA from uninfected vertebrate cells contains nucleotide sequences related to the putative transforming gene of avian myelocytomatosis virus. *J. Virol.*, 31:514–521.

101. Sheiness, D., Vennstrom, B., and Bishop, J. M. (1981): Virus-specific RNAs in cells infected by avian myelocytomatosis virus and avian erythroblastosis virus. *Cell*, 23:291–300.

102. Sheiness, D. K., Hughes, S. H., Stubblefield, E., and Bishop, J. M. (1980): The vertebrate homologue of the putative transforming gene of avian myelocytomatosis virus: Characterization of the DNA locus and its RNA transcript. *Virology*, 105:415–424.

103. Sherr, C. J., Fedele, L. A., Donner, L., and Turek, L. P. (1979): Restriction endonuclease mapping of unintegrated proviral DNA of Snyder-Theilen feline sarcoma virus: Localization of sarcoma specific sequences. *J. Virol.*, 32:860–875.

104. Shibuya, M., Hanafusa, H., and Balduzzi, P. C. (1982): Cellular sequences related to three new *onc* genes of avian sarcoma virus *(fps, yes*, and *ros)* and their expression in normal and transformed cells. *J. Virol.*, 42:143–152.

105. Shimotohno, K., Mizutani, S., and Temin, H. M. (1980): Sequence of retrovirus provirus resembles that of bacterial transposable elements. *Nature*, 185:550–554.

106. Shoemaker, C., Goff, S., Gilboa, E., Paskind, M., Mitra, S. W., and Baltimore, D. (1980): Structure of a cloned circular Moloney leukemia virus DNA molecule containing an inverted segment: implications for retrovirus integration. *Proc. Natl. Acad. Sci. USA*, 77:3932–3936.

107. Shoyab, M., and Baluda, M. A. (1976): Ribonucleotide sequence homology among avian oncoviruses. *J. Virol.*, 17:106–113.

108. Simek, S., and Rice, N. (1980): Analysis of the nucleic acid components in reticuloendotheliosis virus. *J. Virol.*, 33:320–329.

109. Smith, R. E., and Ivanyi, J. (1980): Pathogenesis of virus-induced osteopetrosis in the chicken. *J. Immunol.*, 125:523–530.

110. Southern, E. M. (1975): Detection of specific sequences among DNA fragments separated by gel electrophoresis. *J. Mol. Biol.*, 98:503–517.

111. Spector, D. H., Smith, K., Padgett, T., McCombe, P., Roulland-Dussoix, D., Moscovici, C., Varmus, H. E., and Bishop, J. M. (1978): Uninfected avian cells contain RNA related to the transforming gene of avian sarcoma virus. *Cell*, 13:371–379.

112. Spector, D. H., Varmus, H. E., and Bishop, J. M. (1978): Nucleotide sequences related to the transforming gene of avian sarcoma virus are present in DNA of uninfected vertebrates. *Proc. Natl. Acad. Sci. USA*, 75:4102–4106.

113. Steffen, D., and Weinberg, R. A. (1978): The integrated genome of murine leukemia virus. *Cell*, 15:1003–1010.

114. Stehelin, D., Varmus, H. E., Bishop, J. M., and Vogt, P. K. (1976): DNA related to the transforming gene(s) of avian sarcoma virus is present in normal avian DNA. *Nature*, 260:170–173.

115. Sutcliffe, J. G., Shinnick, T. M., Verma, I. M., and Lerner, R. A. (1980): Nucleotide sequence of Moloney leukemia virus: 3' end reveals details of replication, analogy to bacterial transposons, and an unexpected gene. *Proc. Natl. Acad. Sci. USA*, 73:2356–2360.

116. Swanstrom, R., DeLorbe, W., Bishop, J. M., and Varmus, H. E. (1981): Nucleotide sequence of cloned unintegrated avian sarcoma virus DNA: Viral DNA contains direct and inverted repeats similar to those in transposable elements. *Proc. Natl. Acad. Sci. USA*, 78:124–128.

117. Taylor, J. M., and Illmensee, R. (1975): Site on the RNA of an avian sarcoma virus at which primer is bound. *J. Virol.*, 16:553–558.
118. Taylor, J. M. (1979): DNA intermediates of avian RNA tumor viruses. *Curr. Top. Microbiol. Immunol.*, 87:23–41.
119. Temin, H. M. (1980): Origin of retroviruses from cellular moveable genetic elements. *Cell*, 21:599–600.
120. Temin, H. M., and Mizutani, S. (1970): RNA-dependent DNA polymerase in virions of Rous sarcoma virus. *Nature*, 226:1211–1213.
121. Tsichlis, P. N., and Coffin, J. M. (1980): Recombinants between endogenous and exogenous avian tumor viruses: Role of the c region and other portions of the genome in the control of replication and transformation. *J. Virol.*, 33:238–249.
122. Van Beveren, C., Goddard, J. G., Berns, A., and Verma, I. M. (1980): Structure of Moloney murine leukemia viral DNA: Nucleotide sequence of the 5′ long terminal repeat and adjacent cellular sequences. *Proc. Natl. Acad. Sci. USA*, 77:3307–3311.
123. van der Putten, H., Quint, W., van Raaij, J., Maandag, E. R., Verma, I. M., and Berns, A. (1981): M-MLV-induced leukemogenesis: Integration and structure of recombinant proviruses in tumors. *Cell*, 24:729–740.
124. Wang, L. -H. (1978): The gene order of RNA tumor viruses derived from biochemical analyses of deletion mutants and recombinants. *Ann. Rev. Microbiol.*, 32:561–592.
125. Wang, L. -H., Halpern, C. C., Nadel, M., and Hanafusa, H. (1978): Recombination between viral and cellular sequences generates transforming sarcoma virus. *Proc. Natl. Acad. Sci. USA*, 75:5812–5816.
126. Wang, S. Y., Hayward, W. S., and Hanafusa, H. (1977): Genetic variation in the RNA transcripts of endogenous virus genes in uninfected chicken cells. *J. Virol.*, 24:64–73.
127. Weiss, R. A., and Frisby, D. P. (1981): Are avian endogenous viruses pathogenic? In: *Comparative Research on Leukemia and Related Diseases*, edited by D. S. Yohn. Elsevier-North-Holland, New York *(in press)*.
128. Weiss, S. R., Varmus, H. E., and Bishop, J. M. (1977): The size and genetic composition of virus-specific RNAs in the cytoplasm of cells producing avian sarcoma-leukosis viruses. *Cell*, 12:983–992.
129. Yamamoto, T., Jay, G., and Pastan, I. (1980): Unusual features in the nucleotide sequence of a cDNA clone derived from the constant region of avian sarcoma virus messenger RNA. *Proc. Natl. Acad. Sci. USA*, 77:176–180.
130. Ziff, E. B. (1980): Transcription and RNA processing by DNA tumor viruses. *Nature*, 287:481–499.

Advances in Viral Oncology, Volume 1,
edited by George Klein. Raven Press,
New York © 1982.

Transforming Genes of Nonvirus-Induced Tumors

Robert A. Weinberg

*Center for Cancer Research and Department of Biology, Massachusetts Institute of
Technology, Cambridge, Massachusetts 02139*

The existence of transforming genes of nonvirally induced tumors has been
demonstrated over the past several years by the use of the procedure of gene transfer,
also termed transfection. Gene transfer experiments have made possible the elucidation of the outlines of this group of oncogenes, which in the tumor cell line
have no apparent affiliation with viral genomes. In this chapter, the initially characterized properties of these genes and their possible relationship with transforming
genes of retroviruses are described.

INITIAL DEMONSTRATION OF TRANSFORMING GENES IN DNAs OF CHEMICALLY TRANSFORMED CELLS

The gene transfer procedure of Graham and van der Eb (4) has made possible
the passage of a variety of phenotypes from cell to cell (1–4,10,16). This transfer
may be achieved using naked DNA as the vehicle, and therefore proves that the
phenotypes of interest are encoded directly by the structure of the DNA, and not
by other, nongenetic elements present in the cell. The efficiency of this procedure
is low, but nevertheless adequate to transfer phenotypes encoded by single-copy
genes present in the genome of the donor cell (16).

Among the genetic markers that may be passed from cell to cell by transfection
are those genes that encode transformation. This transfer has been exploited extensively in the field of virology to demonstrate active transforming genes present
in the DNAs of a variety of tumor viruses. With rare exception, these experiments
have involved introduction of these viral genes into recipient fibroblasts cultured
in monolayer. A consequence of the exposure to the viral DNA is the outgrowth
of transformed foci, which are readily distinguishable from the background monolayer. These foci arise *in vitro* in a way that parallels tumor induction by virus
infection *in vivo*. Cells of the foci are able to induce fibrosarcomas in appropriate
hosts, and these cells display a variety of characteristics reminiscent of virus infected, transformed cells.

Application of DNAs of some 3-methyl-cholanthrene- (3-MC) transformed mouse
fibroblast lines to monolayer cultures leads to the induction of foci. This phenom-

enon is not observed in parallel experiments with DNA of four untransformed donor cells (12). By this criterion, the DNA of the 3-MC transformed is structurally altered in relation to normal cellular DNA. Although other structural alterations are not excluded, the alteration being detected by transfection is clearly central to the oncogenic phenotype of the donor cells, since it specifies transformation.

This initial observation has been repeated using DNAs prepared from a variety of transformed donor cells. These experiments demonstrate that many types of tumor cells carry transforming sequences in their DNAs (6,8,11), which are demonstrable by their ability to transform the recipient NIH3T3 mouse fibroblasts. Induction of foci has been observed on transfection of a variety of tumor cell types, which include bladder carcinomas of mouse, rabbit, and humans (6,11), neuroblastomas and gliomas of rat and humans (11; A. Cassill and R. A. Weinberg, *unpublished observations*), and colon and lung carcinomas of humans (8; C. Shih and R. A. Weinberg, *unpublished observations*). Thus the conclusions made initially concerning 3-MC transformed mouse fibroblasts can be extended to include a disparate collection of tumor cell lines.

These data in aggregate indicate that these transforming sequences can act across species and tissue boundaries. A human carcinoma-transforming sequence is as effective as a mouse fibrosarcoma sequence in transforming the recipient NIH3T3 cells. Although each of these sequences functioned originally in a distinct and specialized cellular environment, the sequences are all able to induce the same phenotype when introduced into the common mouse fibroblast recipient cell.

The DNA sequences that impart the transforming competence do not appear to be associated with any readily detectable viral genome. All attempts at rescue of defective transforming retroviruses from the donor cells or from transfectants have been unsuccessful to date (6,11,12). In the absence of any evidence to the contrary, one concludes tentatively that these transforming sequences represent altered variants of normally cellular genes that have become activated as a consequence of carcinogenesis. This conclusion is implicit in much of the following discussion. It will be substantiated in a credible way only after some of these genes are isolated by molecular cloning and analyzed in detail.

MULTIPLICITY OF DIFFERENT TUMOR SEQUENCES

These results described above are compatible with the existence of a single cellular sequence that is able to become activated in various tissue environments, and consequently to induce a different, distinct type of tumor in each of these tissues. For example, one such sequence might become activated in an epithelial cell to induce a carcinoma or in a nerve cell precursor to induce a neuroblastoma. An alternate model is that there are a variety of sequences in the genome, any one of which may become activated to induce transformation in a variety of tissue environments.

Results that bear on this issue are already available. DNAs have been prepared from human tumor cell lines of bladder and colon carcinoma, and promyelocytic leukemia origin (EJ, SW-3, and HL-60). These DNAs have been used to induce foci on mouse fibroblasts. Some of these foci have been grown up, and their DNAs prepared for use in a second round of transfections (8).

The resulting secondary foci have an interesting genetic configuration. Virtually the only human tumor DNA sequence present in these cells are DNA sequences closely associated with the transforming genes whose phenotypes are being scored in these serial transfections. Any remaining human sequences, derived from the original donor tumor cell lines, have been diluted away during the two rounds of transfection.

The human DNA sequences can be detected among the million-fold excess of mouse DNA in these secondary transfectants. This detection is made possible by the fact that the human DNA contains an array of highly repeated sequences of the "Alu family," (5) which are interspersed throughout the entire human genome, and therefore interspersed as well through the limited stretch of human DNA present in these secondary transfectants. These human Alu sequences are detectable specifically amid the mouse background by use of cloned sequence-specific probes that do not cross-react with any sequences present in mouse DNA.

Southern blot analysis (14) of DNAs of a series of secondary transfectants carrying the human colon carcinoma-transforming sequences indicates that all of these independently derived secondary foci carry a common set of restriction fragments reactive with the Alu probe (8). A group of secondary foci deriving from the human bladder carcinoma DNA also carry a spectrum of restriction fragments in common, but this common spectrum is different from that observed on analysis of the colon carcinoma transfectants. Secondary foci produced after transfection of the human promyelocytic leukemia DNA carry a third, distinct set of DNA fragments in common.

Each set of DNA fragments contains DNA sequences that are tightly linked to the transforming gene whose function is being selected in these experiments. Dissociation of these sequences from the gene during transfection can apparently not occur without loss of function. This indicates that each of these three genes is embedded in a distinct array of repeated sequences within the human genome. One concludes that three different transforming sequences are carried by the DNAs of these three different types of human tumors (8).

Each of these sequences behaves in these experiments as if it were a discrete, contiguous DNA stretch, reminiscent in this sense of a gene. We therefore allow ourselves to call these sequences transforming "genes" even though the appropriateness of this term needs a justification that can come only from future experiments.

TRANSFORMING SEQUENCES WITH INDEPENDENTLY TRANSFORMED MOUSE FIBROBLAST LINES

A result contrasting to that described above is obtained in experiments analyzing the DNAs of a series of 3-MC transformed mouse fibroblast lines. The transforming sequences of four independently transformed lines have been analyzed by a different experimental approach. In these experiments, we have probed the structure of these genes by treating various DNAs with restriction enzymes prior to transfection, and ascertained whether the biological activity of the DNAs survives these enzyme treatments. We found that endonuclease EcoRI treatment of the four DNAs inactivated all biological activity. Similarly, HindIII endonuclease treatment prevented focus induction of all four DNAs assayed in subsequent transfection. On the other hand, BamHI, XhoI, and SalI endonucleases spared the biological activity of all four DNAs (13).

The data show that the four different transforming genes from these four, independently transformed lines are associated with the same set of restriction enzyme recognition sites. This identity of behavior is unlikely to result from statistical happenstance, which would occur with a probability of 10^{-4} to 10^{-5} for four arbitrarily chosen genes. Rather, we concluded that the same transforming gene was functioning in these four different lines.

One emerges from this work with an as yet untested hypothesis. Namely, that within a given type of tumor, the same transforming gene is repeatedly activated. However, different types of tumors may carry their own, distinct transforming sequences, each of which is characteristic of that type of specialized tumor.

PROTEINS ENCODED BY THE TRANSFORMING SEQUENCE OF RAT NEUROBLASTOMA

The genes encoding transformation will likely be seen to act by specifying transforming proteins that interact with and perturb cellular metabolism. We have attempted to detect such proteins with an experimental strategy that utilizes the transfected cells. In the example cited here, we have used DNA of ethyl nitrosurea-induced neuroblastomas to derive primary, and then, via serial DNA passage, secondary transfectant cell lines. The serial passage of the neuroblastoma-transforming gene assure that the neuroblastoma-transforming sequence is virtually the only rat sequence present in the secondary foci of transfected NIH3T3 cells, as described earlier. Any protein encoded by this transforming sequence should represent the only xenogeneic protein present in these mouse cells. Clearly, a variety of other novel proteins may be present in these fibroblasts, these other proteins being "neoantigens" of mouse origin that are induced as general consequence of transformation of these cells.

Such transfectants can be used to seed tumors in syngeneic, or quasi-syngeneic NFS mice, in which they grow into fibrosarcomas. The sera of these tumor-bearing animals may exhibit reactivities toward any protein specified by the foreign transforming gene. These sera have been tested in immuneprecipitation reactions with radio-labeled lysates of neuroblastoma cells, of neuroblastoma DNA-derived transfectants, and of untransfected NIH3T3 cells (9).

All antisera from mice bearing these tumors have strong reactivity toward a phosphoprotein of 185,000 daltons, which is found in high levels in the transfectants and in lower level in the parental neuroblastoma. The protein is absent in the untransfected NIH3T3 cells. These sera do not detect this protein in different types of tumor cells, nor in transfectants derived from their DNA. For example, this protein is not detected in cells transformed by DNAs of bladder carcinomas, 3-MC-induced fibroblasts, and a melanoma.

This protein is not, therefore, induced as a general, nonspecific consequence of transformation. Mice bearing tumors grown from a variety of different types of transfectants do not yield sera reactive with this protein unless the tumor they were carrying arose from a neuroblastoma DNA transfectant. The protein is present in all primary and secondary neuroblastoma DNA transfectants and is present as well in a glioblastoma DNA transfectant. It is also present in a neuroblastoma cell line whose DNA was not active in inducing foci on transfection.

These data present a very strong association between this 185K phosphoprotein and the neuroblastoma-transforming gene. The linkage between the presence of the gene and the synthesis of this protein is resistant to a variety of experimental manipulations. It has been concluded that the synthesis of this protein is specifically induced by this gene. The further conclusion that the structure of this protein is actually encoded by the gene depends on results that should be forthcoming (9).

It should be mentioned that all the biologically active rat neuroblastoma DNAs from a series of independently derived tumor cell lines induce the identical protein on transfection. This adds further evidence that the molecular pathways of oncogenesis are identical within a group of tumors of the same tissue type, as discussed in the previous section.

RELATION OF RETROVIRUS *ONC* GENES TO THE TRANSFECTABLE GENES OF NONVIRAL TUMORS

These tumor-transforming sequences appear in many respects to be quite similar to the cellular *onc* sequences that have been acquired by many acutely transforming retrovirus genomes. These similarities may be more apparent than real, since conclusions concerning structural similarities are dependent on experiments not yet fully developed.

The analogies between retrovirus *onc* genes and the nonviral tumor genes relate to several properties of these genetic elements. The first is that both classes appear to derive from normal cellular genes. This conclusion is still based on indirect arguments in the case of the nonviral tumor genes. A second similarity is that each group constitutes a multi-gene family. This conclusion is already well founded in the case of both groups. The third similarity rests from the behavior of these genes on transfection, since members of both families of genes are able to induce foci on application to NIH3T3 monolayers. These similarities between the two groups of genes may be only superficial. Measurements of structural relatedness between the two types of genes will be required to address this directly.

We have attempted to assay structural homologies between the *onc* genes of retroviruses and the nonvirus induced tumor genes. This is being done using cloned, *onc*-specific sequence probes provided us by a number of investigators. These probes are used in a Southern blot analysis of the DNAs of normal and transfected NIH3T3 cells. We have asked whether the transfected cell DNA displays novel DNA fragments that are reactive to the probe in addition to the preexisting, normal cellular endogenous *onc* sequences that are present in all untransfected cells. Detection of a novel DNA fragment in the transfectant would provide strong evidence for homology between the *onc* probe and the acquired tumor gene. A positive, internal control for the efficacy of the procedure is provided by the normal cellular *onc* sequences, which should be detected in all cell DNA samples.

To date, use of a half a dozen different *onc* probes in Southern blot analyses of transfectants deriving from DNAs of as many different tumor types has revealed no cross-reactivity in sequences (L. Parada and R. A. Weinberg, *unpublished observations*). This survey of potential cross-reactivity is being further extended. However, it is already apparent that many of the most frequently studied retrovirus *onc* genes are not homologous with the transforming sequences of the tumor cell types described in earlier sections of this chapter. Given the potentially large size of both groups of oncogenes, it is still possible that many genes represented in both classes will be found.

Isolation of the cellular transforming genes from a spontaneous tumor is proceeding in several laboratories using techniques of molecular cloning. The isolated genes will provide useful reagents for the resolution of a variety of fundamental issues. One will rapidly be able to resolve the structural differences that distinguish the transforming genes from normal cellular counterparts. Such clones will make it possible to characterize any transcripts that serve as templates for the synthesis of transforming proteins. Finally, structural analysis of these clones and recently developed strategies of protein isolation (7,15) will aid in the characterization of these proteins instrumental in the creation of the phenotype of these spontaneous tumors.

ACKNOWLEDGMENTS

This work was supported by NCI grant 26717 to the author and NCI grant 14051 to S. E. Luria.

REFERENCES

1. Andersson, P. (1980): The oncogenic function of mammalian sarcoma viruses. *Adv. Cancer Res.*, 33:109–172.
2. Bacchetti, S., and Graham, F. L. (1977): Transfer of the gene from thymidine kinase to kinase-deficient human cells by purified herpes Simplex viral DNA. *Proc. Natl. Acad. Sci. USA*, 74:1590–1594.
3. Graham, F. L. (1977): Biological activity of tumor virus DNA. *Adv. Cancer Res.*, 25:1–46.
4. Graham, F. L., and van der Eb., A. J. (1973): A new technique of the assay of infectivity of human adenovirus 5 DNA. *Virology*, 52:456–467.
5. Houck, C. M., Rinehart, F. P., and Schmid, C. W. (1979): A ubiquitous family of repeated DNA sequences in the human genome. *J. Mol. Biol.*, 132:289–306.
6. Krontiris, T., and Cooper, G. M. (1981): Transforming activity of human tumor DNAs. *Proc. Natl. Acad. Sci. USA*, 78:1181–1184.
7. Lerner, R. A., Green, N., Alexander, H., Liu, F. T., Sutcliffe, J. G., and Shinnick, T. M. (1981): Chemically synthesized peptides predicted from the nucleotide sequence of the hepatitis B virus

genome elicit antibodies reactive with the native envelope protein of Dane particles. *Proc. Natl. Acad. Sci. USA*, 66:3403–3407.

8. Murray, M., Shilo, B., Shih, C., Cowing, D., Hsu, H. W., and Weinberg, R. A. (1981): Three different human tumor cell lines contain different oncogenes. *Cell*, 25:355–362.

9. Padhy, L. C., Shih, C., and Weinberg, R. A. (1981): A phosphoprotein specifically induced by the transforming gene of rat neuroblastomas. *Cell, (in press)*.

10. Peterson, J. L., and McBride, O. W. (1980): Co-transfer of linked eukaryotic genes and efficient transfer of hypoxanthine phosphoribo-syltransferase by DNA-mediated gene transfer. *Proc. Natl. Acad. Sci. USA*, 77:1583–1587.

11. Shih, C., Padhy, L. C., Murray, M., and Weinberg, R. A. (1981): Introduction of the transforming gene of carcinomas and neuroblastomas into mouse fibroblasts. *Nature*, 290:261–264.

12. Shih, C., Shilo, B., Goldfarb, M. P., Dannenberg, A., and Weinberg, R. A. (1979): Passage of phenotypes of chemically transformed cells via transfection of DNA and chromatin. *Proc. Natl. Acad. Sci. USA*, 76:5714–5718.

13. Shilo, B., and Weinberg, R. A. (1981): Unique transforming gene in carcinogen transformed mouse cells. *Nature*, 289:607–609.

14. Southern, E. M. (1975): Detection of specific sequences among DNA fragments separated by gel electrophoresis. *J. Mol. Biol.*, 98:503–517.

15. Walter, G., Scheidtmann, K. H., Carbone, A., Laudan, A. P., and Doolittle, R. F. (1980): Antibodies specific for the carboxy- and amino-terminal regions of simian virus 40 large tumor antigen. *Proc. Natl. Acad. Sci. USA*, 77:5197–5200.

16. Wigler, M., Pellicer, A., Silverstein, S., and Axel, R. (1978): Biochemical transfer of single-copy eukaryotic genes using total cellular DNA as donor. *Cell*, 14:725–731.

Advances in Viral Oncology, Volume 1, edited by George Klein. Raven Press, New York © 1982.

Analysis of Cellular Transforming Genes by Transfection

Geoffrey M. Cooper, Mary-Ann Lane, Theodore G. Krontiris, and Gerard Goubin

Sidney Farber Cancer Institute and Department of Pathology, Harvard Medical School, Boston, Massachusetts 02115

Transfection by cellular DNAs containing Rous sarcoma virus (RSV) genomes was first reported by Hill and Hillova in 1971 (25,26). Since then, transfection has been used to investigate the biological activity of retrovirus DNAs and, most recently, to analyze transforming genes of uninfected cells. In this chapter we briefly discuss experiments with retrovirus DNAs that illustrate some relevant features of the transfection assay and then describe studies from our laboratory in which transfection has been used to investigate transforming genes of both normal and neoplastic cells. Related experiments from R. A. Weinberg's laboratory are reviewed elsewhere (*this volume*).

TRANSFORMATION BY RETROVIRUS DNAs

Due to the mode of replication of retroviruses, one can envision two general pathways by which transfection with retrovirus DNAs could proceed: (a) direct integration of donor DNA into the genome of recipient cells to form a stably inherited DNA provirus and (b) transcription of donor DNA, possibly without donor DNA integration, resulting in the formation of infectious progeny virus followed by secondary infection of susceptible cells in the DNA-treated recipient culture. Which of these pathways predominates appears to depend on the type of recipient cells employed. For example, transformation of chicken embryo fibroblasts by RSV DNA requires production of infectious progeny virus and secondary virus infection, indicating that transformation does not occur as a direct result of integration of donor DNA into recipient chicken cell genomes (13). In contrast, NIH 3T3 mouse cells, but not most other rodent cell lines, can be efficiently transformed by direct integration of donor DNAs in the absence of virus replication (16,21,32). Consequently, NIH 3T3 cells have been particularly useful recipients for analysis of viral or cellular transforming genes not part of a replication-competent viral genome.

Transformation of NIH 3T3 cells by intact retrovirus DNAs proceeds by one-hit kinetics with efficiencies corresponding to approximately one transforming unit per 10^6 to 10^7 molecules of either integrated, unintegrated, or cloned donor retrovirus

DNAs (4,16,21,22). Integration of donor retrovirus DNAs during transfection of NIH 3T3 cells does not require specific viral DNA sequences and can involve recombinational events within cellular sequences flanking integrated viral DNA or within bacteriophage sequences flanking cloned viral DNA (10,15). The mode of integration of DNA during transfection thus differs from integration of retrovirus DNAs in virus-infected cells, which involves recombinational events at specific sequences at the termini of viral DNAs and resembles integration of transposable elements (18,28,41–45). Instead, integration of retrovirus DNAs during transfection of NIH 3T3 cells probably proceeds by a mechanism similar to integration of cellular DNAs in other rodent cell lines, such as Ltk$^-$ cells, which have been used as recipients for transfection of biochemical markers (47). Recent studies suggest that DNA integration in these cells involves recombination between independent donor DNA molecules followed by integration of recombinant concatamers of donor DNA into chromosomal DNA of the recipient cells (35–37).

Transformation by subgenomic fragments of retrovirus DNAs has contributed to elucidation of the specific genomic regions required for transformation by RSV (17), Moloney sarcoma virus (1,4,8), Harvey sarcoma virus (9,10), and Snyder-Theilen feline sarcoma virus (2). In addition, these experiments have provided data on the role of viral transcriptional promoters, contained within the long terminal repeat (LTR) sequences of retrovirus DNAs (3,48), which have been important in the interpretation of experiments on transfection by cellular transforming genes.

Restriction endonuclease fragments of retrovirus DNAs that contain intact viral transforming genes but do not contain LTR sequences induce transformation with efficiencies that are 100- to 1,000-fold lower than the transforming efficiencies of intact DNAs (4,9,17,34) (Table 1). Ligation of LTR sequences to such DNA fragments restores transforming activity, indicating that efficient transformation requires a transforming gene in association with an active promoter (4,9,34).

The rare cells transformed by viral DNA fragments containing a transforming gene without a viral LTR express the viral transforming gene product in amounts comparable to cells transformed by intact viral genomes (9,17). In addition, DNAs of these transformed cells induce transformation in secondary transfection assays with high efficiencies comparable to the transformation efficiencies of cell DNAs containing intact viral genomes (17) (Table 1). These results suggest that the low

TABLE 1. *Transforming activities of DNAs of RSV-transformed cells*

Donor DNA	Transformant/ μg cell DNA	Transformant/ pmole RSV DNA
Intact RSV genome[a]	2.0	1×10^5
Subgenomic *src* fragment[b]	0.01	5×10^2
Cells transformed by subgenomic *src* fragment[c]	1.0	2×10^6

Data summarized from Copeland et al. (17).

[a]DNA of RSV-transformed chicken embryo fibroblasts (CEF) containing approximately 25 unintegrated RSV DNA molecules per cell (15).

[b]Eco RI-digested DNA of RSV-transformed CEF.

[c]DNA of NIH cells transformed by Eco RI-digested DNA of RSV-transformed CEF.

frequency of transformation induced by viral DNA fragments containing transforming genes without LTR sequences corresponds to the probability of integration of viral DNA fragments in the vicinity of cellular promoter sequences, most likely derived from other donor DNA molecules, resulting in efficient expression of the viral transforming gene. The high efficiency of transformation induced by DNAs of these transformed cells in secondary transfection assays would then result from transfer of the viral transforming gene together with a linked cellular promoter as a single transforming unit.

TRANSFORMING GENES OF NORMAL CELLS

The utility of NIH 3T3 cells as recipients for transfection by viral transforming genes suggested the possibility that transfection could also be used to detect transforming genes of cellular origin. As reviewed elsewhere (chapters by Erikson and Purchio; Goff and Baltimore; Ellis, Lowy, and Skolnick; and Blair and Vande Woude, *this volume*), vertebrate genomes contain normal cellular genes that are closely related to the transforming genes of highly oncogenic retroviruses. However, the level of expression of cellular homologs of retrovirus transforming genes in normal cells is substantially lower than that of viral transforming genes in virus-transformed cells. The findings suggest the possibility that transformation by highly oncogenic retroviruses might be a consequence of abnormal expression of certain cellular genes as a result of insertion of these genes into a viral genome where their expression is regulated by efficient viral transcriptional promoters, instead of by the appropriate cellular sequences that presumably regulate expression of these potential transforming genes in normal cells.

This hypothesis predicts that normal cell DNAs might induce low levels of transformation in transfection assays if transformation could occur as a consequence of DNA rearrangements leading to the integration of potential normal cell transforming genes in the vicinity of inappropriate regulatory sequences that would result in abnormal gene expression. By analogy to transformation by subgenomic fragments of retrovirus DNAs, an example of such rearrangements might be the association of a potential transforming gene with an efficient transcriptional promoter derived from a different donor DNA molecule.

The hypothesis that normal cells contain genes with potential transforming activity was investigated by transfection assays of DNAs of normal chicken embryo fibroblasts, nontransformed mouse cell lines (BALB 3T3 and NIH 3T3 cells), and normal human embryo lung fibroblasts (14; and G. Cooper, *unpublished observations*). Both high molecular weight (> 30 kb) and fragmented (0.5 to 5 kb) DNAs were assayed to investigate the possibility that DNA fragmentation might dissociate potential transforming genes from their normal flanking regulatory sequences, thereby increasing the probability of DNA rearrangements leading to transforming gene activation. Fragments of normal cell DNAs induced transformation with an efficiency of approximately 0.003 transformant/μg DNA (Fig. 1), which was similar to the transformation efficiency of subgenomic DNA fragments of RSV-transformed

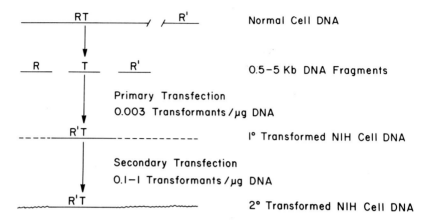

FIG. 1. Model for transformation by normal cell DNAs. Fragmentation of normal cell DNAs results in separation of potential transforming genes *(T)* from regulatory sequences *(R)* that normally control their expression. Transformation occurs at low efficiency (~ 0.003 transformant/µg DNA) as a consequence of recombination between potential transforming genes and inappropriate regulatory sequences *(R')* [probably also derived from donor DNA (35)] resulting in abnormal gene expression. Activated transforming genes of NIH cells transformed by normal cell: DNAs can be transmitted with high efficiencies (0.1 to 1 transformant/µg DNA) in secondary transfection assays. (Data summarized from Cooper et al. ref. 14.)

cells (Table 1). In contrast, high molecular weight normal cell DNAs did not induce transformation detectable above the background level of spontaneous transformation observed in control cultures exposed to fragments of salmon sperm or *Escherichia coli* DNAs ($\sim 3 \times 10^{-4}$ transformant/µg DNA).

To determine whether NIH cells transformed by normal cell DNA fragments contained activated transforming genes that could be efficiently transmitted by transfection, high molecular weight DNAs of these transformed cells were used as donor DNAs in secondary transfection assays. Whereas DNAs of spontaneously transformed NIH cells lacked transforming activity (11,14,16,30), DNAs of NIH cells transformed by normal cell DNA fragments induced transformation with efficiencies of 0.1 to 1 transformant/µg DNA (14) (Fig. 1). These results were analogous to secondary transfection assays of DNAs of NIH cells transformed by subgenomic fragments of RSV DNA (17) (Table 1) and indicated that transformation by fragments of normal cell DNAs resulted in the formation of activated transmissible transforming genes.

Figure 1 summarizes a model for activation of transforming genes of normal cells as a result of DNA rearrangements occurring during transfection. Fragmentation of donor DNA may dissociate potential transforming genes from their normal regulatory sequences and facilitate recombination with inappropriate regulatory sequences (e.g., efficient transcriptional promoters) leading to abnormal gene expression in rare transformed cells. Since extensive recombination occurs between independent donor DNA molecules (35), it is possible that both regulatory and structural sequences are derived from the donor DNA. Activated transforming genes

from transformed cells can then be transmitted at high efficiencies as single transforming units in secondary transfection assays. Studies from G. Vande Woude's
laboratory (34), reviewed elsewhere (Blair and Vande Woude, *this volume*), have
shown that transforming activity of a normal mouse gene homologous to the transforming gene of Moloney sarcoma virus can be activated by similar manipulations
of cloned DNAs.

NIH cells transformed by normal cell DNA fragments are tumorigenic in BALB/c
mice. The transformed cells do not produce retrovirus particles or infectious transforming viruses, nor can transforming viruses be rescued by superinfection with
nontransforming Moloney murine leukemia virus. Moreover, we have to date been
unable to detect exogenous DNA sequences homologous to the transforming genes
of RSV, avian erythroblastosis virus, or avian myelocytomatosis virus strain MC29
in three clones of NIH cells transformed by fragments of chicken DNA and one
clone of NIH cells transformed by fragments of quail DNA.

The transforming genes of three lines of NIH cells transformed by normal chicken
DNA fragments and of two lines of NIH cells transformed by normal human DNA
fragments have been analyzed by determining the sensitivity of the transforming
activities of their DNAs to digestion with restriction endonucleases (Table 2) (14).
The transforming activities of DNAs of two NIH cell lines transformed by chicken
DNA fragments are inactivated by digestion with Bam HI and Kpn I but not by
digestion with Eco RI, Hind III or Xho I. The transforming activities of DNAs of
a third cell line transformed by chicken DNA and of two cell lines transformed by
human DNA display patterns of susceptibility to restriction endonucleases that differ
from each other as well as from the two cell lines described above. These results
are consistent with the possibility that related transforming genes were activated in
two cell lines transformed by chicken DNA, whereas different transforming genes

TABLE 2. *Restriction endonuclease digestion of DNAs of NIH cells
transformed by normal cell DNA fragments*[a]

DNA	Transforming activity after digestion				
	Bam HI	Eco RI	Hind III	Kpn I	Xho I
NIH (CEF DNA)					
cl 1	+	+	−	+	+
cl 2	−	+	+	−	+
cl 3	−	+	+	−	+
NIH (HEF DNA)					
cl 1	−	+	−	N.D.	N.D.
cl 2	+	+	+	N.D.	+

[a]The transforming activities of DNAs of three lines of NIH cells transformed by fragments of normal chicken embryo fibroblast DNA and two
lines of NIH cells transformed by fragments of normal human embryo fibroblast DNA were assayed after digestion with the indicated restriction
endonucleases. +, retention of transforming activity after digestion; −,
loss of transforming activity after digestion.
Data from Cooper et al. (14), and G. Cooper, *unpublished observations*.

were activated in a third cell line transformed by chicken DNA and in two cell lines transformed by human DNA.

ACTIVATED TRANSFORMING GENES OF NEOPLASTIC CELLS

The activation of normal cell transforming genes by transfection suggested that oncogenic events in some tumors might involve dominant mutations or gene rearrangements resulting in the activation of transforming genes, which would then be detectable by induction of high efficiency transformation on transfection of high molecular weight DNAs. Shih et al. (39) initially demonstrated efficient transformation by high molecular weight DNAs of 5 out of 15 chemically transformed mouse fibroblast cell lines. We have investigated the transforming activities of DNAs of a variety of virally induced, chemically induced, and spontaneously occurring tumors of avian, murine, and human origin. Results of these experiments are reviewed here.

Virus-Induced Tumors

In contrast to the highly oncogenic sarcoma and acute leukemia viruses, many retroviruses do not appear to contain specific viral transforming genes. Although these viruses do not transform cells in culture, some viruses of this type do induce tumors after long latent periods in infected animals. Since the genetic basis for oncogenicity of these viruses is unclear, we investigated the possibility that tumors induced by two such viruses—avian lymphoid leukosis virus (LLV) and mouse mammary tumor virus (MMTV)—contained activated cellular transforming genes detectable by transfection.

High molecular weight DNAs of seven LLV-induced chicken tumors, including one nephroblastoma, four metastatic bursal lymphomas, and two premetastatic bursal nodules, induced transformation of NIH 3T3 with efficiencies of approximately 0.1 transformant/μg DNA (11) (Table 3). Similarly, DNAs of five MMTV-induced mammary carcinomas of C3H mice (5) induced transformation of NIH 3T3 cells with efficiencies of approximately 0.2 transformants/μg DNA (31) (Table 3). In contrast, DNAs of LLV- and MMTV-infected nonneoplastic tissues lacked transforming activity (11,31).

TABLE 3. *Transformation by DNAs of virus-induced tumors*

Tumor type	Fraction positive tumors
LLV-induced	
Metastatic lymphomas	4/4
Bursal nodules	2/2
Nephroblastoma	1/1
MMTV-induced mammary carcinoma	5/5
Total	12/12

Data summarized from Cooper and Neiman (11) and Lane et al. (31).

DNAs of NIH cells transformed by DNAs of LLV- and MMTV-induced tumors induced transformation in secondary transfection assays with efficiencies comparable to the primary transfection efficiencies of the tumor DNAs (11,31). To determine whether the transforming genes of these tumors were linked to viral DNA sequences, DNAs of transformed NIH cells were hybridized to ^{32}P-DNA probes either representative of the viral genomes or specific for the viral LTR sequences. No viral DNA sequences were detectable with either probe in 6 NIH cell lines transformed by DNAs of 4 different LLV-induced tumors (11) or in 10 NIH cell lines transformed by DNAs of 5 different MMTV-induced tumors (31).

These results indicate that neoplasms induced by either LLV or MMTV contain activated cellular transforming genes that are not linked to viral DNA. Since activation of cellular transforming genes was detected in all 12 tumors studied, it would appear that this represents a significant event in oncogenesis by these viruses.

Recent studies by Hayward et al. (24) have revealed that LLV-induced metastatic lymphomas contain viral LTR sequences integrated in the vicinity of the chicken gene (c-*myc*) homologous to the presumed transforming gene of the highly oncogenic acute leukemia virus MC29. Integration of viral LTR sequences, which contain the viral transcriptional promoter, apparently results in increased expression of c-*myc* (24). We have confirmed that LTR sequences are integrated in the vicinity of c-*myc* in the LLV-induced neoplasms used for transfection assays, including the bursal nodules and nephroblastoma (12). However, analysis of the DNAs of transformed NIH cells indicates that c-*myc* sequences (in addition to viral LTR sequences) are not transferred to NIH cells transformed by LLV-induced tumor DNAs (12). LLV-induced tumors thus appear to contain at least two different genes with potential oncogenic activity: (a) a c-*myc* gene activated by integration of viral LTR sequences and (b) a distinct cellular gene, not linked to viral DNA, which is capable of efficiently transforming NIH 3T3 cells.

The long latent period and the pathogenesis of tumors induced by LLV and MMTV suggests a multi-step process that might be expected to involve more than a single transformation event. In the case of LLV-induced lymphomas, preneoplastic-transformed follicles can be observed in bursas of most birds (10 to 100 transformed follicles per bursa) within approximately 40 days after LLV-infection (33). Most of these transformed follicles regress, but a small fraction (approximately 2%) appear to develop into progressively growing neoplastic bursal nodules, which are the presumed precursors of metastatic lymphomas (33). These observations suggest that proliferation of preneoplastic-transformed follicles is a relatively frequent early event in the disease process and that a second event occurs in some cells of this population to result in neoplasia. It is thus possible that viral activation of c-*myc* is involved in a stage of tumor development that precedes or complements the activation of cellular transforming genes detected by transfection. As one specific possibility, viral activation of c-*myc* might lead to proliferation of preneoplastic-transformed follicles and mutations or gene rearrangements within some cells of this proliferative population might then result in activation of the cellular transforming genes detected by transfection. Further studies will be required to define the roles of these potential transforming genes in the disease process.

Chemically Induced Tumors

DNA of one chemically induced mouse mammary carcinoma has been found to induce transformation of NIH 3T3 cells with high efficiencies (0.1 transformant/μg DNA) (31), whereas DNAs of nine other chemically induced tumors and transformed cell lines that we have studied lack significant transforming activity (Table 4) (14,31; and N. Copeland, D. Shalloway, T. Krontiris, and G. Cooper, *unpublished observations*). More extensive studies of chemically transformed cells by Weinberg and his colleagues indicate that DNAs of some chemically transformed mouse fibroblast cell lines, mouse bladder carcinomas, and rat neuroblastomas efficiently transform NIH 3T3 cells (38,39). It thus appears that a fraction of chemically induced transformation events involve dominant mutations or gene rearrangements resulting in the activation of cellular transforming genes that are then detectable by transfection. It is of interest that the two chemically induced mammary carcinomas we have studied resulted from dimethylbenzanthracene treatment of the same hormonally induced preneoplastic nodule outgrowth (23). The finding that one of these tumors contained an activated transmissible transforming gene whereas the other did not (31) (Table 4) therefore suggests that transformation may have occurred by different mechanisms in two chemically induced tumors derived from the same preneoplastic cell population.

Human Tumors

High molecular weight DNAs of 36 human tumors and tumor cell lines have been assayed for transforming activity on NIH 3T3 cells (30,31; and T. Krontiris *unpublished observations*). DNAs of 3 of these tumors—2 bladder carcinomas and 1 mammary carcinoma—induced transformation with high efficiencies (~ 0.2 transformant/μg DNA), whereas DNAs of the other 33 tumors studied lacked significant transforming activity (Table 5). Transforming activity of one of these

TABLE 4. *Transformation by DNAs of chemically induced tumors*

Tumor type	Fraction positive tumors
Sarcomas	
Chicken	0/1
Quail	0/3
Rat neuroblastoma	0/1
Mouse bladder carcinomas	0/2
Mouse mammary carcinomas	1/2
Total	1/9

Data summarized from Cooper et al. (14), Lane et al. (31), and N. Copeland et al., *unpublished observations*.

TABLE 5. *Transformation by DNAs of human tumors*

Tumor type	Fraction positive tumors
Lymphomas	0/6
Leukemias	0/11
Neuroblastomas	0/3
Melanomas	0/2
Sarcoma	0/1
Carcinomas	
Bladder	2/4
Mammary	1/2
Lung	0/2
Ovary	0/2
Colon	0/1
Esophagus	0/1
Squamous cell	0/1
Total	3/36

Data summarized from Krontiris and Cooper (30), Lane et al. (31), and T. Krontiris, *unpublished observations.*

bladder carcinoma DNAs has also been reported by Shih et al. (38). DNAs of NIH cells transformed by human tumor DNAs induced transformation in secondary transfection with efficiencies of 0.2 to 0.6 transformant/μg DNA (30,31). These efficiencies were similar to the initial efficiencies of transformation by the tumor DNAs, as expected for serial transfer of a transforming gene activated in the tumors. NIH cells transformed by both bladder and mammary carcinoma DNAs induced undifferentiated fibrosarcomas in BALB/c mice.

NIH cells transformed by both human bladder and mammary carcinoma DNAs contained human DNA sequences detectable by hybridization of restriction endo-nuclease-digested DNAs to a probe containing a human *Alu* family sequence. The *Alu* family sequences are interspersed repetitive sequences of 300 nucleotides present in approximately 300,000 copies per genome (27). The presence of these human sequences in NIH cells transformed by human carcinoma DNAs provides biochemical evidence that transformation was mediated by human DNA.

These results indicate that a small fraction ($\sim$ 10%) of the human tumors thus far examined contain activated transforming genes that induce transformation of NIH 3T3 mouse cells with high efficiencies. Carcinogenesis in these tumors is therefore likely to have involved a dominant genetic alteration, either by mutation or gene rearrangement, which resulted in transforming gene activation.

TISSUE SPECIFICITY OF TRANSFORMING GENES ACTIVATED IN TUMORS

The activated transforming genes of human bladder carcinomas and human and mouse mammary carcinomas have been characterized by investigating the sensitivity of transforming activities of their DNAs to digestion with restriction endonucleases.

Transforming activities of DNAs of both human bladder carcinoma cell lines are inactivated by digestion with all of the restriction endonucleases which have been tested (30; and T. Krontiris *unpublished observations*) (Table 6). Consistent with these results, preliminary analysis of the effects of random shearing on the transforming activities of these DNAs suggests that the transforming genes are about 10 kb.

In contrast to these results, the transforming activities of both mouse and human mammary carcinoma DNAs displayed a distinctive pattern of susceptibility to digestion with seven different restriction endonucleases (31). The transforming activities of DNAs of five MMTV-induced tumors, a dimethylbenzanthracene-induced mouse mammary tumor, and the human mammary tumor cell line MCF-7 were inactivated by digestion with Pvu II and Sac I but not by Bam HI, Eco RI, Hind III, Kpn I, and Xho I (31) (Table 6). This pattern differs from that of the human bladder carcinomas described above, from five lines of NIH cells transformed by normal chicken and human DNA fragments (Table 2) and from chemically transformed mouse fibroblasts (40) (Table 6).

The probability of different genes yielding the same pattern of sensitivity to restriction endonucleases observed for the mammary carcinoma DNAs can be estimated by the Poisson distribution from the average cleavage frequency of the restriction enzymes used in total cellular DNA. Bam HI, Eco RI, Hind III, Pvu II, Sac I, and Xho I cleave cellular DNAs at average intervals of approximately 4 kb, and Kpn I cleaves at average intervals of approximately 15 kb. Assuming a gene size of 4 kb, the probability of inactivation by Bam HI, Eco RI, Hind III, Pvu II, Sac I, or Xho I is approximately 0.63 and the probability of inactivation by Kpn I is approximately 0.2. The probability of two different 4 kb genes displaying the pattern observed for the mammary carcinoma DNAs is therefore $(0.37)^4 (0.63)^2 (0.8) = 0.006$. The probability of all seven tumor DNAs displaying this pattern by chance is $(0.006)^6 = 4 \times 10^{-14}$. The maximum likelihood of two genes displaying the observed pattern by chance would occur if the gene size was 1.6 kb. In this case, the probability of all seven tumor DNAs displaying the pattern is approximately 10^{-10}. It thus appears that the same or closely related transforming genes were activated in all seven mammary carcinomas.

TABLE 6. *Restriction endonuclease digestion of tumor and transformed cell DNAs*

Tumor (number)	Transforming activity after digestion				
	Bam HI	Eco RI	Hind III	Kpn I	Xho I
Human bladder carcinomas (2)[a]	N.D.	−	−	−	−
Mouse and human mammary carcinomas (7)[b]	+	+	+	+	+
Chemically transformed mouse fibroblasts (4)[c]	+	−	−	N.D.	+

[a]T. Krontiris and G. Cooper (30); *unpublished observations.*
[b]Lane et al. (31).
[c]Shilo and Weinberg (40).
Data summarized as in Table 2.

To determine whether the expected evolutionary divergence between human and mouse genes was inconsistent with the identical pattern of sensitivity to seven restriction endonucleases observed for human and mouse mammary carcinoma DNAs, computer analysis of DNA sequences was used to compare the sensitivity of human and mouse β-globin and Kappa constant region genes to cleavage by 18 six-base recognition restriction endonucleases. In both gene pairs, 14 of these enzymes yielded the same pattern of cleavage sensitivity for the human and mouse gene homologs. It is, therefore, not extraordinary to obtain an identical pattern of sensitivity to 7 enzymes in homologous genes activated in human and mouse mammary carcinomas.

Activation of related transforming genes in mouse mammary carcinomas induced by both viral and chemical carcinogens and in a cell line derived from a spontaneous human mammary carcinoma suggests the possibility that specific transforming genes are activated in neoplasms of particular tissue types. Recent studies of Shilo and Weinberg (40), indicating that the transforming genes activated in four chemically transformed lines of mouse fibroblasts were related to each other, are also consistent with this notion. One hypothesis suggested by these observations is that, in some differentiated cell types, only one or a few of the total number of cellular genes with potential transforming activity are susceptible targets for mutations or DNA rearrangements resulting in transforming gene activation. Alternatively, the total set of genes with potential transforming activity might be susceptible targets for activation in differentiated cells, but the state of differentiation of some cell types might render the cells phenotypically sensitive to the effects of only one or a few of these genes. In either case, it will be of interest to test the possibility that genes involved in transformation of particular differentiated cell types might be normally involved in growth control of those cells.

SUMMARY

The results of transfection assays of both normal and tumor cell DNAs are summarized in Fig. 2. Two general conclusions are indicated: (a) potential transforming genes of normal cells can be activated after transfection and then transmitted with high efficiencies in secondary transfection assays of transformed cell DNAs and (b) some neoplasms contain activated transforming genes that can be transmitted with high efficiencies in both primary and secondary transfection assays. The transforming activity of normal cell DNAs suggests that DNA rearrangements can result in transformation, presumably as a consequence of abnormal gene expression. Current evidence suggesting that some naturally occurring carcinogenic events may involve DNA rearrangements rather than somatic mutations has recently been reviewed by Cairns (7), and it is possible that the activation of cellular transforming genes in tumors results from DNA rearrangements analogous to those occurring during the activation of normal cell transforming genes by transfection. Alternatively, the activation of cellular transforming genes in tumors could be a consequence of dominant mutations in either structural genes or *cis*-acting regulatory sequences.

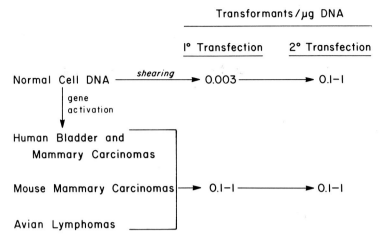

FIG. 2. Summary of transforming activities of normal and tumor cell DNAs. Potential transforming genes of normal cells can be activated with low efficiencies during transfection and then transmitted at high efficiencies in secondary transfection assays. In some neoplasms, transforming genes are activated as a consequence of dominant mutations or gene rearrangements and are then transmissible at high efficiencies in both primary and secondary transfection assays.

Activated cellular transforming genes detectable by transfection of NIH 3T3 cells have been found in all virus-induced tumors studied, but in only a fraction of chemically induced or spontaneously occurring tumors. The nature of oncogenic changes in those tumors that do not contain activated transforming genes detectable in this assay is unclear. It is possible that these tumors contain activated transforming genes that do not induce transformation of the NIH 3T3 cells used as recipients. Alternatively, the lesions resulting in oncogenic transformation in these tumors may have involved epigenetic changes (29), recessive mutations, or alterations in multiple unlinked genes required for transformation.

Analysis of the susceptibility of activated transforming genes to digestion with restriction endonucleases suggests that (a) a number of different transforming genes can be detected by transfection of NIH 3T3 cells and (b) specific transforming genes may be activated in neoplasms of particular differentiated cell types. For example, closely related or identical transforming genes were activated in mouse mammary carcinomas induced by either a viral or a chemical carcinogen and in a human mammary carcinoma cell line (31). However, activated transforming genes were not detected in two other mammary carcinomas studies (30,31). A unifying, although at present speculative, hypothesis is that normal cells contain a number of genes with potential transforming activity. Neoplasms of particular differentiated cell types might result from abnormal expression of a specific subset of these genes. Such abnormal gene expression could occur by two general mechanisms: (a) dominant mutations or gene rearrangements leading to the formation of an activated transforming gene detectable by transfection or (b) recessive mutations or epigenetic changes that might affect expression of the same gene without resulting in an alteration detectable in the transfection assay.

Finally, it should be noted that carcinogenesis in a variety of systems appears to involve a series of progressive changes rather than a single event (6,19,20,29,33,46). The NIH 3T3 cells that have been used as recipients in transfection assays are a permanent heteroploid mouse cell line that may have already undergone some of the carcinogenic events involved in transformation of normal cells. Consequently, transfection in this system may identify only those genes involved in stages of the neoplastic process required for final oncogenic transformation of NIH 3T3 cells. The finding that LLV-induced tumors contain at least two different genes with potential oncogenic activity may be an example of this complexity.

The ability to detect cellular transforming genes by transfection provides an approach to the isolation of these genes by molecular cloning. Such studies are underway in both our own and other laboratories and can be expected to lead to the analysis of cellular transformation at the molecular level.

ACKNOWLEDGMENTS

We are grateful to D. M. Livingston for many stimulating discussions and critical reading of the manuscript. Work from our laboratory was supported by NIH grants CA18689, CA21802, and CA26825 and by a Faculty Research Award to the first author from the American Cancer Society.

REFERENCES

1. Andersson, P., Goldfarb, M. P., and Weinberg, R. A. (1979): A defined subgenomic fragment of *in vitro* synthesized Moloney sarcoma virus DNA can induce cell transformation upon transfection. *Cell*, 16:63–75.
2. Barbacid, M. (1981): Cellular transformation by subgenomic feline sarcoma virus DNA. *J. Virol.*, 37:518–523.
3. Benz, E. W., Wydro, R. M., Nadal-Ginard, B., and Dina, D. (1980): Moloney murine sarcoma proviral DNA is a transcriptional unit. *Nature*, 288:665–669.
4. Blair, D. G., McClements, W. L., Oskarsson, M. K., Fischinger, P. J., and Vande Woude, G. F. (1980): Biological activity of cloned Moloney sarcoma virus DNA: Terminally redundant sequences may enhance transformation efficiency. *Proc. Natl. Acad. Sci. USA*, 77:3504–3508.
5. Blair, P. B. (1968): The mammary tumor virus. *Curr. Top. Microbiol. Immunol.*, 45:1–69.
6. Boutwell, R. K. (1977): The role of the induction of ornithine decarboxylase in tumor promotion. In: *Origins of Human Cancer*, edited by H. H. Hiatt, J. D. Watson, and J. A. Winsten, pp. 773–783. Cold Spring Harbor Laboratory, New York.
7. Cairns, J. (1981): The origin of human cancers. *Nature*, 289:353–357.
8. Canaani, E., Robbins, K. C., and Aaronson, S. A. (1979): The transforming gene of Moloney murine sarcoma virus. *Nature*, 282:378–383.
9. Chang, E. H., Ellis, R. W., Scolnick, E. M., and Lowy, D. R. (1980): Transformation by cloned Harvey murine sarcoma virus DNA: Efficiency increased by long terminal repeat DNA. *Science*, 210:1249–1251.
10. Chang, E. H., Maryak, J. M., Wei, C. -M., Shih, T. Y., Shober, R., Cheung, H. L., Ellis, R. W., Hager, G. L., Scolnick, E. M., and Lowy, D. R. (1980): Functional organization of the Harvey murine sarcoma virus genome. *J. Virol.*, 35:76–92.
11. Cooper, G. M., and Neiman, P. E. (1980): Transforming genes of neoplasms induced by avian lymphoid leukosis viruses. *Nature*, 287:656–659.
12. Cooper, G. M., and Neiman, P. E. (1981): Two distinct candidate transforming genes of lymphoid leukosis virus-induced neoplasms. *Nature*, 292:857–858.
13. Cooper, G. M., and Okenquist, S. (1978): Mechanism of transfection of chicken embryo fibroblasts by Rous sarcoma virus DNA. *J. Virol.*, 28:45–52.

14. Cooper, G. M., Okenquist, S., and Silverman, L. (1980): Transforming activity of DNA of chemically-transformed and normal cells. *Nature*, 284:418–421.
15. Copeland, N. G., Jenkins, N. A., and Cooper, G. M. (1981): Integration of Rous sarcoma virus DNA during transfection. *Cell*, 23:51–60.
16. Copeland, N. G., Zelenetz, A. D., and Cooper, G. M. (1979): Transformation of NIH 3T3 mouse cells by DNA of Rous sarcoma virus. *Cell*, 17:993–1002.
17. Copeland, N. G., Zelenetz, A. D., and Cooper, G. M. (1980): Transformation by subgenomic fragments of Rous sarcoma virus DNA. *Cell*, 19:863–870.
18. Dhar, R., McClements, W. L., Enquist, L. W., and Vande Woude, G. (1980): Nucleotide sequences of integrated Moloney sarcoma provirus long terminal repeats and their host and viral junctions. *Proc. Natl. Acad. Sci. USA*, 77:3937–3941.
19. Doll, R. (1978): An epidemiological perspective of the biology of cancer. *Cancer Res.*, 38:3573–3583.
20. Fernandez, A., Mondal, S., and Heidelberger, C. (1980): Probabilistic view of the transformation of cultured C3H 10T½ mouse embryo fibroblasts by methylcholanthrene. *Proc. Natl. Acad. Sci. USA*, 77:7272–7276.
21. Goldfarb, M. P., and Weinberg, R. A. (1979): Physical map of Harvey sarcoma virus unintegrated linear DNA. *J. Virol.*, 32:30–39.
22. Hager, G. L., Chang, E. H., Chan, H. W., Garon, C. F., Israel, M. A., Martin, M. A., Scolnick, E. M., and Lowy, D. R. (1979): Molecular cloning of the Harvey sarcoma virus closed circular DNA intermediates: Initial structural and biological characterization. *J. Virol.*, 31:795–809.
23. Halpin, Z. T., Vaage, J., and Blair, P. (1972): Lack of antigenicity of mammary tumors induced by carcinogens in a nonantigenic preneoplastic lesion. *Cancer Res.*, 32:2197–2200.
24. Hayward, W. S., Neel, B. G., and Astrin, S. M. (1981): Activation of a cellular *onc* gene by promoter insertion in ALV-induced lymphoid leukosis. *Nature*, 290:475–480.
25. Hill, M., and Hillova, J. (1971): Production virale dans les fibroblastes de poule traités par l'acide desoxyribonucleique de cellules XC de rat transformées par le virus de Rous. *C. R. Acad. Sci. [Paris D.]*, 272:3094–3097.
26. Hill, M., and Hillova, J. (1972): Virus recovery in chicken cells tested with Rous sarcoma cell DNA. *Nature New Biol.*, 237:35–39.
27. Jelinek, W. R., Toomey, T. P., Leinwand, L., Duncan C. H., Biro, P. A., Choudary, P. V., Weissman, S. M., Rubin, C. M., Houck, C. M., Deininger, P. L., and Schmid, C. W. (1980): Ubiquitous, interspersed repeated sequences in mammalian genomes. *Proc. Natl. Acad. Sci. USA*, 77:1398–1402.
28. Ju, G., and Skalka, A. M. (1980): Nucleotide sequence analysis of the long terminal repeat (LTR) of avian retroviruses: Structural similarities with transposable elements. *Cell*, 22:379–386.
29. Kennedy, A. R., Fox, M., Murphy, G., and Little, J. B. (1980): Relationship between X-ray exposure and malignant transformation in C3H 10T½ cells. *Proc. Natl. Acad. Sci. USA*, 77:7262–7266.
30. Krontiris, T. G., and Cooper, G. M. (1981): Transforming activity of human tumor DNAs. *Proc. Natl. Acad. Sci. USA*, 78:1181–1184.
31. Lane, M. A., Sainten, A., and Cooper, G. M. (1981): Activation of related transforming genes in mouse and human mammary carcinomas. *Proc. Natl. Acad. Sci. USA*, 78:5185–5189.
32. Lowy, D. R., Rands, E., and Scolnick, E. M. (1978): Helper-independent transformation by unintegrated Harvey sarcoma virus DNA. *J. Virol.*, 26:291–298.
33. Neiman, P. E., Payne, L. N., Jordan, L., and Weiss, R. A. (1980): Malignant lymphoma of the bursa of Farbricius: Analysis of early transformation. *Cold Spring Harbor Conf. Cell Prolif.*, 7:519–528.
34. Oskarsson, M., McClements, W. L., Blair, D. G., Maizel, J. V., and Vande Woude, G. F. (1980): Properties of a normal mouse cell DNA sequence (sarc) homologous to the src sequence of Moloney sarcoma virus. *Science*, 207:1222–1224.
35. Perucho, M., Hanahan, D., and Wigler, M. (1980): Genetic and physical linkage of exogenous sequences in transformed cells. *Cell*, 22:309–317.
36. Robins, D. M., Ripley, S., Henderson, A. S., and Axel, R. (1981): Transforming DNA integrates into the host chromosome. *Cell*, 23:29–39.
37. Scangos, G. A., Huttner, K. M., Juricek, D. K., and Ruddle, F. H. (1981): Deoxyribonucleic acid-mediated gene transfer in mammalian cells: Molecular analysis of unstable transformants and their progression to stability. *Mol. Cell Biol.*, 1:111–120.

38. Shih, C., Padhy, L. C., Murray, M., and Weinberg, R. A. (1981): Transforming genes of carcinomas and neuroblastomas introduced into mouse fibroblasts. *Nature*, 290:261–264.
39. Shih, C., Shilo, B. -Z., Goldfarb, M. P., Dannenberg, A., and Weinberg, R. A. (1979): Passage of phenotypes of chemically-transformed cells via transfection of DNA and chromatin. *Proc. Natl. Acad. Sci. USA*, 76:5714–5718.
40. Shilo, B. -Z., and Weinberg, R. A. (1981): Unique transforming gene in carcinogen-transformed mouse cells. *Nature*, 289:607–609.
41. Shimotohno, K., Mizutani, S., and Temin, H. M. (1980): Sequence of retrovirus provirus resembles that of bacterial transposable elements. *Nature*, 285:550–554.
42. Shoemaker, C., Goff, S., Gilboa, E., Paskind, M., Mitra, S. W., and Baltimore, D. (1980): Structure of a cloned circular Moloney murine leukemia virus DNA molecule containing an inverted segment: Implications for retrovirus integration. *Proc. Natl. Acad. Sci. USA*, 77:3932–3936.
43. Sutcliffe, J. G., Shinnick, T. M., Verma, I. M., and Lerner, R. A. (1980): Nucleotide sequence of Moloney leukemia virus: 3′ end reveals details of replication, analogy to bacterial transposons, and an unexpected gene. *Proc. Natl. Acad. Sci. USA*, 77:3302–3306.
44. Swanstrom, R., DeLorbe, W. J., Bishop, J. M., and Varmus, H. E. (1981): Nucleotide sequence of cloned unintegrated avian sarcoma virus DNA: Viral DNA contains direct and inverted repeats similar to those in transposable elements. *Proc. Natl. Acad. Sci. USA*, 78:124–128.
45. Van Beveren, C., Goddard, J. G., Berns, A., and Verma, I. M. (1980): Structure of Moloney leukemia viral DNA: Nucleotide sequence of the 5′ long terminal repeat and adjacent cellular sequences. *Proc. Natl. Acad. Sci. USA*, 77:3307–3311.
46. Weinstein, I. B., Wigler, M., and Pietropaolo, C. (1977): The action of tumor-promoting agents in cell culture. In: *Origins of Human Cancer*, edited by H. H. Hiatt, J. D. Watson, and J. A. Winsten, pp. 751–772. Cold Spring Harbor Laboratory, New York.
47. Wigler, M., Pellicer, A., Silverstein, S., and Axel, R. (1978): Biochemical transfer of single-copy eucaryotic genes using total cellular DNA as donor. *Cell*, 14:725–731.
48. Yamamoto, T., de Crombrugghe, B., and Pastan, I. (1980): Identification of a functional promoter in the long terminal repeat of Rous sarcoma virus. *Cell*, 22:787–797.

Subject Index